AF535078

SPEECH PATHOLOGY FOR TRACHEOSTOMIZED AND VENTILATOR DEPENDENT PATIENTS

Mary F. Mason, M.S., C.C.C.-SLP

With Contributors

1993

Voicing! • Newport Beach • California

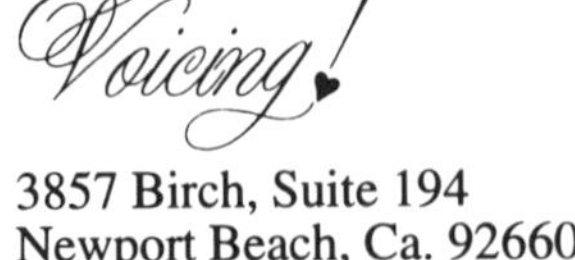

3857 Birch, Suite 194
Newport Beach, Ca. 92660

Library of Congress Catalog Number: 93-94984

Mason, Mary F.

**Speech Pathology
for
Tracheostomized and
Ventilator Dependent
Patients**

ISBN 0-9633596-0-6

The authors have made every effort to ensure the accuracy of the information herein, however, appropriate information sources should be consulted, especially for new or unfamiliar procedures. It is the responsibility of every practitioner to evaluate the appropriateness of a particular opinion in the context of actual clinical situations and with due consideration to new developments.

Speech Pathology for Tracheostomized and Ventilator Dependent Patients

ISBN 0-9633596-0-6

"The ability to communicate is what makes us human."

Stephen Hawking
September 27, 1993

Stephen Hawking, CBE, FRS
Lucasian Professor of Mathematics
Department of Applied Mathematics and Theoretical Physics
University of Cambridge
Cambridge, England

Author of
A Brief History of Time
and
Black Holes and Baby Universes and Other Essays

I gratefully acknowledge Dr. Hawking's eloquent contribution to this text.

Mary F. Mason

"The contents of this book can teach us to bring tracheostomized and ventilator dependent patients out of the dark and back to life again. When we can't communicate we are separated from each other — as Helen Keller said, 'Deafness is darker by far than blindness.' Don't be deaf to the needs of these people, allow them to come out of their darkness and speak to us."

Bernie S. Siegel
October 2, 1993

Bernie S. Siegel, M.D.
Author of
Love, Medicine, and Miracles
and
Peace, Love and Healing

I am most grateful to Dr. Siegel for understanding my goals in writing this book and for expressing so compassionately the essence of the challenges and the spirit of the achievements with these patients.

Mary F. Mason

ACKNOWLEDGMENTS

I have been fortunate in the past few years to have experienced the continued support of several people who have encouraged and assisted me in my professional growth in this specialized field of tracheostomized and ventilator dependent patients. It is with their understanding and advocacy of my professional pursuits that I have been able to develop this book.

I wish to acknowledge the many patients, families, nurses, respiratory therapists, and physicians who have inspired my work in this area. I have been blessed with two very important colleagues: Lynn, whose editing expertise improved the quality of my work immensely, and Louise whose commitment to this project and to my professional goals over the years has helped me to accomplish beyond my expectations. After the writing comes the arduous task of typing and organizing the production of the book. To these behind the scene creators of reality, Lydia, Ann, and Lee, I express my gratitude for the long hours and the lost weekends. I extend appreciation and recognition to Christopher for his countless hours and determination in assuring the quality of the final printed text. To the entire staff who rose to the challenge and gave the best of themselves, I am grateful.

I am indebted to the many contributors, editors, and reviewers for their acuity and judicious examination of the text as well as for their kindness in supporting this endeavor. A special thank you to my husband, Mike, and my son, Benjamin, for walking through the commitment with me.

This book was accomplished through a team effort with people who have given generously and with enthusiasm in the hope that through this book silent patients will be able to experience voicing and an enhanced quality of life.

MARY F. MASON

Contents

CHAPTER III
TRACHEOSTOMY AND TRACHEOSTOMY TUBES

CHAPTER IV
RESPIRATORY CARE

CHAPTER V
TRANSDISCIPLINARY TEAM CONCEPT

CHAPTER VII
VOCAL TREATMENT STRATEGIES

CHAPTER VIII
PEDIATRICS

CONTRIBUTORS, EDITORS, AND REVIEWERS

CHAPTER I
ANATOMY AND PHYSIOLOGY

Contributors: **Mary F. Mason, M.S., C.C.C.-SLP**
President
Voicing! Inc.
Newport Beach, California
Private Practice
Professional Speech Services, Inc.
Columbus, Ohio
Director
Speech-Language Pathology Services
Americare Marion
Marion, Ohio
Coordinator
Speech-Language Pathology Services
Health Care Plus
Columbus, Ohio
Americare Circleville
Circleville, Ohio
Marion General Home Care
MedCenter Hospital
Marion General Hospital
Marion, Ohio

Lori Stewart Gonzalez, Ph.D., C.C.C.-SLP
Assistant Professor
Division of Communication Disorders
University of Kentucky
Lexington, Kentucky

Editors: **J. David Garrett, Ph.D.**
Chief, Speech Pathology Services
Methodist Hospital
Assistant Professor
Otolaryngology Department
Baylor College of Medicine
Houston, Texas

Thomas L. Layton, Ph.D., C.C.C.-SLP
Associate Professor
Division of Speech and Hearing Sciences
Department of Medical Allied Health Problems
The School of Medicine
University of North Carolina at Chapel Hill
Chapel Hill, North Carolina

Chapter II
AIRWAY ISSUES

Contributor: **Mary F. Mason, M.S., C.C.C.-SLP**

Editors:

Barbara M. Baker, Ph.D.
Associate Professor of Surgery
Division of Communicative Disorders
University of Louisville School of Medicine
Private Practice
University Speech Pathology Associates
Louisville, Kentucky

Lauren D. Holinger, M.D., F.A.C.S.
Head, Division Pediatric Otolaryngology
The Children's Memorial Hospital
Professor
Department of Otolaryngology-Head and Neck Surgery
Northwestern University Medical School
Chicago, Illinois

Reviewers:

Robin Cotton, M.D.
Director
Pediatric Otolaryngology and Maxillofacial Surgery
Children's Hospital Medical Center
Professor
Department of Otolaryngology
College of Medicine
University of Cincinnati
Cincinnati, Ohio

Martha Langston, C.R.T.T.
Supervisor
Respiratory Care Department
The Institute for Rehabilitation and Research
Texas Medical Center
Houston, Texas

Kaye Meehan, R.N.C.S., A.N.P., C.O.R.L.N.
Certified Adult Nurse Practitioner
Department of Otolaryngology–Head and Neck Surgery
Carle Clinic Association
Urbana, Illinois

Donna Wilson, M.S.N., R.N., R.R.T.
Pulmonary Clinical Nurse Specialist
Memorial Sloan Kettering Cancer Center
New York, New York

Chapter III
TRACHEOSTOMY AND TRACHEOSTOMY TUBES

Contributors: **Mary F. Mason, M.S., C.C.C.-SLP**

Kaye Meehan, R.N.C.S., A.N.P., C.O.R.L.N.
Certified Adult Nurse Practitioner
Department of Otolaryngology-Head and Neck Surgery
Carle Clinic Association
Urbana, Illinois

Editor: **Lauren D. Holinger, M.D., F.A.C.S.**
Head, Division Pediatric Otolaryngology
The Children's Memorial Hospital
Chicago, Illinois
Professor
Department of Otolaryngology-Head and Neck Surgery
Northwestern University Medical School
Chicago, Illinois

Reviewers: **Craig Davis, R.R.T.**
Assistant Director
Respiratory Therapy Department
Centerburg Nursing Center
Centerburg, Ohio

Joan Davis, R.N.
Assistant Director
Department of Nursing
Centerburg Nursing Center
Centerburg, Ohio

Tony Hilton, R.N., M.P.H., C.R.R.N.
Pulmonary Rehabilitation
Clinical Nurse Specialist
Loma Linda University Medical Center
Loma Linda, California

Lisa Kohlenberger, M.A., C.C.C.-SLP
Department of Speech Pathology
USC University Hospital
Los Angeles, California

Martha Langston, C.R.T.T
Supervisor
Respiratory Care Department
The Institute for Rehabilitation and Research
Houston, Texas

Kitty Reid, R.N.C.
ENT Clinician
Scott and White Clinic
Scott and White Memorial Hospital
Texas A & M University College of Medicine
Temple, Texas

Mary Speights, R.N., B.S.N.
Head and Neck Cancer Nurse Clinician
Coordinator
Scott and White Clinic
Scott and White Memorial Hospital
Texas A & M University College of Medicine
Temple, Texas

Chapter IV
RESPIRATORY CARE

Contributors: **Mary F. Mason, M.S., C.C.C.-SLP**

Jo Ann Irene Frey, B.S.N., R.N., C., C.R.R.N.
Pulmonary Nurse Clinician
Pulmonary Rehabilitation Coordinator
Pulmonary Rehabilitation, Pulmonary Services
Good Samaritan Hospital
Cincinnati, Ohio

Beverly Fornoff, B.S., R.R.T.
R. Adams Cowley Shock Trauma Center
Maryland Institute for Emergency Medical Services Systems
University of Maryland Medical System
Baltimore, Maryland

Editors:

Edward Anthony Oppenheimer, M.D., F.A.C.P., F.C.C.P.
Chief, Pulmonary Medicine
Los Angeles Kaiser Permanente Medical Center
Physician Coordinator of Kaiser Permanente Regional Ventilator Home Care Program
Associate Professor of Medicine
University of California School of Medicine, Los Angeles
Los Angeles, California

Pope L. Moseley, M.D., M.S.
Associate Professor
Department of Internal Medicine
Division of Pulmonary, Critical Care, and Occupational Medicine and the Department of Exercise Science
University of Iowa
Iowa City, Iowa

Reviewers:

Sharon Davids, R.R.T., R.E.M.T.
South Miami Hospital
ihs at Green Briar
Miami, Florida

Nicolas Dawson, R.C.P., C.R.T.T.
Staff Respiratory Care Practitioner
Howard County General Hospital
Baltimore, Maryland

Joseph P. Lynott, M.H.A., R.R.T.
Director
Respiratory Care Services
The National Rehabilitation Hospital
Washington, D.C.

Chapter V
TRANSDISCIPLINARY TEAM CONCEPT

Contributors: **Marta S. Kazandjian, M.A., C.C.C.-SLP**
Co-Director
Speech Pathology
Long Beach Memorial Hospital
Long Island, New York
Director
Speech Pathology
Village Nursing Home
New York, New York
Consultant
Silvercrest Extended Care Facility
Jamaica, New York
Executive Director
Communication Independence for Neurologically Impaired
New York, New York

Karen Dikeman, M.A., C.C.C.-SLP
Co-Director
Speech Pathology
Long Beach Memorial Hospital
Long Island, New York
Consultant
Silvercrest Extended Care Facility
Jamaica, New York
Consultant
Mary Manning Walsh Home
New York, New York

Editors: **Theronne B. Singletary, M.S., C.C.C.-SLP**
Director
Speech-Language Pathology Services
University of Tennessee Medical Center at Knoxville
Instructor
Department of Audiology and Speech Pathology
University of Tennessee
Knoxville, Tennessee

Ahmet Baydur, M.D., F.A.C.P., F.C.C.P.
Director
Chest Medicine Service
Rancho Los Amigos Medical Center
Downey, California
Associate Professor of Clinical Medicine
University of Southern California School of Medicine
Los Angeles, California

Reviewers:

Sharon Davids, R.R.T., R.E.M.T.
South Miami Hospital
ihs at Green Briar
Miami, Florida

Barbara M. Baker, Ph.D.
Associate Professor of Surgery
Division of Communicative Disorders
University of Louisville School of Medicine
Private Practice
University Speech Pathology Associates
Louisville, Kentucky

Rita Crabtree-Kampe, M.S., C.C.C.-SLP
Clinical Specialist
Motor Speech Disorders
Communication Disorders Department
Rancho Los Amigos Medical Center
Downey, California

Beverly Fornoff, B.S., R.R.T.
R. Adams Cowley Shock Trauma Center
Maryland Institute for Emergency
Medical Services Systems
University of Maryland Medical System
Baltimore, Maryland

Derinda R. Lewis, M.A., C.C.C.-SLP
Acute Care Specialist/Educational Consultant
Department of Rehabilitation Services
The Moses H. Cone Memorial Hospital
Greensboro, North Carolina

Chapter VI
NONVOCAL TREATMENT

Contributors:

Lisa Adams, M.A., C.C.C.-SLP
Clinical Supervisor
Queens College of the City
University of New York
New York, New York

Maria A. Connolly, D.N.Sc., C.C.R.N.
Assistant Professor of Nursing
Department of Medical-Surgical Nursing
Niehoff School of Nursing
Loyola University of Chicago
Chicago, Illinois

Editors:

Carole Oglesby, M.S., C.C.C.-SLP
University Speech Pathology Associates
Louisville, Kentucky

Mary F. Mason, M.S., C.C.C.-SLP

Reviewers:

Molly Doyle, M.S., C.C.C.-SLP
Clinical Specialist
Augmentative/Alternative Communication
Communication Disorders Department
Rancho Los Amigos Medical Center
Downey, California

Jo Ann Irene Frey, B.S.N., R.N.C., C.R.R.N.
Pulmonary Nurse Clinician
Pulmonary Rehabilitation Coordinator
Pulmonary Rehabilitation, Pulmonary Services
Good Samaritan Hospital
Cincinnati, Ohio

Marta S. Kazandjian, M.A., C.C.C.-SLP
Co-Director
Speech Pathology
Long Beach Memorial Hospital
Director
Speech Pathology
Village Nursing Home
New York, New York
Consultant
Silvercrest Extended Care Facility
Jamaica, New York
Executive Director
Communication Independence for Neurologically Impaired
New York, New York

Chapter VII
VOCAL TREATMENT STRATEGIES

Contributor: **Mary F. Mason, M.S., C.C.C.-SLP**

Editors: **Kris Ward, M.S., C.C.C.-SLP**
Pulmonary Rehabilitation Program
Tustin Rehabilitation Hospital
Tustin, California

Roxann Diez Gross, M.A., C.C.C.-SLP
The Eye and Ear Institute
Department of Otolaryngology
University of Pittsburgh Medical Center
Pittsburgh, Pennsylvania

Reviewers: **Augusta Alba, M.D.**
Director of Rehabilitation Medicine
Goldwater Memorial Hospital
Professor of Clinical Rehabilitation Medicine
New York University
New York, New York

John R. Bach, M.D., F.R.C.P.C.
Associate Professor and Vice Chairman
Department of Physical Medicine and Rehabilitation
UMD-New Jersey Medical School
Director of Research and Associate Medical Director
Department of Physical Medicine and Rehabilitation
University Hospital
Co-Director
Jerry Lewis MDA Clinic
UMD-New Jersey Medical School
Newark, New Jersey
Medical Director
Center for Ventilator Management
Alternatives and Pulmonary Rehabilitation
Kessler Institute for Rehabilitation
West Orange, New Jersey

Robert J. Byrick, M.D., F.R.C.P.C.
Professor and Chairman
Department of Anaesthesia
St. Michael's Hospital
University of Toronto
Toronto, Ontario

Mary A. Cherepski, M.S., C.C.C.-SLP
Supervisor
Speech Pathology Services
St. Vincent Infirmary Medical Center
Little Rock, Arkansas

Jo Ann Irene Frey, B.S.N., R.N., C., C.R.R.N.
Pulmonary Nurse Clinician
Pulmonary Rehabilitation Coordinator
Pulmonary Rehabilitation, Pulmonary Services
Good Samaritan Hospital
Cincinnati, Ohio

Stan Martinkosky, Ph.D.
Clinical Associate Professor
Division of Otolaryngology
Department of Surgery
University of North Carolina School of Medicine
Chapel Hill, North Carolina

Diana Powell, M.S., C.C.C.-SLP
Director, Speech Pathology
Department of Rehabilitation Services
Stanford University Hospital
Stanford, California

Michael Ries, M.D., F.C.C.P.
Assistant Professor of Medicine
Pulmonary and Critical Care Medicine
Rush Medical College
Rush-Presbyterian-St. Luke's Medical Center
Chicago, Illinois
Co-Director
Residency Training Program
Rush North Shore Medical Center
Skokie, Illinois
Medical Director
Imperial Ventilator Center
Chicago, Illinois

Chapter VIII
PEDIATRICS

Contributors:

Stefanie Albamonte, M.S., C.C.C.-SLP
Clinical Coordinator of Speech and Hearing
Children's Specialized Hospital
Mountainside, New Jersey

Angela M. Jerome, R.N., M.S.N.
Pediatric Pulmonary Nurse Specialist
Children's Home Health
Pediatric Clinical Nurse Specialist
Adjunct Clinical Instructor
Old Dominion University
Norfolk, Virginia

Editors:

Varada Diwadkar, M.D.
Private Practice
Pediatric Pulmonology
Scottish Rite Children's Medical Center
Kennestone Hospital
Atlanta, Georgia

Allan B. Seid, M.D., F.A.C.S., F.A.A.P.
Attending Pediatric Otolaryngologist
Children's Hospital and Health Center
Associate Clinical Professor
Otolaryngology–Head and Neck Surgery
University of California, San Diego
San Diego, California

Reviewers:

Linda Hill, M.A., C.C.C.-SLP
Certified in Neurodevelopmental Treatment
Providence Speech and Hearing Center
Children's Hospital of Orange County
Orange, California

Julie A. McDougal, R.R.T., M.A.E.
Assistant Professor of Pediatrics
Pediatric Pulmonary Division
The University of Alabama at Birmingham
Birmingham, Alabama

Phyllis M. Palmer, M.S., C.C.C.-SLP
The Department of Speech Pathology and Audiology
University of Iowa
Iowa City, Iowa

Jenni L. Raake, R.R.T.
Clinical Therapist II
Children's Hospital Medical Center
Cincinnati, Ohio

Kitty Reid, R.N.C.
ENT Clinician
Scott and White Clinic
Scott and White Memorial Hospital
Texas A & M University College of Medicine
Temple, Texas

Mary Speights, R.N., B.S.N.
Head and Neck Cancer Nurse Clinician
Coordinator
Scott and White Clinic
Scott and White Memorial Hospital
Texas A & M University College of Medicine
Temple, Texas

Geralyn Timler, M.S., C.C.C.-SLP
Clinical Supervisor, Speech Pathologist
Speech Pathology Associates
Irvine, California

Cynthia Vance, M.A., C.C.C.-SLP
Department of Speech, Language and Learning Disorders
Texas Children's Hospital
Houston, Texas

Chapter IX
PSYCHOSOCIAL

Contributors: **Jeffrey L. Santee, Ph.D.**
Licensed Clinical Psychologist
Private Practice
Behavioral Medicine
Wheaton, Illinois
Consultant
Ventilator Support Center
Suburban Hospital
Hinsdale, Illinois

John Connors, D.M.D.
Private Practice
Huntington, Connecticut

Karen Bither
Parent
Anderson, California

Julia Almand, R.N.
Texarkana, Texas

Lori A. Hinderer
President
Ability 2000
St. Louis, Missouri

David Muir
Inventor
Passy-Muir Tracheostomy Speaking Valves

Angela Vangalis
Parent
Irvine, California

Tedde Scharf, M.A.
Associate Director
Disabled Student Resources
Arizona State University
Tempe, Arizona

Chapter X
DYSPHAGIA

Contributors: **Jo Puntil, M.S., C.C.C.-SLP**
Dysphagia Clinical Specialist
Private Practice
Seal Beach, California

Mary F. Mason, M.S., C.C.C.-SLP

Editor: **Melissa Scott, M.A., C.C.C.-SLP**
Specialist in Ventilator Dependent Patients
Private Practice
La Grange, Illinois

Reviewers: **Michael E. Groher, Ph.D.**
Chief
Audiology/Speech Pathology
James A. Haley Veterans Administration Hospital
Tampa, Florida

Michael Crary, Ph.D.
Professor and Chief
Speech and Language Pathology
Department of Communicative Disorders
University of Florida Health Science Center
Gainsville, Florida

Lisa Kohlenberger, M.A., C.C.C.-SLP
Department of Speech Pathology
USC University Hospital
Los Angeles, California

Diana Powell, M.S., C.C.C.-SLP
Director
Speech Pathology
Department of Rehabilitation Services
Stanford University Hospital
Stanford, California

LIST OF ILLUSTRATIONS

List of Figures

List of Tables

PREFACE

The advancements made in medical technology and treatment procedures have dramatically increased the survival rate of people who experience serious illness and injury.

Sophisticated life support systems are maintaining life for neonatal and geriatric populations far beyond what was ever anticipated. These advanced lifesaving procedures have created a challenging environment for many health professionals in their effort to enhance and ensure their patients' quality of life through rehabilitative therapies.

There has also been a major transformation in the roles of allied health professionals including respiratory therapists, nurses, physical and occupational therapists, speech-language pathologists and dieticians who are working with patients whose lives have been extended because of state-of-the-art medical interventions. No longer do these allied health specialists deliver care in isolation but instead they have begun to coordinate their efforts. This practice has evolved into today's transdisciplinary team approach.

In the past ten years, there has been an increase in the number of tracheostomized and ventilator dependent patients found not only in hospital intensive care units (ICUs), but also in long-term care facilities and home care settings. This fragile and complicated patient population presents a challenging opportunity for the speech-language pathologist to participate as a vital member of the transdisciplinary team in the identification and delivery of early intervention strategies for communication disorders and dysphagia.

The services of the speech-language pathologist in health care are no longer limited to the neurologically impaired patient on the rehabilitation or general hospital unit. The need for these services is now apparent for patients in other areas of the hospital including the ICU, pediatric nursery, burn unit, cardiac unit, oncology unit, spinal cord injury unit, and pulmonary unit. Currently, the speech-language pathologist can be found working closely with respiratory therapists and pulmonologists in the implementation of ventilator weaning therapies that facilitate a patient's recovery and successful discharge from the hospital. Tracheostomy and ventilator dependent patients who in the past were forced to suffer in silence are now voicing with the interventions provided to them by the speech-language pathologist. In addition, even the most critical and/or terminal patient can be provided a few crucial moments to express his or her thoughts, to facilitate closure on crucial personal matters and to express their "I love you's" and "good-byes."

The speech-language pathologist is becoming increasingly more involved in the process of transitioning and mainstreaming into school and/or home environments individuals who are expected to be long-term or permanently tracheostomized or ventilator dependent.

As speech-language pathologists, we should recognize that the doors of opportunity are open and technology is now available to enable us to provide therapeutic interventions that can make a significant difference in the well-being and recovery of tracheostomized and ventilator dependent patients. The lack of education and training currently available to speech-language pathologists in the area of respiratory disorders and their impact upon effective communication and swallowing function has significantly impeded our therapy efforts. The motivation and inspiration to write this book came from my own personal struggles to identify the most successful communication and dysphagia treatment strategies for the tracheostomy and ventilator dependent patients with whom I work.

While there has been an increase over the past few years in research, articles, and presentations on the subject of treatment interventions with tracheostomized and ventilator dependent patients, no comprehensive textbook providing the speech-language pathologist with an in-depth discussion of this patient population has been available. I have therefore endeavored to develop a text that will provide the speech-language pathologist with necessary background information as well as the tools to implement successful assessment and intervention strategies with tracheostomy and ventilator dependent patients. It has been my experience that the difference between success and failure in therapeutic intervention with these patients is often dependent upon whether a transdisciplinary team approach has been utilized. Consequently, in writing this text, I have involved individuals representing several disciplines. I have solicited the expertise of colleagues in the area of speech-language pathology, experienced respiratory and nursing specialists, as well as several of the most accomplished professionals in pulmonary and otolaryngology medicine. I gratefully acknowledge the assistance of these professionals who, because they are involved in the day-to-day challenges of working with this patient population, have contributed what I believe to be state-of-the-art educational material regarding effective transdisciplinary treatment approaches for the tracheostomy and ventilator dependent patient.

It is my hope that this text will provide the speech-language pathologist with the information needed to facilitate successful transition of tracheostomized and ventilator dependent patients from frustration and isolation to a quality of life that restores their dignity and independence. If I have been successful in this endeavor, it is directly related to the expertise and participation of my co-contributors, editors, and reviewers; any deficiencies are mine.

SPEECH PATHOLOGY FOR TRACHEOSTOMIZED AND VENTILATOR DEPENDENT PATIENTS

CHAPTER I

ANATOMY AND PHYSIOLOGY

Mary F. Mason, *M.S., C.C.C.-SLP*

Lori Gonzalez, *Ph.D., C.C.C.-SLP*
Assistant Professor
Division of Communication Disorders
University of Kentucky
Lexington, Kentucky

Edited by:

J. David Garrett, *Ph.D.*
Chief, Speech Pathology Services
Methodist Hospital
Assistant Professor, Otolaryngology Department
Baylor College of Medicine
Houston, Texas

Thomas L. Layton, *Ph.D.*
Associate Professor
Division of Speech and Hearing Sciences
Department of Medical Allied Health Problems
The School of Medicine
University of North Carolina at Chapel Hill
Chapel Hill, North Carolina

INTRODUCTION

In this chapter, the anatomy and physiology of pertinent systems are reviewed in order to better understand the changes associated with tracheostomized and ventilator dependent patients.

All body systems are related both anatomically and functionally. This interrelationship is especially true for the respiratory system (Figure 1-1), the larynx, and the articulatory system. For example, we now know that with tracheostomy placement, mucus production increases, vocal fold abduction during inspiration is reduced, and the swallow is often affected. Reduction of airflow to the olfactory receptors in the nasal cavity affects the sense of smell and the ability to taste. In addition, as a result of tracheostomy placement, the ability to oxygenate efficiently is often reduced due to the lack of resistance to the airstream normally produced by the upper airway. With ventilator dependency, there are additional effects on systems which may include heart rate, blood pressure, intracranial pressure, upper and lower airway tissue alteration, renal system changes, and electrolyte fluctation.

BONES AND MUSCULATURE OF THE HEAD AND NECK

In this portion of the chapter the anatomy and physiology of the head and neck are reviewed. A complete understanding of these structures is critical when working with tracheostomized and ventilator dependent patients. Accurate diagnosis and treatment procedures are dependent on the clinician's knowledge of anatomy and their ability to understand how a deficit in one structure affects the remaining structures. Many disorders the speech-language pathologist works with affect one, or more of the structures discussed in this chapter.

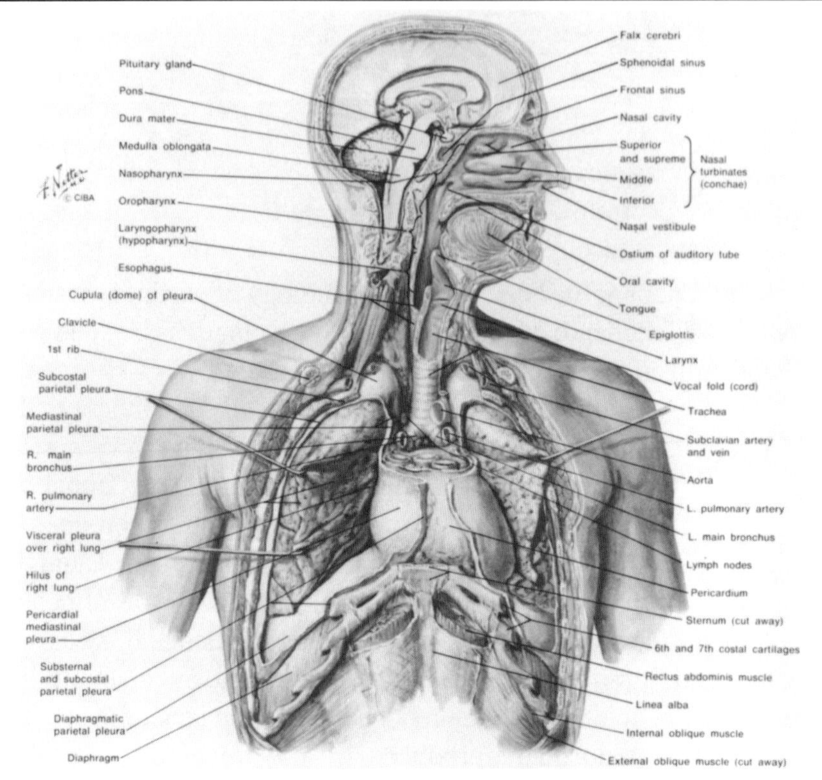

Figure 1-1 Respiratory system. (Copyright 1988 CIBA-GEIGY Corporation. Reproduced with permission from the CIBA COLLECTION OF MEDICAL ILLUSTRATIONS *by Frank H. Netter, M.D., West Caldwell, NJ, All rights reserved.*

Fascia and Muscles of the Scalp

Superficial fascia
Epicranius
Temporoparietalis
Occipitofrontalis

Fascia refers to the connective tissue of body structures associated with the muscles, bones, and organs. Superficial fascia covers the facial muscles, superficial blood vessels, and nerves. It contains a rich blood supply and varies in thickness depending on its location on the scalp. The superficial fascia connects directly to facial fascia.

The epicranius (Figure 1-2) is a muscular and tendinous layer that extends from the top and sides of the skull from the occipital bone to the eyebrow (frontal bone) and extends laterally to the squamae of the temporal bones. The epicranius associates with the occipitofrontalis, the galea aponeurotica (Figures 1-2 and 1-3), and two temporoparietalis muscles. The occipitofrontalis muscles (Figures 1-2 and 1-3) contain four thin, broad, muscular bellies, two frontal and two occipital. These muscle bellies are connected by the galea aponeurotica, which serves to attach these muscles groups but still allows movement of the scalp freely over the underlying calvaria of the skull. The occipitofrontalis draws back the scalp to wrinkle the forehead and raise the eyebrows (expression of surprise). The temporoparietalis muscle is a variable

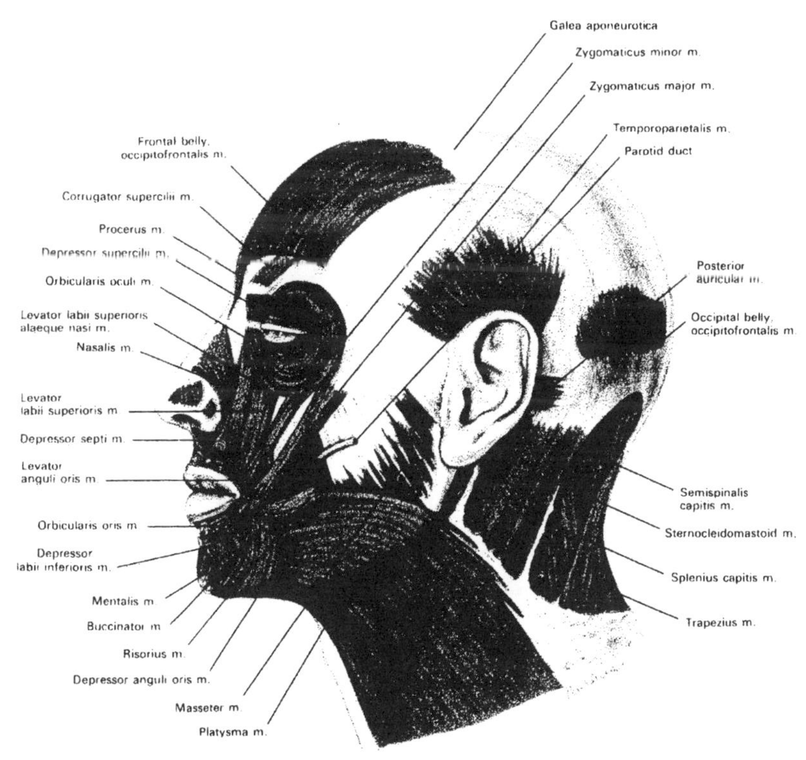

Figure 1-2 Superficial muscles of the face, scalp, and neck; left lateral view. (From Gray, H., Gray's Anatomy, *Philadelphia: Lea & Febiger, 1985.)*

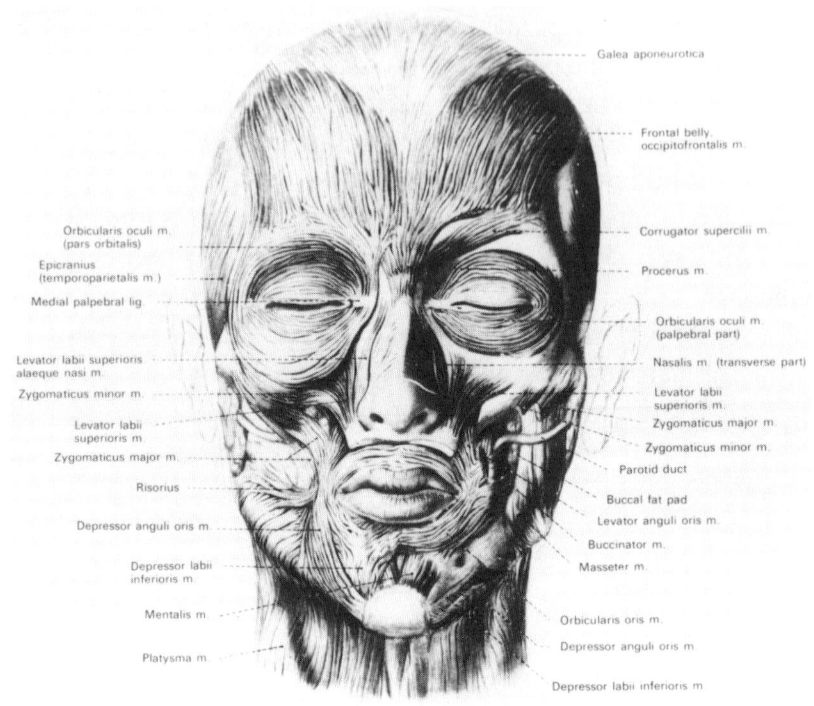

Figure 1-3 The facial muscles; anterior view. On the right (reader's left) is shown the more superficial layer, while on the left are the deeper muscles. (From Gray, H., Gray's Anatomy, *Philadelphia: Lea & Febiger, 1985.)*

muscle sheet that tightens the scalp, draws back the skin of the temples, and combines with the occipitofrontalis to widen the eyes (expression of fright) or wrinkle the forehead.

These muscles are innervated by the temporal and zygomatic branches of the facial nerve.

Muscles of the Nose

Procerus
Nasalis
Depressor Septi

Muscles of the nose include the procerus, nasalis, and depressor septi (Figures 1-2 and 1-3). The procerus and nasalis muscle fibers decussate with the frontal belly of the occipitofrontalis muscles. The procerus nasalis extends from the skin of the forehead between the eyebrows and reaches superiorly over the bridge of the nose, covering the upper part of the lateral nasal cartilage and the lower part of the nasal bone; it is a small pyramidal slip arising on each side by tendinous fibers from the covering fascia. The procerus acts to bring down the medial angle of the eyebrows to produce wrinkles across the nose bridge. The nasalis muscle contains the transverse and alar muscles. The transverse part (compressor naris) depresses the cartilaginous part of the nose and brings the ala toward the septum. The alar part of the nasalis increases the size of the nares openings, serving to avoid closure, but it can contract severely in strong emotions (e.g., anger) as well as with difficult breathing. The depressor septi constricts the opening of the nares by bringing the ala downward. Innervation for these structures is provided by the buccal branch of the facial nerve.

Muscles of the Mouth

Levator labii superioris
Levator labii superioris alaeque nasi
Levator anguli oris
Zygomaticus minor
Zygomaticus major
Risorius zygomaticus major
Depressor labii inferioris
Depressor anguli oris
Transversus menti
Buccinator orbicularis oris

The *levator labii superioris* (Figures 1-2 and 1-3) begins immediately above the infraorbital foramen with some attachment to the maxilla and zygomatic bones from the lower portion of the orbit. These muscle fibers unite with the muscles of the upper lip located between the levator anguli oris and the levator labii superioris alaeque nasi. The levator labii superioris is a thin quadrangular muscle that raises the upper lip and brings it somewhat forward. The levator anguli oris is a quadrilateral flat muscle below the infraorbital foramen; it extends from the canine fossa and unites with the mouth's depressor anguli, zygomatic major (Figures 1-2 and 1-3), and orbicularis oris to form expressions of contempt or disdain with the nose and mouth. The levator labii superioris alaeque nasi dilates the nares and raises the upper lip. It extends from the upper portion of the maxillary frontal process and obliquely passes laterally and downward, dividing into two slips. One slip blends with the *levator labii superioris* in the upper lip; the other slip of the levator labii superioris inserts into the greater alar cartilage of the nose.

The *zygomaticus minor* (Figures 1-2 and 1-3) is a small muscle fiber bundle extending from the malar surface of the zygomatic bone directly behind the zygomatic maxillary structure traveling medially and downward as a slip and inserts into the upper lip between the levator labii superioris and the *zygomaticus major*. During laughter the zygomaticus minor brings the mouth angle upward and back.

The zygomaticus major extends from the zygomatic bone and descends medially and obliquely to connect to the angle of the mouth, attaching to the depressor and levator anguli oris as well as the orbicularis oris muscle. The previous five muscles (levator labii superioris, levator labii superioris alaeque nasi, levator anguli oris, zygomaticus minor, and zygomaticus major) are innervated by the buccal branches of the facial nerve.

Varying in size, the *risorius* (Figures 1-2 and 1-3) extends from the parotid fascia, passing forward horizontally across the platysma and superficially connecting at the angle of the mouth into the skin. Its function is to retract the mouth angle.

The *depressor labii inferioris* (Figure 1-3) brings the lower lip directly downward with some lateral movement. The depressor labii inferioris begins in the platysma muscle at the oblique line of the mandible and contains fat in its fibers. It extends upward medially into the skin of the lower lip where it unites with the orbicularis oris and depressor labii inferioris of the opposite side.

The *depressor anguli oris* (Figures 1-3 and 1-4) muscle begins from the oblique line of the mandible below and lateral to the depressor labii inferioris. It is the antagonist of the levator anguli oris and zygomaticus major and brings the mouth angle medial. The depressor anguli oris muscle fibers are curved and connect to the narrow fasciculus of the angle of the mouth.

The mentalis is a small and conical fasciculus located at the side of the frenulum below the lower lip. It begins at the mandible and extends downward to connect to the chin integument. The transverse menti muscle is small and extends across the midline portion of the chin. It serves to protrude the lower lip and wrinkle the chin as in pouting or expression of doubt. The transverse menti muscle is usually aligned with the depressor anguli oris. All of these muscles of the lower lip are innervated by the buccal and mandibular branches of the facial nerve.

The orbicularis oris (Figures 1-3 and 1-4) is innervated by the facial nerve and surrounds the orifice of the mouth. It contains many strata of muscular fibers. In addition to its intrinsic fibers, it incorporates fibers from surrounding muscles, including the buccinator, levator labii superioris, zygomaticus major, and depressor labii inferioris. Its lateral band is the incisivus labii superioris, located in the upper lip. The medial band is the nasolabialis muscle, which attaches the upper lip with the septum of the nose. The philtrum is the

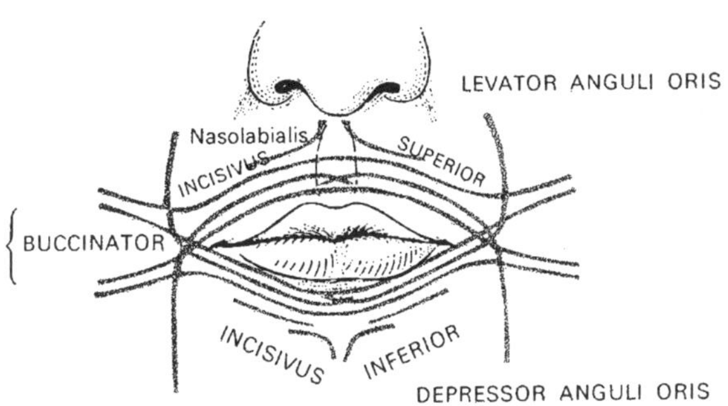

Figure 1-4 Diagram showing arrangement of fibers of the orbicularis oris. (From Gray, H., Gray's Anatomy, *Philadelphia: Lea & Febiger, 1985.)*

depression of the upper lip under the nose between the two nasolabialis muscle bands. Forming the lower lip is the incisivus labii inferior, which begins at the mandible lateral to the mentalis, joining with the other muscles of the mouth. All of these components of the orbicularis oris are of importance to this text because it is this musculature that assists speech articulation with movements of the lips and mouth. The orbicularis oris also keeps the mouth closed and close to the teeth and alveolar arches, which is most important in feeding and drinking. The orbicularis oris is innervated by the facial nerve.

The buccinator is one of the deepest facial muscles. It forms the lateral walls of the oral cavity and is the primary muscle of the cheek. It is located lateral to the teeth and extends from the mandible and maxilla. Posteriorly, the buccinator attaches to the pterygomandibular raphe. The pterygomandibular raphe is a tendinous structure that provides anterior origin to the buccinator and posterior origin to the pharyngeal constrictor. It extends and becomes continuous with the orbicularis oris. The buccinator is covered superficially by the buccopharyngeal fascia and buccal fat pad. Deeper, it is connected to the buccal glands and mucus membranes of the mouth. It is also penetrated by the duct of the parotid gland located by the upper second molar tooth. The buccinator compresses the cheek, allowing for blowing or the forcing of air out through the lips as with playing wind instruments. The buccinator is an important accessory muscle to mastication as it can compress the cheek, holding food closely against the teeth for deglutition. Innervation is supplied by the lower buccal branches of the facial nerve. The buccal fat pad is an encapsulated mass that lies superficial to the buccinator and anterior borders of the masseter muscle. In infants, this mass is supportive to the buccinator and thought to aid in sucking (suctorial pad). The buccal fat pad in infants is larger in anatomical relation than in the adult.

The pterygomandibular raphe is a tendinous structure that extends superiorly from the medial pterygoid plate hamulus to the mylohyoid line posterior end. It is the origin for the buccinator and pharyngeal constrictor muscles. Its medial surface is covered by the mucus membrane of the oral cavity and its lateral surface is covered by adipose tissue of the buccal fat pad. The buccopharyngeal fascia is the lateral covering of the raphe and superior pharyngeal and constrictor muscles. The buccopharyngeal fascia provides a cleft between these muscles and superficial structures, allowing them to move freely.

Muscles of Mastication

Muscles of mastication are for the movement of the mandible during the primary function of chewing. However, there is a great deal of mandibular movement during the production of speech. These muscles include the temporalis, masseter, medial pterygoid, mandibular sling, and lateral pterygoid. The fascia of mastication includes the temporal fascia, parotid-masseteric fascia, and pterygoid fascia.

The temporalis muscle (Figure 1-5) is positioned on the side of the head and is a wide, broad muscle that radiates or fans out over the side of the skull. It originates from the deep temporal fascia and the whole of the temporal fossa. The temporalis muscle fibers descend into a tendon that passes under the zygomatic arch. This tendon inserts to the coronoid process, and the anterior ramus of the mandibular. The function of the temporalis muscle is to elevate the mandible and close the jaws, retracting the mandible with its posterior fibers. It is innervated by the deep anterior and posterior temporal nerves of the anterior trunk of the mandibular division of the trigeminal nerve.

The masseter muscle (Figure 1-5) contains three divisions: superficial, intermediate, and deep. The largest division is the superficial part, which originates as a thick, tendinous aponeurosis from the zygomatic process of the maxilla and the anterior inferior border of the zygomatic arch. These muscle fibers course inferiorly and posteriorly and insert into the angle and lower portion of the lateral surface of the ramus of the mandible. The intermediate portion of the masseter muscles begins at the inner anterior surface of the zygomatic arch and inserts into the ramus of the mandible. The deep part originates from the posterior inner surface of the zygomatic arch and, with the intermediate part courses anteriorly and inferiorly and inserts into the superior portion of the ramus of the mandible. The function of the masseter muscle is to elevate the mandible and close the jaws. It is innervated by the masseteric branch of the mandibular division of the trigeminal nerve.

The medial pterygoid muscle (Figure 1-6) is located on the inner

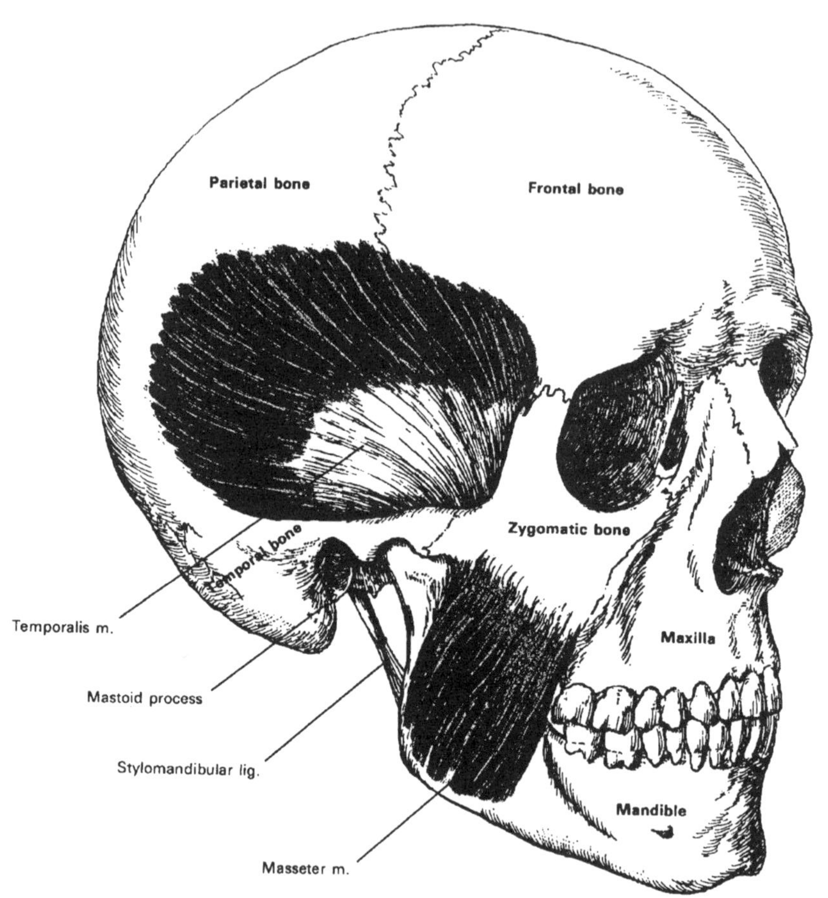

Figure 1-5 A lateral view of the skull showing the origin and insertion of the masseter muscle, as well as those of the temporalis muscle and the stylomandibular ligament. (From Gray, H., Gray's Anatomy, *Philadelphia: Lea & Febiger, 1985.)*

portion of the ramus of the mandible, in contrast to the masseter muscle, which is located on the outer portion. It is a thick and quadrilateral muscle that is vital in the chewing of food. It works in conjunction with the lateral pterygoid muscles in chewing. As the jaw moves from side to side the alternate opposing lateral pterygoid assists in this type of movement. It is attached by strong tendinous lamina into the lower anterior portion of the medial surface of the ramus and the angle of the mandible. It is innervated by the medial pterygoid branch of the mandibular division of the trigeminal nerve.

The mandibular sling refers to the suspension of the mandible by the coordination and positioning of the medial pterygoid and masseter muscles. The mandibular sling is attached to the sphenomandibular ligament which acts as a guide to its range of motion.

The lateral pterygoid muscle (Figure 1-6) is a thick, short muscle with two ends or heads. It extends horizontally between the condyle of the mandible and the infratemporal fossa. This first head, or superior head, begins from the infratemporal crest and inferior part of the lateral surface of the great wing of the sphenoid bone. The inferior head begins at the lateral surface of the pterygoid plate. These muscle fibers extend backward horizontally and laterally and then are inserted into a depression in the anterior portion of the neck at the condyle of the mandible and into the anterior margin of the articular disc of the temporomandibular joint. The lateral pterygoid muscle opens the mouth and in coordination with the elevator muscle of the

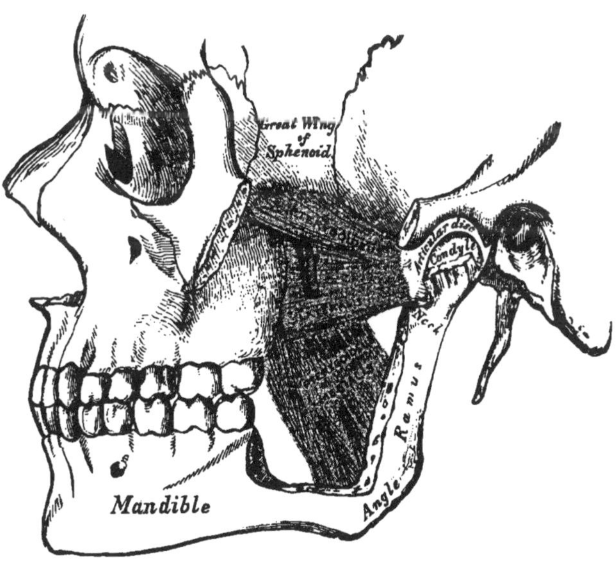

Figure 1-6 The lateral and medial pterygoid muscles; left side, lateral view. The zygomatic arch and a portion of the ramus of the mandible have been removed to show the position of the maxillary artery. (From Gray, H., Gray's Anatomy, *Philadelphia: Lea & Febiger, 1985.)*

mandible can extend the jaw forward. It also assists in chewing action. It is innervated by the mandibular division of the trigeminal nerve.

Group muscles that provide action for mastication include the temporalis, medial pterygoid, and masseter muscles to close the jaws. Biting is performed with the medial pterygoid and masseter, with some action contributed by the temporalis. Chewing requires all three of these muscles to act. Jaw opening is primarily the function of the lateral pterygoid. Suprahyoid and infrahyoid muscles of the neck also contribute to jaw opening.

Major fascia for the muscles of mastication include the temporal fascia, parotid masseteric fascia, and pterygoid fascia (Figure 1-7). The temporal fascia is a strong fibrous sheeting that is aponeurotic and covers the temporalis and attaches to it with fibers. It is the deepest cranial extension of fascia. The parotid-masseteric fascia converts the masseter muscle and divides to close the parotid gland. This fascia extends from the zygomatic arch to attach the mandible anteriorly, posteriorly, and inferiorly. The pterygoid fascia covers the lateral and medial pterygoid muscles. It follows below the mandible and attaches deep internally to the spine.

Muscles of the Neck

For the purpose of this text neck muscles are described as they affect respiration, phonation, and swallowing. Some of these muscles will be discussed again later in the portion of the text that describes muscles involved with ventilation.

Muscles of the Larynx

Because the ability to speak requires movement of the articulators as well as laryngeal function, we will briefly review some laryngeal muscles that produce phonation by primarily controlling changes in frequency, as well as the muscles that close the airway during swallowing (Figures 1-8 and 1-9). The thyroarytenoid and cricoarytenoid muscles provide several functions in the control of motion of the vocal folds. The posterior cricoarytenoid muscles act as abduc-

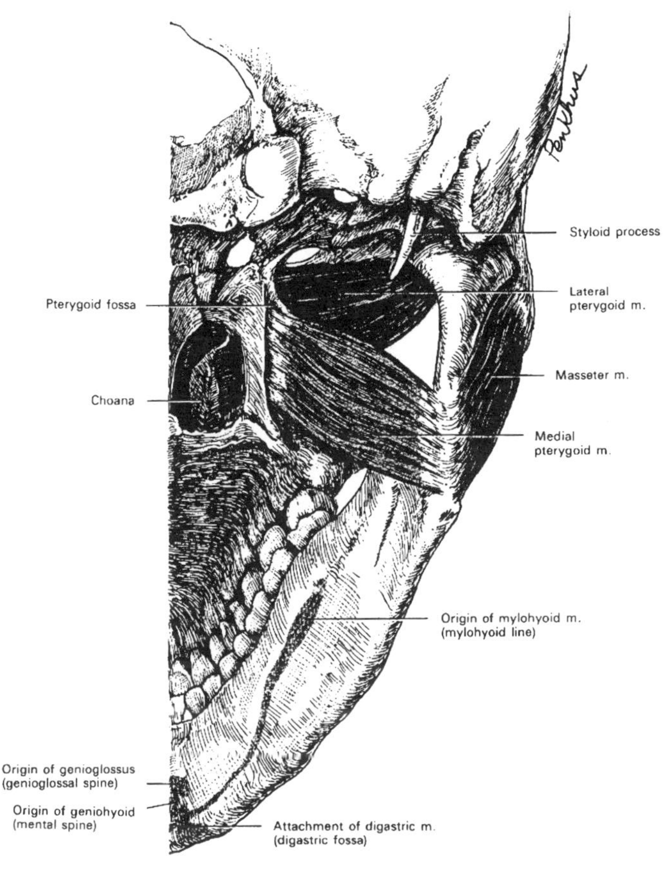

Figure 1-7 The pterygoid and masseter muscles viewed from below, showing how the medial pterygoid and masseter form a sling suspending the angle of the mandible. (From Gray, H., Gray's Anatomy, *Philadelphia: Lea & Febiger, 1985.)*

tors, pulling the vocal folds open. The lateral cricoarytenoid muscles function as adductors, bringing vocal folds together. The thyroarytenoid muscles are within the vocal folds and provide longitudinal tension. These two muscles work together to manipulate vocal fold function rapidly and with great precision. Also providing this coordination of function are both the transverse and oblique interarytenoid muscles. Aryepiglottic muscle fibers connect epiglottic structures to the lower arytenoid housing of the vocal folds. (Figure 1-8 and 1-9).

Suprahyoid Muscles

The suprahyoid muscles (Figure 1-10) are located superior to the hyoid bone and include the stylohyoid, mylohyoid, geniohyoid and digastric muscles.

The stylohyoid muscle retracts and elevates the hyoid bone, which causes the floor of the oral cavity to elongate. It is innervated by the facial nerve. It is a slim muscle located superiorly and anteriorly to the digastric muscles. Anteriorly it passes and inferiorly attaches to the greater horn of the hyoid bone.

The mylohyoid is a triangular, flat muscle, located superiorly to the digastric muscle (Figures 1-10 and 1-11). It causes the floor of the oral cavity to rise during swallowing or with tongue protrusion. It is capable of depressing the mandible and assists in mastication. It is

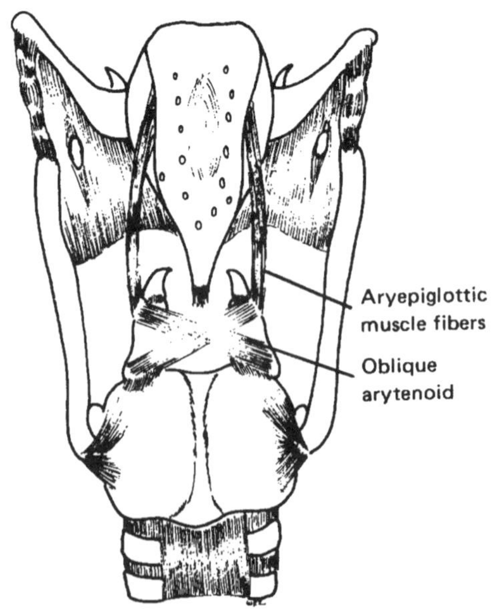

Figure 1-8 Schematic of the oblique and aryepiglottic fibers of the interarytenoid muscle. (From Willard R. Zemlin, SPEECH AND HEARING SCIENCE, *2/E, (c) 1981, p. 166. Reprinted by permission of Prentice-Hall, Inc., Englewood Cliffs, NJ.)*

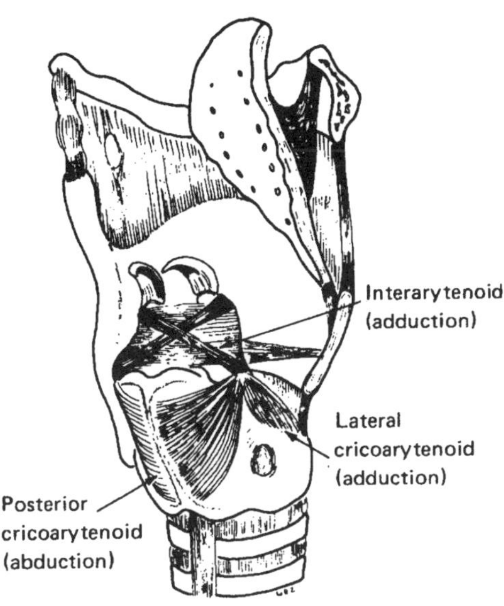

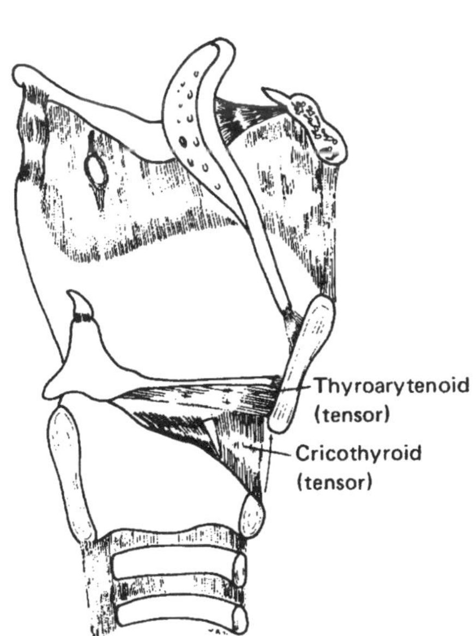

Figure 1-9 Schematic summary of the actions of the intrinsic laryngeal muscles. (From Willard R. Zemlin, SPEECH AND HEARING SCIENCE, *2/E, (c) 1981, p. 168. Reprinted by permission of Prentice-Hall, Inc., Englewood Cliffs, NJ.)*

innervated by the later mandibular division of the trigeminal nerve, which forms the inferior alveolar nerve and provides for mylohyoid nerve branching.

This muscle is a deep neck muscle and attaches from the anterior portion of the hyoid and extends to attach to the inferior mental spine (Figures 1-10 and 1-13). Its functions include movement of the hyoid bone slightly upward and forward to facilitate the reception of food into the oral cavity by shortening the floor of the mouth. It also assists in the retraction and depression of the mandible to facilitate mastication. The innervation source for the geniohyoid muscle is from the first cervical nerve.

The digastric muscle assists in lowering the mandible for feeding, along with the pterygoid muscle (Figure 1-10 and 1-11). The digastric muscle has two bellies: posterior and anterior. The posterior

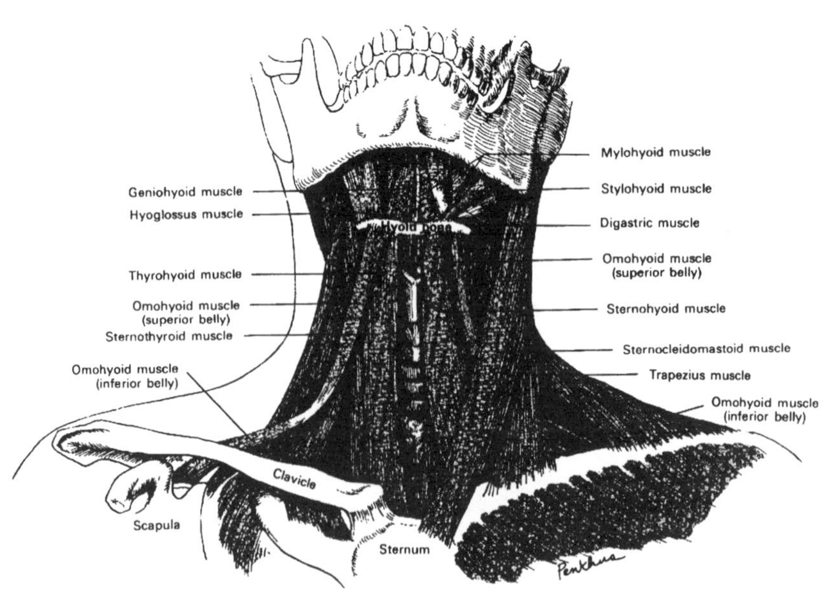

Figure 1-10 Muscles of the neck; anterior view. (From Gray, H., Gray's Anatomy, *Philadelphia: Lea & Febiger, 1985.)*

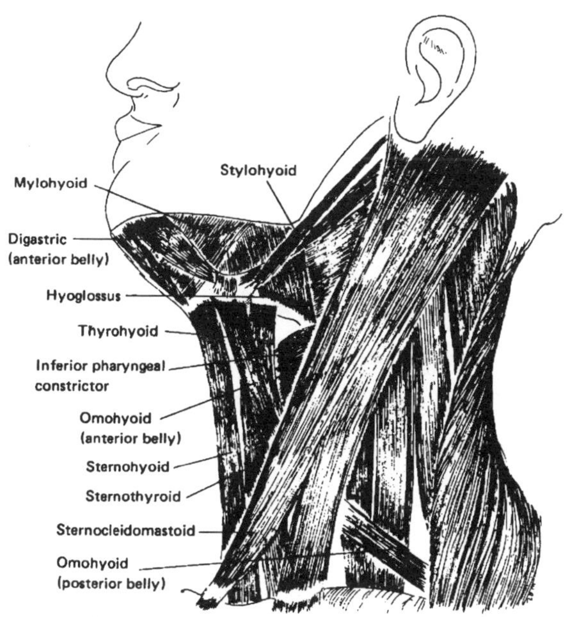

Figure 1-11 Muscles of the neck that can influence the position of and behavior of the larynx. (From Willard R. Zemlin, SPEECH AND HEARING SCIENCE, *2/E, (c) 1981, p. 152, Reprinted by permission of Prentice-Hall, Inc., Englewood Cliffs, NJ.)*

belly begins at the temporal bone mastoid notch. The anterior belly begins at the inner side of the mandible at the inferior border depression. Both bellies end in a tendon that attaches to the stylohyoid muscle and to the greater horn of the hyoid bone. The digastric muscle is innervated by the inferior alveolar branch mandibular division of the trigeminal nerve.

Infrahyoid Muscles

Additional muscles of the neck include the infrahyoid muscles located inferiorly to the hyoid bone. These are the sternohyoid, sternothyroid, thyrohyoid and omohyoid muscles. These infrahyoid muscles play a role in swallowing function and movement of the hyoid bone. The sternohyoid is a narrow strip of muscle that depresses the hyoid bone after swallow and acts as an antagonist of the elevators of hyoid bone and larynx. The sternothyroid muscles draw the larynx

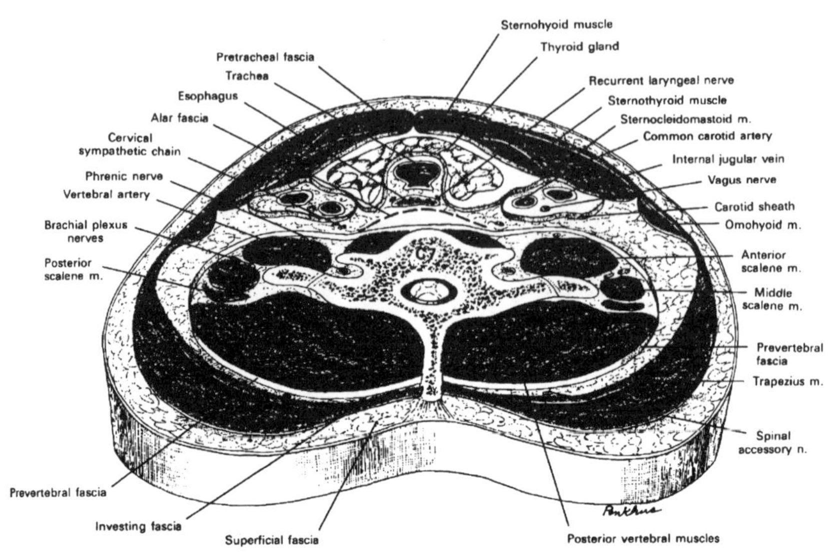

Figure 1-12 Cross section of the neck at the level of the seventh cervical vertebra. Observe the superficial fascia and the layers of deep cervical fascia. (From Gray, H., Gray's Anatomy, *Philadelphia: Lea & Febiger, 1985.)*

downward after it has been elevated after swallow. The thyrohyoid muscle depresses the hyoid bone; if the hyoid is in a fixed position it will draw the thyroid cartilage superiorly. The omohyoid depresses the hyoid bone after it has been elevated.

Anterolateral Vertebral Muscles

Anterolateral vertebral muscles include the: longus colli, longus capitis, rectus capitis anterior, rectus capitis lateralis and are used for head control and neck flexion. Laterally, vertebral muscles include the scalenus anterior, scalenus medius, and scalenus posterior, which move the neck and may assist as accessory breathing muscles by lifting the first and/or second ribs.

Triangles of the Neck

The sternocleidomastoid muscles divide the cervical region into posterior and anterior triangles (Figures 1-12 and 1-14). The borders

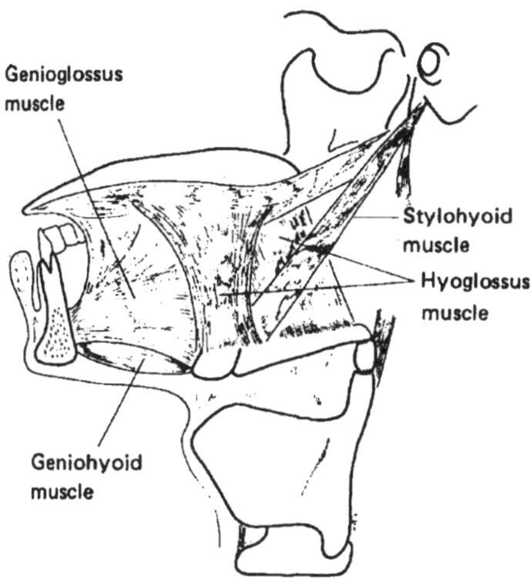

Figure 1-13 Schematic of the extrinsic tongue muscles, showing their relationship to the laryngeal structures. (From Willard R. Zemlin, SPEECH AND HEARING SCIENCE, *2/E, (c) 1981, p. 155, Reprinted by permission of Prentice-Hall, Inc., Englewood Cliffs, NJ.)*

of the triangle are defined by the lower edge of the mandible and the anterior edge of the sternocleidomastoid muscle. It divides further into three more triangles. The first is the submandibular triangle above the hyoid bone, which is defined by the mandible at its inferior border and both posteriorly and anteriorly by the corresponding digastric muscle bellies. The second is the carotid triangle, which is defined by the anterior edge of the sternocleidomastoid posteriorly and to the superior belly of the omohyoid muscle inferiorly; superiorly it is defined by the digastric posterior belly, located below and above the hyoid bone. The third triangle is the muscular triangle below the hyoid bone, which is defined superiorly to the omohyoid superior belly and the anterior edge of the sternocleidomastoid and medially to the anterior midline of the neck.

The posterior triangle of the neck is attached below the clavicle and to the trapezius and sternocleidomastoid muscles. It contains two triangular subdivisions: the occipital triangle and the omoclavicular triangle. The occipital triangle attaches inferiorly to the omohyoid, posteriorly to the trapezius, and anteriorly to the sternocleidomastoid muscle. The omoclavicular triangle, also known as the subclavian or

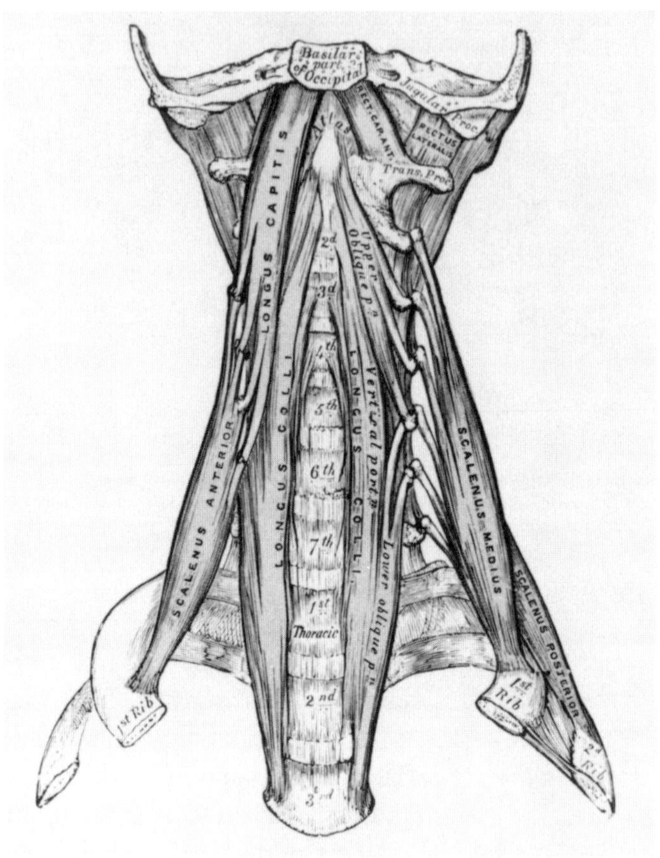

Figure 1-14 The anterior and lateral vertebral muscles. (From Gray, H., Gray's Anatomy, *Philadelphia : Lea & Febiger, 1985.)*

supraclavicular triangle, is located below the omohyoid anterior to the sternocleidomastoid muscle.

Neck Fascia

Fascial planes of the neck include superficial fascia, superficial cervical fascia, and deep cervical fascia. Superficial fascia is a loose layer that holds the platysma muscle. The superficial layer (Figure 1-12) of the deep cervical fascia is a sheet completely surrounding or enveloping the neck. It passes over the sternocleidomastoid muscle, splitting to form a sheath of the sternocleidomastoid, and splits again prior to its vertebral attachment, to envelop the trapezius muscle.

Anteriorly, at the midline, the superficial layer of the deep cervical fascia (Figure 1-12) divides into posterior and anterior sheets, attaching to the manubrium to form the suprasternal space of Burns, which is located just over the manubrium of the sternum. Venous channels (right and left sides) run between the suprasternal space. The jugular veins are located anteriorly and externally within the anterior surface layer of the deep cervical fascia.

The next layer of fascial sheeting is the deep cervical fascia (middle layer), composed of three layers: the deepest is the visceral layer (pretracheal [Figure 1-12] or buccopharyngeal), followed by the sternohyoid-omohyoid layer, and then the sternothyroid-thyrohyoid layer. Fusing with the anterior wall of carotid sheathing is the sternothyroid-thyrohyoid fascia. This fascia crosses anteriorly at the midline, surrounding the sternothyroid and thyrohyoid muscles. Crossing midline and surrounding the sternothyroid-omohyoid muscles bilaterally is the sternohyoid-omohyoid layer of fascia. The visceral fascia is the deepest layer of the cervical fascia. It envelopes the thyroid gland, trachea, and esophagus completely. This is also known as buccopharyngeal and pretracheal fascia.

Eventually, the visceral fascia (Figure 1-12) joins with the alar fascia of the carotid sheath at the root of the neck. With the fibrous pericardium, the alar fascia of the carotid sheath extends caudally. The thyroid gland, esophagus, and trachea are encapsulated in the space formed by the visceral fascia.

Bones of the Skull

The bones of the skull are made up of 22 bones that in the adult are all rigidly joined together except for the mandible. They are typically divided into the cranial skeleton (cranium), the facial skeleton, and the ear ossicula. The cranial skeleton (Figure 1-15) is made up of the eight bones that function to protect the brain.

The frontal bone forms the forehead and extends back to form the roofs of the orbital and nasal cavities. The parietal bones shape the rounded upper sides of the cranium. The temporal bones form the

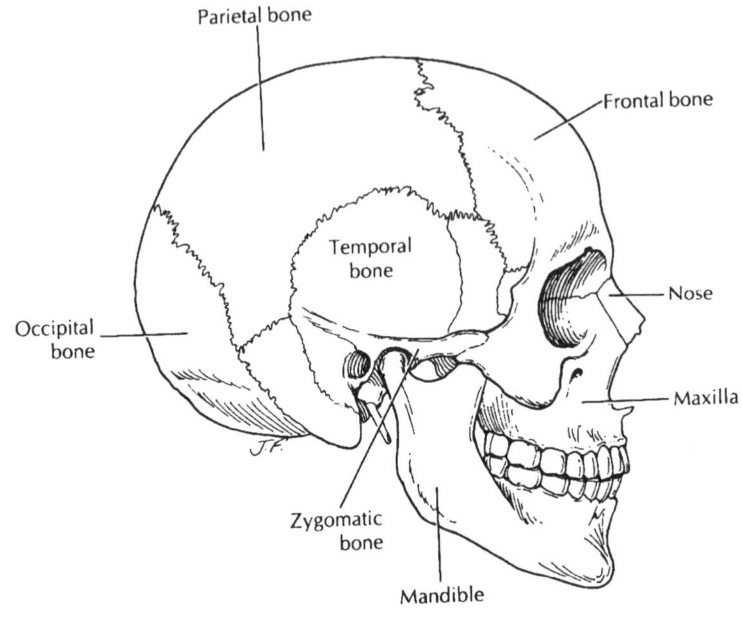

Figure 1-15 Bones of the skull. (From Eubanks, D., and Bone, R.C., Comprehensive Respiratory Care: A Learning System, *2nd Edition, St Louis: The C.V. Mosby Company, 1990.)*

lateral sides of the cranium and house the middle and inner ear. The back portion of the cranium is made up of the occipital bone, which articulates laterally with the parietal and temporal bones and extends to the base of the skull where the spinal cord exits the cranium. The sphenoid bone is a complex-shaped bone. The pterygoid plates of the sphenoid are important because they are the bony attachments for several articulatory muscles. The ethmoid bone is an irregularly-shaped bone that is located at the roof of the nasal cavity. It is perforated to allow the passage to the olfactory nerves from the cranium to the upper nasal cavity.

There are 14 bones that form the facial skeleton. The maxilla is the primary foundation for the facial bones. The maxilla contains the alveolar process that houses the upper teeth and forms the anterior 3/4ths of the hard palate. The posterior part of the hard palate is made up of the palatine bones. Both the maxilla and the zygomatic bones form the cheek bones. The nasal bone is the upper portion of the nose bridge. The bony nasal septum is made up of the ethmoid bone and vomer bone. The portion of the nose extending from the skull is made up of cartilage and tissue. The lower lateral walls of the nasal cavity are made up of the inferior conchae.

The lacrimal bones are located at the lower inside of the orbit (eye socket). It contains a canal or duct that extends from the corners of the eye to inside of the nasal cavity. The fluids of the eye (tears) are drained through the lacrimal duct to the nasal cavity. Normally the fluids are incorporated into the nasal mucus and are passed to the back of the throat where they are swallowed. The "runny nose" that occurs when one cries is due to the excess amounts of fluid that is passed through the lacrimal duct to the nasal cavity.

The mandible is the only bone of the skull that is not rigidly fixed in the adult. It is the lower jaw and it contains an alveolar process that houses the lower teeth. The mandible articulates with the temporal bone in the temporomandibular joint (TMJ). This joint can be felt just in front of the ear canal by opening and closing the mouth.

The hyoid bone is not considered a part of the skull because it does not articulate with any other bone. It is a U-shaped bone that can be felt in the midline at the angle where the underside of the chin meets with the neck. It is held in place strictly by the ligaments and muscles that attach to it.

Behind and below the external ear is the bony protuberance of the mastoid process. The inner part of this bone is hollowed out (honey-combed) with air cells; the superior and anterior portions communicate with the inner ear, the tympanic cavity.

NOSE

The portion of the nose extending from the skull is made up of cartilage and tissue. The nasal cavity is separated into two passages by the nasal septum. Inside the skull, the bony nasal septum is made up of two bones. The anterior nares are the lower portion of these passageways and provide the entry to the respiratory system. The anterior nares are flared. Just beyond the nares are the vestibules of the nose, which are lined with stratified squamous epithelium (the same type as found in the skin). This tough stratified squamous epithelium can withstand aggressive rubbing. Vibrissae are coarse hairs that arise from the walls of the internal nose and extend into the vestibules. The vibrissae serve a filtering function by helping to prevent large particles from entering the nasal cavities. Superior to the vestibules are the nasal fossae, the pathways through the nose within the hollow nasal cavity.

Bones that line the nasal cavity consist of the nasal bones, sphenoid bone, ethmoid bone, frontal bone, palatine bone, and maxillary bone. The two bones of the septum are the perpendicular plate of the ethmoid bone, which descends from the roof of the nasal cavity, and the thin vomer bone, which forms the lower portion of the bony nasal septum. The conchae are the shelves of bones extending medially along the lateral walls of the nasal cavity. The conchae (Figure 1-16) are also referred to as *turbinates*. There are three sets of conchae, or turbinates, known as the superior, the middle, and inferior conchae. The middle and superior conchae are part of the ethmoid bone, whereas the inferior conchae are distinct and separate bones. The meati channel into the conchae, dividing them into the superior

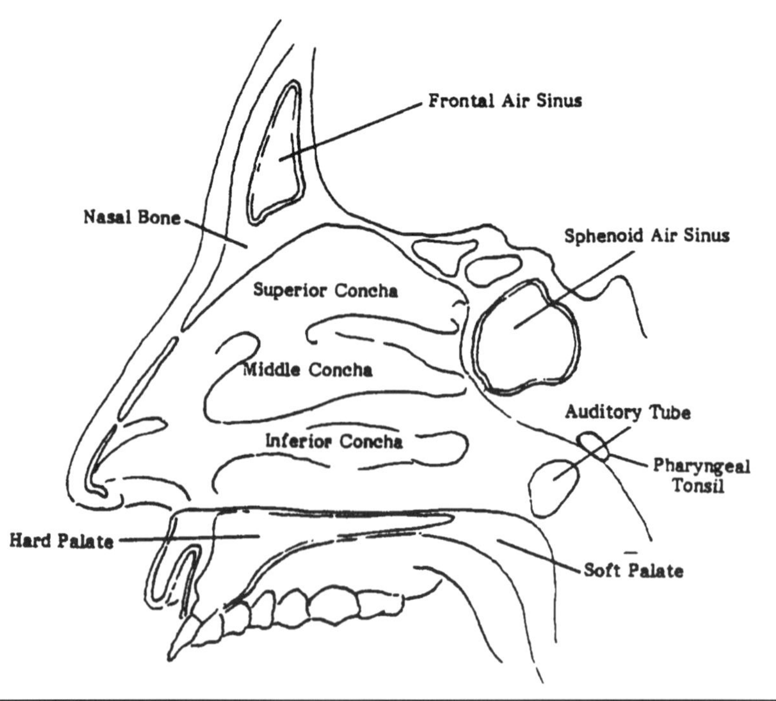

Figure 1-16 Sagittal section of the nasal cavity. (From California College for Health Sciences, Entry Level Respiratory Therapy Program, *Vol. 1, Fig. 2-1, p. [RTT 102] 2-3, National City, CA, 1985.)*

meati. The superior meati form the channel between the superior and middle conchae. The inferior meati are the channels between the inferior conchae and the floor of the nasal cavity. Sphenoethmoidal recesses are the spaces between the roof of the nasal cavity and the superior conchae.

Nasal Mucosa

The lining of the nasal cavity is mucosal. This mucosal tissue secretes mucus and serves as a lining for a hollow structure or organ. It is made of pseudostratified ciliated columnar epithelium that contains goblet cells. This type of mucosa is found throughout the respiratory system and is also referred to as *respiratory epithelium.* (Figure 1-17). Goblet cells are column-shaped cells that produce mucus. Pseudostratified ciliated columnar epithelium cells are column-shaped and stacked upon each other, with only lower cells attaching to the basement membrane. In actuality, all of these cells connect to the basement membrane with a very thin filament that slips between lower cells. Numerous cilia protrude from the epithelium. They are flexible rods that are responsible for the movement of material and mucus towards the back of the throat for swallow or expectoration. These cilia have an extremely important function in the movement of material and mucus in the respiratory system towards the back of the throat for swallow or expectoration.

Lamina Propria

The layer below the mucus layer is the lamina propria, where mucus-producing glands and the serous glands are located. Serous glands produce an enzyme-rich, watery fluid that helps to fight bacteria. For example, lysozyme and the watery secretions help to dilute thickened mucus.

Paranasal Sinuses

The paranasal sinuses are lined with pseudostratified ciliated columnar epithelium and also have serous glands, mucus glands, and goblet cells, although these are fewer in number. The paranasal sinuses are bone pockets that surround the nasal cavity and open into the nasal fossae. Each of these sinuses is named for the bone from which it originates, including the frontal paranasal sinuses, sphenoid, ethmoid, and maxillary bones. Secretions from these surrounding structures eventually drain into the nasal fossae.

In addition to the action of the cilia, mucus aids in the filtration of air as particles touch against the walls of the nasal fossae and conchae and become entrapped in the sticky substance. In addition, the sharp angle of entry into the nasal fossae and conchae helps airborne particles to become heavier with inertia than the lighter gas molecules with which they are traveling. This results in a filtering action as these particles attach to the mucus layer and later are expelled by the action of the cilia. The active rod-like cilia move with rhythmic motion to move mucus out of the nasal cavity into the pharynx where it can be swallowed and eliminated with other unused materials through the digestive system.

Mucus

In the normal adult, 100 ml of mucus are secreted each day. Mucus normally contains water and a few glycoproteins. These glycoproteins give mucus a thick and sticky texture. Due to constant evaporation, the mucus layer is constantly losing water and becomes thickened. The gel layer is on the thicker, outer mucus layer. If mucus becomes too thick, it is difficult for cilia (Figure 1-17) to move the mucus layer. Thus, serous cells (Figure 1-17) in the lamina propria must release their thinning watery enzymes into the layer just below the mucus layer to the cilia to thin the mucus. This watery layer is called the sol layer. In extreme environments, even the sol layer can become dry and form a crust.

Nasolacrimal Canals

The drainage ducts of the eyes are called *nasolacrimal canals* and empty into the nasal fossae. Tears help the serous watery secretions thin mucus. Tears form in the lacrimal glands in the upper lateral corner of the eye. They pass over the surface of the eye, collect in the

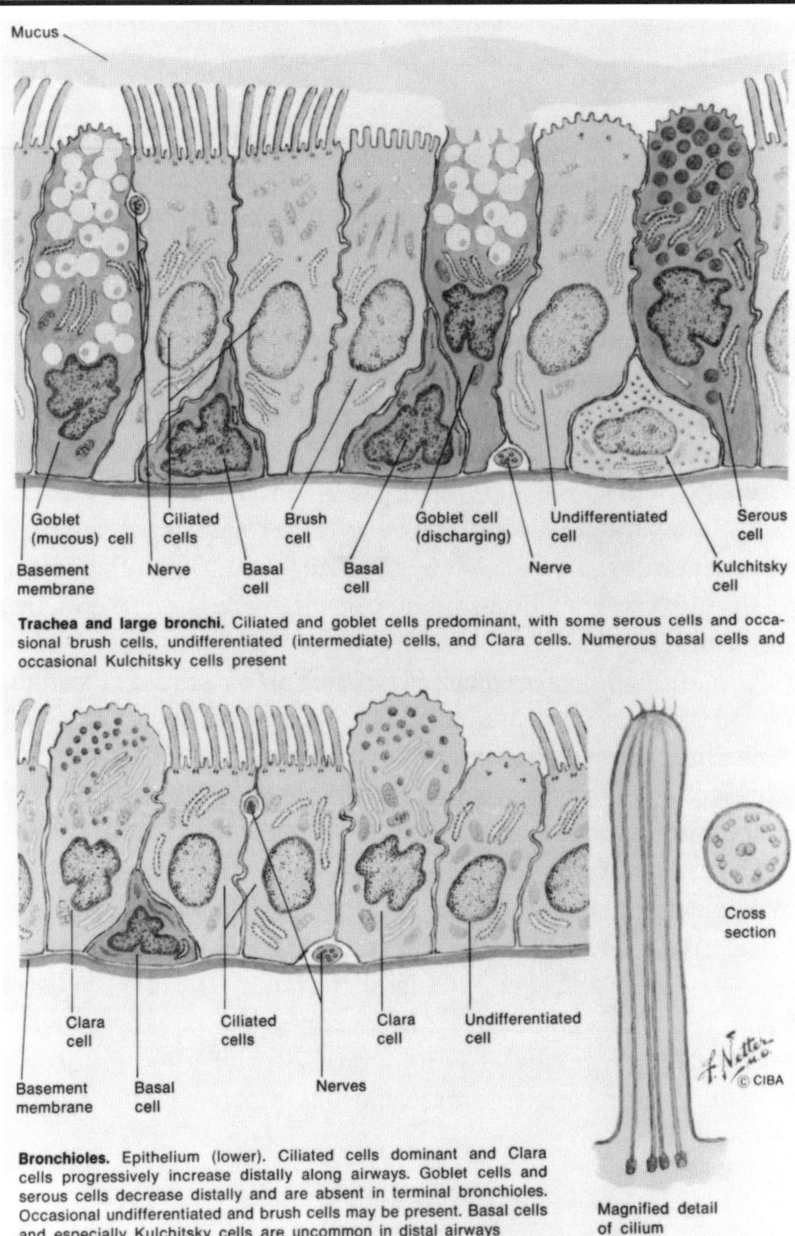

Figure 1-17 Ultrastructure of respiratory epithelium. (Copyright 1988 CIBA-GEIGY Corporation. Reproduced with permission from the CIBA COLLECTION OF MEDICAL ILLUSTRATIONS *by Frank H. Netter, M.D., West Caldwell, NJ, All rights reserved.)*

medial corner of the eye, empty into the nasolacrimal canals, and drain into the nasal fossae.

Nasal Fossae

The nasal fossae serve as passageways for olfaction and respiration. All the passageways in the nasal cavity and nasal fossae serve as airways and provide humidification to the air before it enters the lungs. Olfactory cells high in the nasal cavity detect odors.

Humidification of airflow into the respiratory passageways is one of the most important functions of the nasal fossae. One breath of air takes approximately 0.25 second to pass from the anterior nares to the posterior nares. In this brief period of time, due to the exquisite architecture of the nose, air is rapidly warmed to within a few degrees of body temperature despite changes in outside temperature. In addition, even dry ambient air is humidified to 75 to 85% of saturation. Also, during this time, most foreign particles have been filtered from inspired air.

Humidification takes place as entering air passes over the mucus layer and picks up moisture, increasing the humidity of inspired air. The swelling lamina propria also aid in increasing surface area for humidification purposes. Also, tears from the nasolacrimal canals can aid in humidification.

The rapid warming of the air is due to the rich supply of blood vessels under the lamina propria. The lamina propria is the thin layer of connective tissue directly beneath the surface epithelium of mucus membranes. With each pulse of blood, the lamina propria swells and shrinks. When the lamina propria stretches, the covering mucosa increases its surface area, making it easier for heat to be lost from blood as air passes though the meati and thus allowing for the warming of inspired air.

OROPHARYNX

The oral cavity includes the opening of the lips, teeth (dentes), and tongue. Directly behind the oral cavity (mouth) is the oropharynx. It is located from the nasopharynx to the root of the tongue. It can be seen when you look into the mouth. The oropharynx is shared by the respiratory and digestive systems and is typically what we think of as the mouth. The oral cavity connects to the oropharynx via the faucial pillars or arches. The lateral walls of the fauces are formed by two folds of tissue. The palatoglossal muscle and mucosal tissue form the anterior faucial arches. The column of lymphatic tissue called the *palatine tonsils* are located between the anterior and posterior faucial arches. Lingual tonsils are embedded in the root of the tongue, giving it a rough appearance of diffuse masses of lymphatic tissue. The adenoids, or pharyngeal tonsils are located at the back of the pharyngeal wall. All of the tonsils collectively form a complete ring around the entrances of the respiratory and digestive systems and are made of lymphatic tissues. The palatopharyngeal muscle and the mucosal tissue form the posterior faucial arches.

NASOPHARYNX

The nasopharynx is the posterior portion of the mouth and extends from the roof of the mouth to the part of the pharynx directly above the conchae. The soft palate prevents food from entering the nasopharynx by contracting and closing the velopharyngeal port (opening to the nasal cavity). The mucosa of the nasopharynx is most like that of the nasal cavity as it also contains pseudostratified ciliated columnar epithelium. The soft palate extends down from the posterior part of the roof of the mouth.

From the middle ear the eustachian tube, or auditory tube, opens into the nasopharynx. As air pressures change, these tubes open to equalize the pressure in the middle ear cavity.

The pharynx is a muscular tube shared by both the respiratory system and the digestive system. In respiration it allows for air passage. In digestion the pharynx is vital to swallowing (deglutition). Located on the posterior walls of the pharynx are the pharyngeal tonsils, or adenoids. These are composed of lymphatic tissues.

LARYNGOPHARYNX

Just inferior to the oropharynx is the laryngeal pharynx, or laryngopharynx. This portion of the pharynx extends from the oropharynx to the entrances of the larynx and esophagus. As with the oropharynx, the laryngopharynx is shared by the digestive and respiratory systems and is lined with tough mucosa. This mucosa is lined

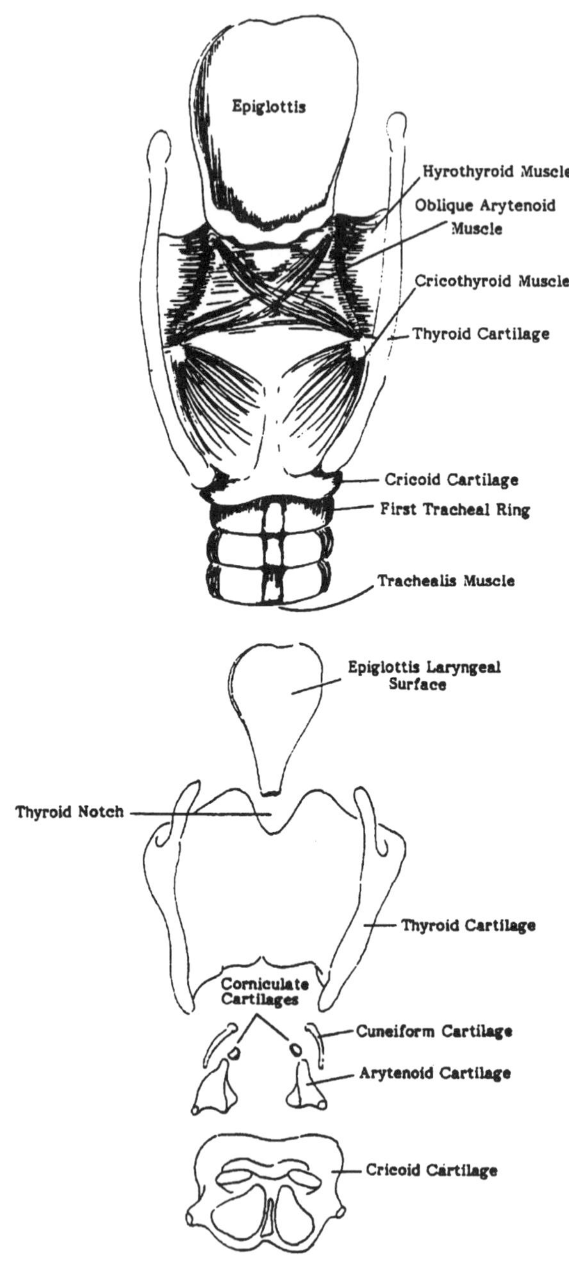

Figure 1-18 Posterior views of the larynx. (From California College for Health Sciences, Entry Level Respiratory Therapy Program, Vol.1, *Fig 2-2 p. [RRT 102] 2-8 and Figure 2-3 p. [RRT 102] 2-9. National City, CA; 1985.)*

with stratified squamous epithelium and lacks cilia.

The larynx contains nine cartilages: three paired cartilages (Figure 1-18) and three single cartilages. The cricoid cartilage is the most inferior cartilage and forms a full ring. The next structure, the thyroid cartilage, has two portions that unite to form a V-shape. It is the anterior portion of the thyroid cartilage that juts forward in males, causing the subcutaneous protrusion called the Adam's apple. The upper edge of the thyroid cartilage attaches to the hyoid bone by the thyrohyoid ligament. The thyroid notch is at the superior edge of the thyroid cartilage.

The valleculae are depressions between the root of the tongue and epiglottis. The epiglottis a broad, thin, and round elastic cartilage, connected to the thyroepiglottic ligament. The epiglottis is partially shielded by the thyroid cartilage (Figure 1-18). The epiglottic cartilage protects the opening to the airway during deglutition as it swings down to cover the glottis. The glottis is the opening between the vocal folds.

The arytenoid cartilages are two small pyramid-shaped structures (Figure 1-18) to which the vocal folds and intrinsic laryngeal muscles are attached. The arytenoid cartilage apices, or tips, each have a tiny cone-shaped cartilage, the corniculate cartilage. Forming the entrance to the larynx are the aryepiglottic folds, composed of mucus membrane. These folds extend from sides of the epiglottis to the apexes of the arytenoid cartilages. Long, thin, cuneiform cartilages are embedded within the aryepiglottic folds.

The true vocal ligaments are bands of fibroelastic tissue along the edge of the vocal folds and are enveloped in stratified squamous epithelium. Air flows through the glottic opening between the vocal folds and causes the vocal folds to vibrate, resulting in sound. The vocal folds also serve to protect the lower airway from the inhalation of secretions, fluid, and food material.

In addition to protecting the lower airways, the larynx provides for phonation. The false vocal folds, or ventricular folds, are located just above the true vocal folds. The ventricular folds are not involved in production of phonation but serve to help protect the lower airway during swallowing, as do the true folds and epiglottis. In addition, the velum (soft palate) can be raised, sending sound out the mouth, or lowered, for nasal sounds, sending sound out through the nasopharynx. The respiratory system provides the pressure needed to initiate vocal fold vibration. Each time the vocal folds open and close, a small puff of air escapes through the glottis. These periodic puffs produce a buzz-like sound that is modified by the articulators to form vowels and voiced consonants.

The larynx is a vital component of the cough response. The cough is produced by a rapid inhalation, followed by sealing off the airway by tight closure of the vocal and ventricular folds. The expiratory muscles then contract, producing an extremely high subglottic pressure. The pressure is then rapidly released. The combination of high pressure and high resistance creates an extremely high airflow that shears mucus off of the walls of the larynx and trachea. Typically, the mucus is projected into the pharynx, where it is swallowed.

The normal cough response is significantly compromised in patients with a tracheostomy because the airstream is directed outward prior to entering the larynx. This means that it is difficult, if not impossible, to produce the same high pressures, resistances, and airflow. Therefore, the ability to generate the shearing forces needed to remove the mucus is significantly diminished. This is especially important since the insertion of a tube in the trachea irritates the tracheal lining, resulting in a much higher production of mucus. Patients with non-cuffed tubes that are smaller than the lumen of the trachea may be able to cover the external hole of the tube in order to allow the participation of the larynx to reestablish a more normal physiological cough.

Phonation requires articulation in order to generate repeatable patterns of sound for speech. These sounds are grouped into two major categories: consonants and vowels. Vowels require phonation (voicing) (Tables 1-1, 1-2, and 1-3) and provide the carrying power of the voice. The tongue forms contours in the front, middle, and back that vary with different vowels. Consonant production (Tables 1-1, 1-2, and 1-3) requires greater precision in placement of the tongue and air control than does vowel production. Children learn vowel production before consonant production.

There are seven points of articulation:

Bilabial: This is made with the lips creating /b/, /m/, /p/ sounds.

Labiodental: This requires placement of the upper teeth on the lower lip and the blowing of air through the narrow slit, creating /f/ and /v/ sounds.

Linguadental: This requires placement of the tongue tip between the teeth, creating a narrow slit used to produce the voiced and voiceless "th," as in "thin" and "them."

Alveolar: This requires placement of the tongue against the upper gum or alveolar ridge. More sounds are produced this way than any other.

Palatal: The tongue tip must be placed up to the hard palate, producing the "sh" and "zh" sounds as in "ship," and "azure."

Velar: This is made by lifting the back of the tongue up toward the soft palate or velum used to produce these sounds, /g/ and /k/.

Glottal: This is the only sound in the English language made by blowing air through the glottic opening. It is used to produce the sound /h/ in the English language.

	NASALS	GLIDES	LATERAL	FRICATIVES	AFFRICATES	PLOSIVES
Bilabials	m	w hw				p b
Labiodentals				f v		
Dentals				υð		
Alveolar	n		l	s z	tʃ dʒ	t d
Palatal		j(l)r		ʃ ʒ		
Velar	ŋ					k g
Glottal				h		

Table 1-1 Classification of Consonant Sounds. (From C.V. Riper and L. Emerick, SPEECH CORRECTION: AN INTRODUCTION TO SPEECH PATHOLOGY AND AUDIOLOGY, *(c) 1990, p. 72. Reprinted by permission of Prentice-Hall, Inc., Englewood Cliffs, NJ.)*

Vowels, Phonemic Diphthongs, and Syllabics		Consonants	
Phonetic Symbol	Key Word	Phonetic Symbol	Key Word
i	peat	m	sum
ɪ	pit	n	sun
e	pate	ŋ	sung
ɛ	pet	p	pot
æ	pat	b	bob
ɑ	pot	t	tot
ɔ	pall	d	dot
o	poll	g	got
u	pool	k	cot
ʊ	pull	f	fine
ɝ ɜ	purr	v	vine
ɚ ə	putter	θ	ether
ʌ	putt	ð	either
ɔɪ	coy	s	seal
au	cow	z	zeal
aɪ	my	ʃ	bash
ɪu	mew	ʒ	beige
n̩	button	h	hump
l̩	saddle	tʃ	chump
m̩	chasm	dʒ	jump
		l	led
		r	red
		w	wet
		j	yet

Table 1-2 Phonetic Symbols. (From Shames, G.H., and Wiig, E.H., Human Communication Disorders: An Introduction,*Columbus, OH: Charles Merrill Publishing Co., 1982; Table 2.1, p. 28.)*

Consonants are grouped into various categories based on how they are made (Table 1-2):

Nasal: These are made by occluding the oral cavity at the lips or palate and leaving the velopharyngeal port open. This directs the air stream through the nasal cavity, producing nasal resonance. The nasal sounds are "m," "n", and "-ing."

Glides: These are made while the mouth is in motion as in the production of the /w/ in "we." These sounds are made during transition.

Lateral: This is a half consonant and half vowel sound. There is only one used in the English language: /l/. The front of the tongue maintains contact with the palate while air travels around its sides.

Fricatives: These sounds are produced by forcing the airstream through a constriction. This produces turbulence to the airstream, which creates random noise (similar to the hiss of steam escaping from a radiator). In English,

PHONETIC SYMBOL	Key Words		PHONETIC SYMBOL	Key Words	
	ENGLISH	PHONETIC		ENGLISH	PHONETIC
			CONSONANTS		
b	back, cab	bæk kæb	p	pig, sap	pig sæp
d	dig, red	dɪg, rɛd	r	rat, poor	ræt pur
f	feel, leaf	fil lif	s	so, miss	so mɪs
g	go, egg	go ɛg	t	to, wit	tu wɪt
dʒ	just, edge	dʒʌst ɛdʒ	ʃ	she, wish	ʃi wɪʃ
h	he behaves	hi bɪhevz	tʃ	chin, itch	tʃɪn ɪtʃ
k	keep, track	kip træk	θ	think truth	θɪŋk truθ
l	low, ball	lo bɔl	ð	then, bathe	ðɛn beð
l̩	simple, fable	simpl febl	v	vest, live	vɛst lɪv
m	my, aim	maɪ em	w	we, swim	wi swɪm
m̩	kingdom madam	kɪŋdm̩ mædm	hw	where, when	hwɛr hwɛn
n	not, any	nɑt ɛnɪ	j	yell, young	jɛl, jʌŋ
n̩	action, mission	æk ʃn mɪ ʃn̩	ʒ	measure, version	mɛʒɚ vɝʒn
ŋ	sing, uncle	sɪŋ ʌŋkl̩	z	zebra, ozone	zibrə ozon
ʔ	oh oh!	ʔo ʔo			
			VOWELS		
a*	far, sad	far sad	ɒ*	law, wrong	lɒrɒŋ
ɑ	father, mop	fɑðɚ mɑp	ɝ	early, bird	ɜlɪ bɜd
e	great, ache	gret ek	ɜ*	early bird	ɜlɪ b ɜd
æ	sad, sack	sæd sæk	ɚ	perhaps, never	pɚ hæps nɛvɚ
i	intrigue, me	intrig mi	u	to, you	tu ju
ɛ	head, rest	hɛd rɛst	u	pudding, cook	pudɪŋ kuk
ɪ	his, itch	hɪz ɪtʃ	ʌ	mother, drug	mʌðɚ drʌg
o	own, bone	on bon	ə	above, suppose	əbʌv səpoz
ɔ	all, dog	ɔl dɔg			
			DIPHTHONGS		
aɪ	my, eye	maɪ aɪ	ɔɪ	toy, boil	tɔɪ b ɔɪl
au	cow, about	kau əbaut			
			CENTERING DIPHTHONGS		
ɛr	wear, fair	wɛr fɛr	Ir	beer, weird	bɪr wɪrd
ɑr	barn, far	bɑrn, fɑr	aɪr	wire, tire	waɪr taɪr
ur	lure, moor	lur mur	aur	hour, flower	aur flaur
ɔr	shore, born	ʃɔr bɔrn			

*These vowels are heard in Eastern and Southern speech.

Table 1-3 The Phonetic Alphabet. (From C.V. Riper and L. Emerick, SPEECH CORRECTION: AN INTRODUCTION TO SPEECH PATHOLOGY AND AUDIOLOGY, *(c) 1990, p. 72. Reprinted by permission of Prentice-Hall, Inc., Englewood Cliffs, NJ.)*

there are four primary places where these constrictions can be made: labiodental, linguadental, alveolar, and palatal (Table 1-2).

Affricates: These are simply a plosive (stop consonant) with a fricative release. The two affricates are "t" + "sh", such as in "chair" and "d" + "zh", as in "jar".

Plosives: The airstream is briefly blocked and then released. The built-up pressure is rapidly released, producing the plosive, or stop consonant. These are the /p/, /b/, /t/, /d/, /g/, and /k/ sounds.

Voicing is a complex mechanism requiring the delicate orchestration of respiration, resonation, articulation, and phonation. Normally all of these processes combine effortlessly and automatically, to enable us to emit sound and to communicate.

The upper airway, with the exception of the vocal folds, is covered with mucus producing pseudostratified ciliated columnar epithelium with goblet cells. The false folds, or ventricular folds are located directly above the vocal folds. In between the two sets of folds is the laryngeal ventrical. The laryngeal ventrical is lined with mucus producing glands that dump mucus into the ventrical. Movement of the folds allows the mucus to flow over the vocal folds, providing the lubrication needed to maintain vocal fold vibration.

The thyroid cartilage is above the cricoid cartilage and the trachea is attached directly to the cricoid. The thyroid gland is located anterior to the thyroid and cricoid cartilages.

TRACHEA

The trachea extends from the larynx to the upper thorax where it bifurcates into the mainstem bronchi (Figure 1-19). The trachea contains 16 to 20 C-shaped cartilage rings joined by connective tissue. This structure of cartilage serves to keep the trachea open during respiration, especially during expiration when airway passages are more likely to collapse. The tracheal wall is lined with

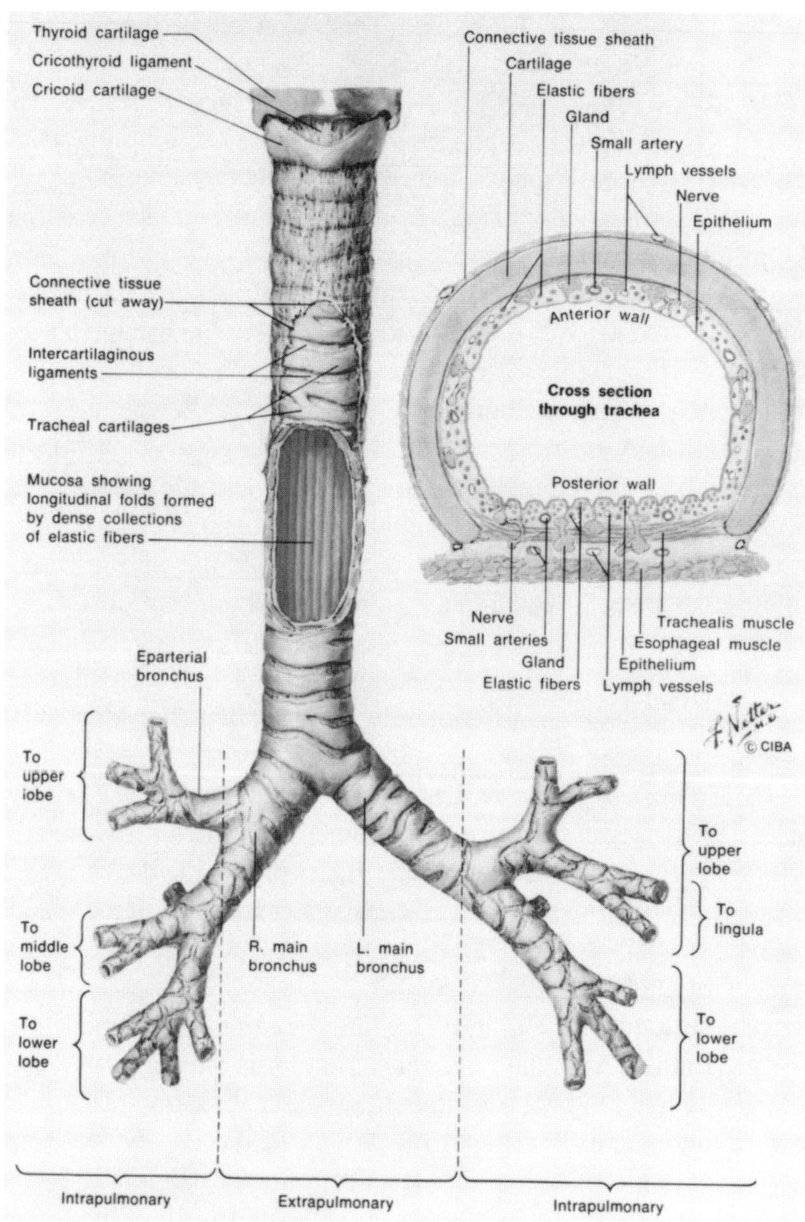

Figure 1-19 Structure of the trachea and major bronchi. (Copyright 1988 CIBA-GEIGY Corporation. Reproduced with permission from the CIBA COLLECTION OF MEDICAL ILLUSTRATIONS *by Frank H. Netter, M.D., West Caldwell, NJ; All rights reserved.)*

pseudostratified ciliated columnar epithelium with numerous goblet cells and mucus glands. Along its C-shaped structure the trachea is supported by the membranous posterior wall adjoining the esophagus and both the trachea and the esophagus share this common wall. During swallowing the esophagus may bulge into the lumen of the trachea. The trachealis muscle interconnects the C-shaped cartilages with elastic fibers of smooth muscle. This muscle contracts, constricting the lumen of the trachea and increasing the velocity of airflow. The lower end of the trachea bifurcates into two branches, the primary bronchi. The point of this bifurcation is called the *carina* and is located at the level of the fifth thoracic vertebra. With expiration, the carina may rise to the fourth thoracic vertebral level, and with inspiration it may be pulled down to the level of the sixth thoracic vertebra. The joint between the manubrium and the body of the sternum is a useful landmark for obtaining the location of the carina. The carina is lined with many nerve endings and may cause violent coughing or bronchospasm. In addition, touching any part of the trachea can elicit coughing.

Although men tend to have larger tracheas than women, averages sizes in adults are approximately 11 cm in length and 2.5 cm in diameter, varying in individual anatomies.

Differences of the trachea in infants include more than relative size; differences also exist in the relationship of structures within the airway (Figures 1-20, 1-21, and 1-22). In the infant, the larynx is high in the neck at birth, with the cricoid cartilage, at the level of the second or third cervical vertebra. The thyroid cartilage sits immediately under the hyoid bone. It is more difficult to establish the location of laryngeal structures in children due to the softness and mobility of cartilage. In the infant, the laryngeal structure is only slightly wider than the tracheal lumen. At birth the laryngeal structure has a much wider funnel shape. With age, the larynx descends and becomes straight, more elongated, and vertically funneled (Figure 1-20) in alignment to the trachea. The angle of the posterior tilt of the larynx in children results in the subglottic airway extending more inferiorly and posteriorly than in adult airways. This angle can present difficulties in visualization and intubation of the airway. In addition, the angle between the epiglottis and vocal folds is sharper (more acute), adding to difficulties in visualization but allowing for airway protection during nursing. With age, the relationship of airway structure change in each child must be assessed individually.

LOWER AIRWAYS

Gross Lung Anatomy

The lungs are contained within the thoracic cavity and enclosed by the rib cage. The diaphragm muscle forms the base of the thoracic cavity. The lungs are shaped like blunted cones. The tops of the lungs are the rounded apices or cupolas, and the bases of the lungs are wider and more concave and rest on the superior portion of the diaphragm muscle. The hilum is the medial indentation where the root of the lung enters. The space between the two lungs is called the *mediastinum.* The mediastinum is where the heart and major blood vessels of the heart are located. Also sharing the space of the mediastinum are the thymus gland, esophagus, several major nerves, and other structures. The bulk of the heart is to the left side of the mediastinum, which causes the left lung to be smaller than the right lung.

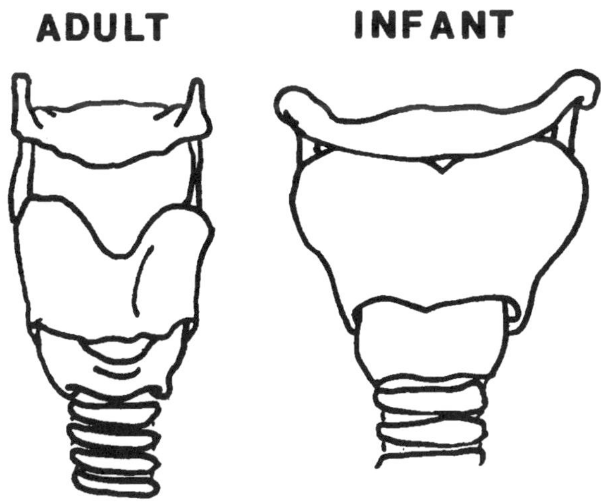

Figure 1-20 Adult and infant larynges shown in equal proportion. Note the absence of a space between the cricoid and thyroid cartilages. (From Myers, E.N., Stool, S.E., and Johnson, J.T., Tracheotomy, *New York: Churchill Livingstone, Inc. Fig. 5-4.)*

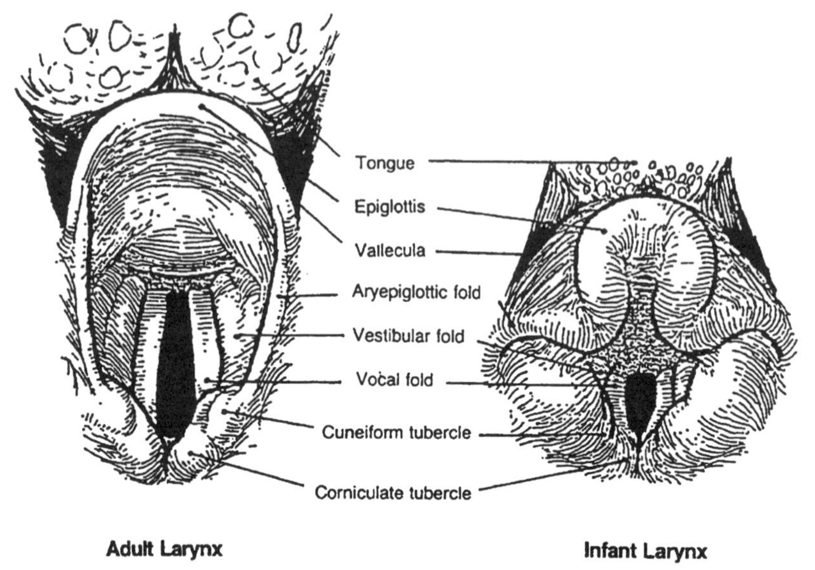

Figure 1-21 Comparison of the anatomies of the adult and pediatric larynges. (From Dickison, Anne E., Respiratory Management, *V20, #2, "Child with Upper Airway Obstruction, Part 1", Boston: Little Brown & Co., 1982: Fig.1.)*

The pleura is the lining of the inner wall of the thoracic cavity. The pleura is a thin, tough membrane made of connective tissue and epithelial tissue. The connective tissue gives the pleural membrane strength, and the epithelial tissue secretes serous fluid, which forms the pleural fluid that keeps the pleural membrane moist. The pleural membrane is termed the *parietal pleura*, and it forms upward on either side of the mediastinum to create sacs. These are the pleural sacs, which contain the lungs. As the parietal pleura forms over the roots of the lungs it combines with the visceral pleura. The visceral pleura is another connective and epithelial tissue that adheres so closely to the lungs that it is considered the outer layer of the lungs. The outer layer of visceral pleura also secretes serous fluid, as does the parietal pleura. The surfaces of the visceral pleura and parietal pleura face each other and are in contact with each other. The thin film of serous fluid that forms pleural fluid lubricates and reduces surface tension between the two pleura so that the thoracic wall and lungs do not abrade during ventilation. This film of thin pleural fluid normally fills the intrapleu-

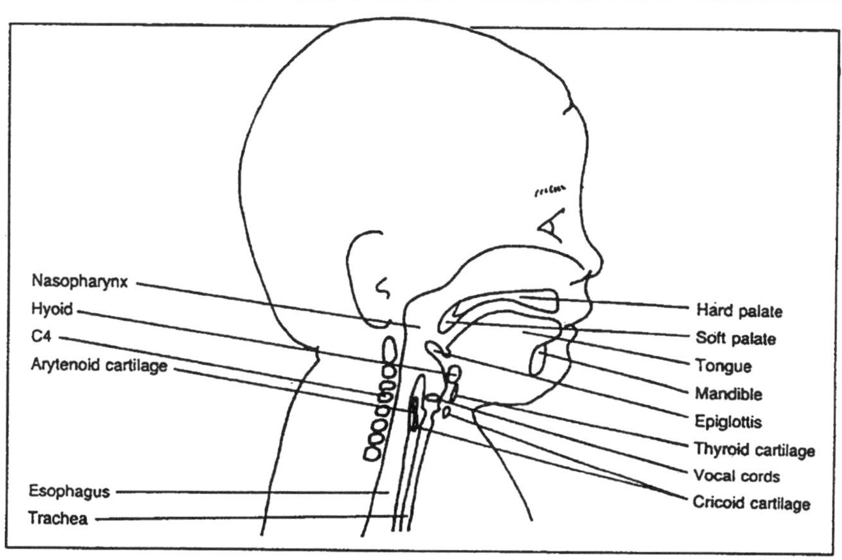

Figure 1-22 The pediatric airway. (From Dickison, Anne E., Respiratory Management, *V20, #2, "Child with Upper Airway Obstruction, Part 1," Boston: Little Brown & Co., 1982: Fig. 2.)*

ral space. The thin space between the outer layer of the lungs and the inner layer of the chest wall is called the *interplural space.* Normally, there is a negative pressure in this space, which keeps the lungs attached to the inside wall of the thorax. If this negative pressure is not present, the elastic properties of the lungs will cause them to collapse.

Bronchopulmonary Segments and Segmental Bronchi

The lungs are divided into five lobes (Figure 1-23), the right upper, middle, and lower lobes and the left upper and lower lobes. The lobes divide into bronchopulmonary segments. The right lung divides into ten bronchopulmonary segments, three in the right upper lobe, two in the middle lobe, and five in the lower lobe. The left lung contains eight bronchopulmonary segments. The lobes of the lungs are separated by fissures. The oblique fissure separates the two lobes of the left lung. The upper lobe of the left lung is the superior lobe and the lower lobe is the inferior lobe. The right lung contains three lobes. The inferior lobes are also divided by an oblique fissure, while the medial lobe is separated by a horizontal fissure from the upper and lower lobes. The visceral pleura also forms the outer layer of the lung lobes and helps to keep them separated.

Bronchopulmonary segments are supported by the connective tissue of the visceral pleural septa. Bronchopulmonary segments are as follows:

Right superior:	apical, posterior, anterior
Right medial:	lateral and medial
Right inferior:	apical, medial basal, anterior basal, lateral basal, posterior basal

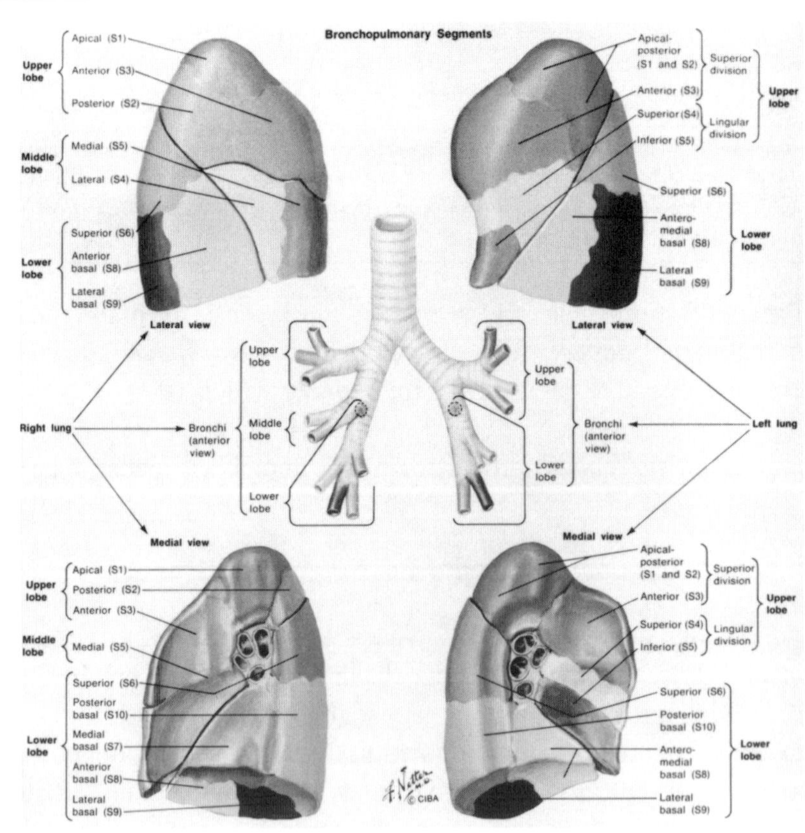

Figure 1-23 Bronchopulmonary segments. (Copyright 1988 CIBA-GEIGY Corporation. Reproduced with permission from the CIBA COLLECTION OF MEDICAL ILLUSTRATIONS *by Frank H. Netter, M.D., West Caldwell, NJ; All rights reserved.)*

Some schools of thought suggest that the medial basal and anterior basal form one segment.

The left upper and lower lobes contain four or five bronchopulmonary segments each:

Left lung:	Left superior lobe: apical, posterior, anterior
Lingular division:	superior lingular, inferior lingular
Left inferior lobe:	apical or superior, medial basal or cardiac, anterior basal, lateral basal, posterior basal

Some believe that apical and posterior bronchopulmonary segments form one segment. A portion of the lower lobe of the left lung is analogous to the middle lobe of the right lung.

Bronchi

The mainstem bronchi branch from the trachea and share a similar (Figures 1-24 and 1-25) lining of pseudostratified ciliated columnar epithelium with goblet cells. The right mainstem bronchus is shorter and wider than the left mainstem bronchus and runs downward from the trachea at a straight angle. Because of this angle, objects can be more readily lodged in the right mainstem bronchus. Narrower and longer, the left mainstem bronchus runs perpendicular. The mainstem bronchi serve as airway passages to lung tissues. The mainstem bronchi divide further as they get closer to lung tissue. The right mainstem bronchus divides into three bronchi: the upper, middle, and lower lung lobes. The left mainstem bronchus divides into two bronchi: the upper and lower lobes.

The roots of the lungs include the mainstem bronchi, pulmonary arteries, pulmonary veins and lymphatic vessels that come from the lungs, and lung nerves.

Segmental bronchi also continue to branch into generations of bronchi (Figures 1-24 to 1-27). They continue to branch, becoming smaller and smaller in diameter until the cartilage in their walls decreases and is eventually completely replaced by smooth muscle. This happens somewhere between the ninth and eleventh generation of branching. As a bronchus becomes all smooth muscle, it becomes possible to contract and close it. These bronchi are called *bronchioles* and are about 1 mm or less in diameter. The bronchioles continue to branch, and when they are approximately 0.5 mm in diameter, they are

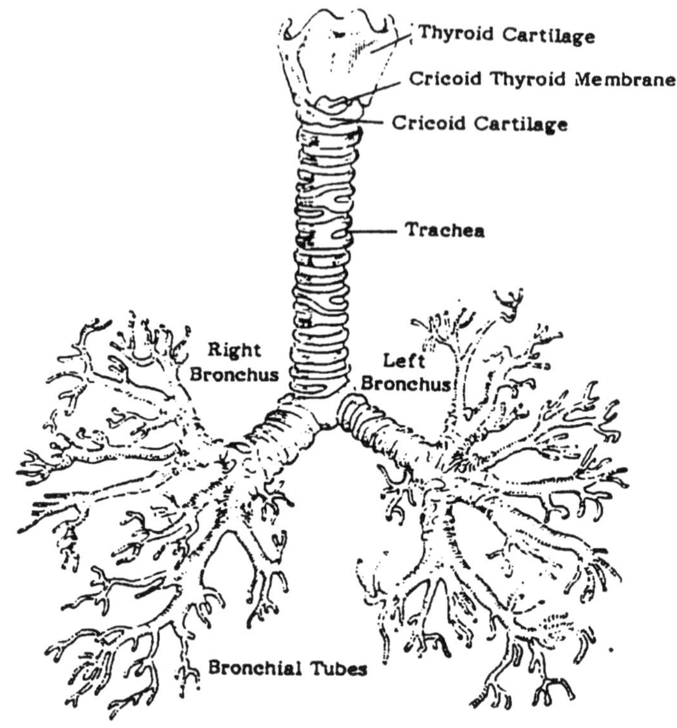

Figure 1-24 Tracheobronchial tree. (From California College for Health Sciences, Entry Level Respiratory Therapy Program, *Vol.1, Figure 2-4 p. [RRT 102] 2-10. National City, California, 1985.)*

called *terminal bronchioles* (Figure 1-27). Terminal bronchioles do not have goblet cells in their mucosa or mucus producing cells in their lamina propria. Their mucosa are cuboidal in shape, and not all cells have cilia. As air in the terminal bronchioles is not available for gas exchange, the volume of this air is called *deadspace volume*.

Terminal Respiratory Units

Distal to the terminal bronchioles are the terminal respiratory units (TRUs) (Figure 1-27). These structures are also termed *pulmonary acini* or *primary lobules*. Terminal respiratory units consist of two to five orders of branching respiratory bronchioles and two to five orders of alveolar ducts. In addition, there are 10 to 16 alveoli per alveolar duct.

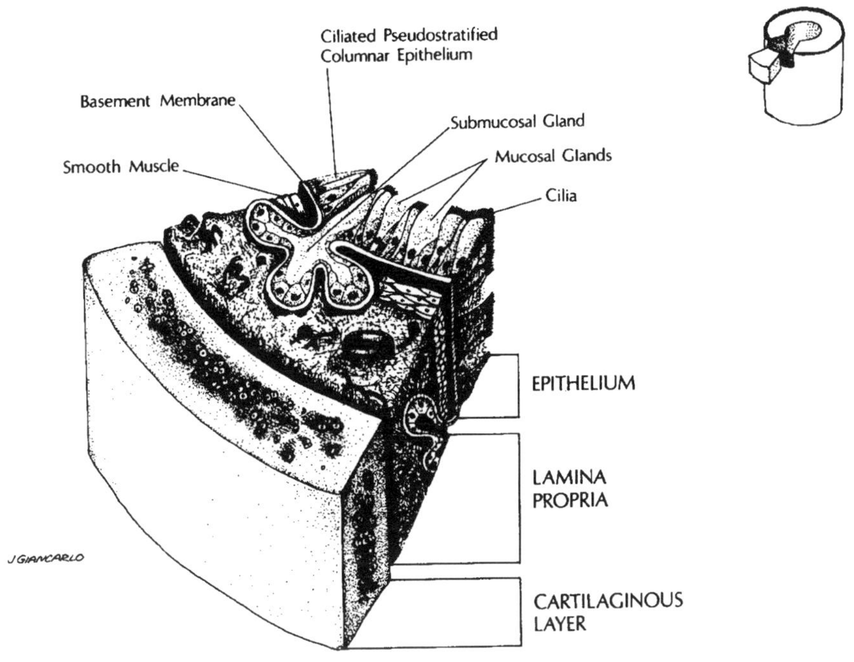

Figure 1-25 Model concept of the three major layers of the tracheobronchial wall. (From Shapiro, B.A., Clinical Application of Respiratory Care, *4th Edition, St. Louis, Mosby -Year Book, 1991.)*

Lung parenchyma consist of clusters of TRUs (or lobules) containing 300 million alveoli. The terminal bronchioles contain alveoli in their walls. Alveolarization increases as terminal bronchioles continue to the periphery and divide further to establish from one to five alveolar ducts. The walls of the alveolar ducts are alveolarized and are smooth muscle fibers (epithelium) that can narrow or shorten alveolar ducts. As an individual grows, the number of alveoli increases. This may be due to a relationship to the person's height. The alveoli are lined with thin epithelium membrane surrounded by numerous thin-walled pulmonary capillaries, forming the site for direct gas exchange (Figure 1-28). It is due to this thin capillary membrane, 0.01 to 0.05 microns in width, that gases can easily diffuse back and forth between alveolar air and pulmonary capillary blood. This network of pulmonary capillaries carries blood, allowing for gas

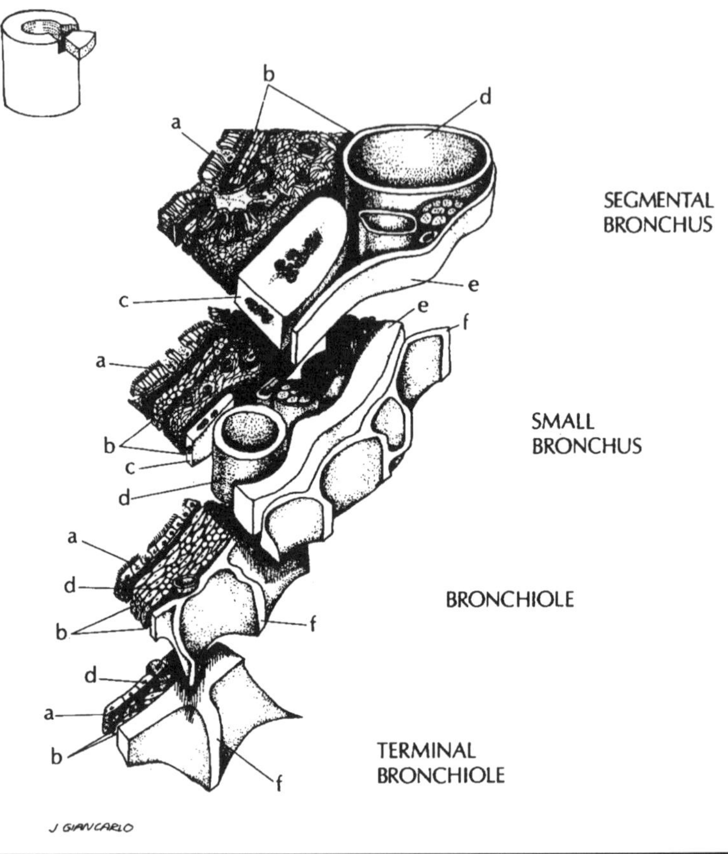

Figure 1-26 Relationship of the tracheobronchial components at various levels; ***A****, Pulmonary mucosa:* ***B****, Lamina propria (smooth muscle component);* ***C****, Cartilage;* ***D****, Blood vessels;* ***E****, Peribronchial connective tissue; and* ***F****, Lung parenchyma. (From Shapiro, B.A.,* Clinical Application of Respiratory Care, *4th Edition, St. Louis, Mosby-Year Book, 1991.)*

exchange. These capillary walls are made up of thin squamous endothelial cells with a basement membrane.

All of these layers form a composite barrier approximately 1 micron thick, allowing for gas diffusion to take place in less than 0.75 second. The exchange of carbon dioxide and oxygen is termed *respiration*. This exchange between the alveoli and blood is termed *external gas exchange. Internal gas exchange* occurs at the tissue level when oxygenated blood diffuses through the capillary wall (Figure 1-29) into the interstitial extracellular fluid and through the

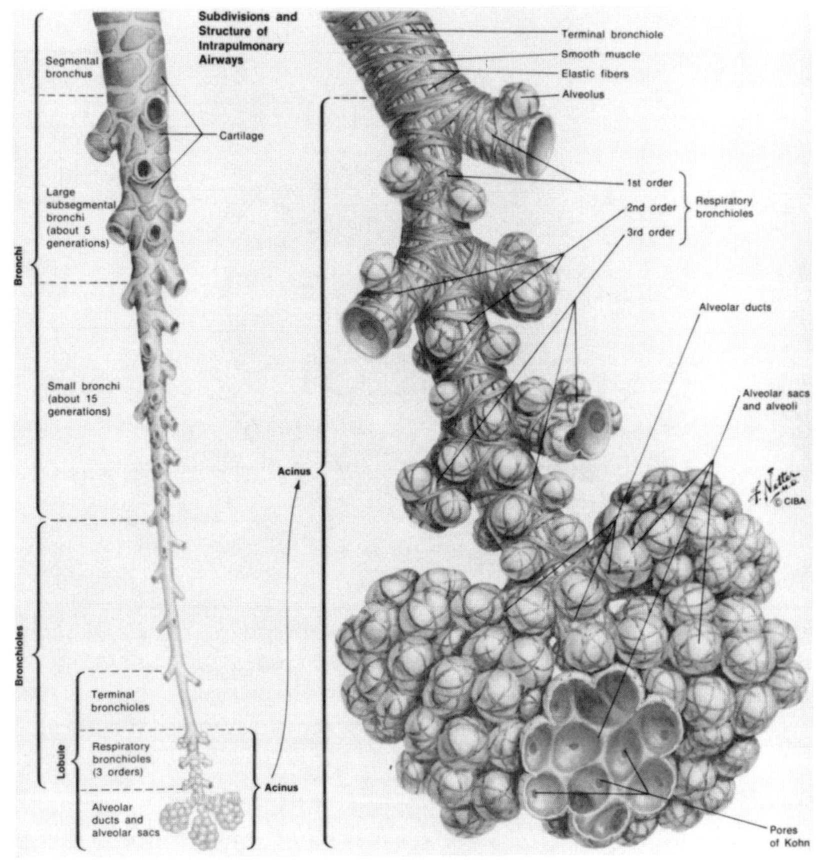

Figure 1-27 Subdivisions and structure of intrapulmonary airways. (Copyright 1988 CIBA-GEIGY Corporation. Reproduced with permission from the CIBA COLLECTION OF MEDICAL ILLUSTRATIONS *by Frank H. Netter, M.D. All rights reserved.)*

plasma membranes of cells, where it is used in the metabolic processes of the cells. Carbon dioxide exists in the cells as the by-product of metabolism. It diffuses from the cell into the interstitial fluid and through the capillaries of the blood, completing internal gas exchange. As it enters plasma, blood oxygen passes through a thin layer of water and surfactant, then through the epithelial cells of the wall of the alveolus and through the basement membrane of the alveolar epithelium entering the basement membrane of the capillary epithelium, into the capillary cells.

The thin epithelium membrane of the alveoli contains two types

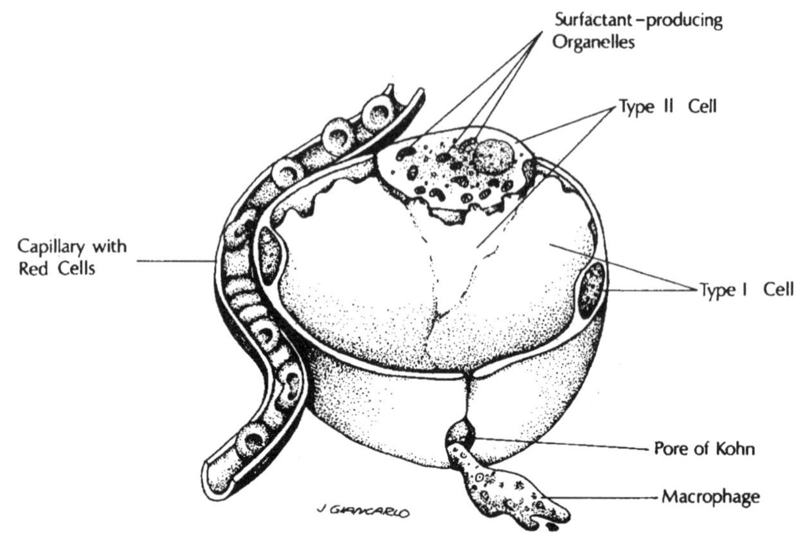

Figure 1-28 Schematic representation of alveolar epithelium. (From Shapiro, B.A., Clinical Application of Respiratory Care, *4th Edition, St. Louis, Mosby-Year Book, 1991.)*

of cells: Type I and Type II. Type I cells are simple, thin, flat, squamous epithelial cells. Type II cells have a more cuboidal shape and have been documented to secrete surfactant. Surfactant is an important substance shown to prevent alveolar wall collapse during expiration. Surfactant lowers the surface tension of alveolar fluid to prevent alveolar walls from sticking together during expiration and allowing them to readily fill with air upon inspiration.

There are mobile cells called macrophages that reside on the alveolar walls. These cells contain phagocytes which engulf foreign particles that have escaped the filtration of the nasal cavity.

The walls of the alveoli between lobules of alveoli and the intervening capillaries form the inter-alveolar septa. The inter-alveolar septa contain pores or openings that allow air to pass between two adjacent lobules if one becomes blocked. The openings are called the *alveolar pores of Kohn* (Figure 1-28). The alveolar pores of Kohn ensure that function of a blocked lobule will not be totally lost. Providing a similar function between alveolar ducts are openings called the *channels of Lambert.*

The alveolar epithelium requires a basement membrane or basal lamina of connective tissue to supply a foundation for attachment of epithelial cells. This basement membrane is filled with connective tissue fibers that contribute to the important elastic behavior of the lungs. These fibers are reduced in quantity and function in patients with pulmonary emphysema.

The walls of the alveoli exchange gases through passive diffusion from the side of higher partial pressure to the side of lower partial pressure. The law of diffusion requires higher pressures to be attracted to lower pressures.

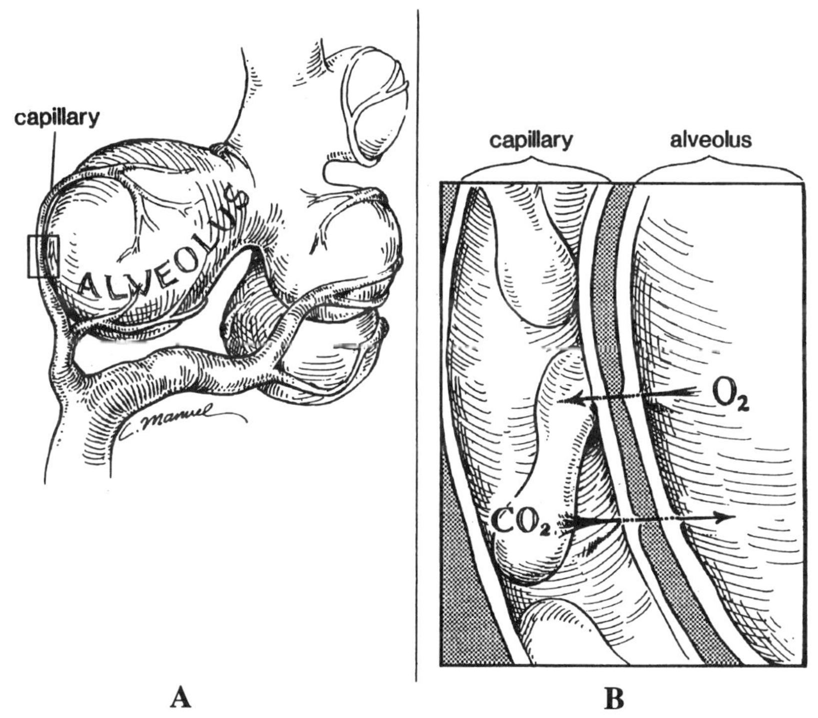

Figure 1-29 The inspired oxygen passes through the tissues of the alveoli, which are rich with capillary arteries. ***A****, From there, the oxygen is carried through the bloodstream to the cells, where oxidation occurs. The process is reversed during exhalation. Carbon dioxide from the capillaries of the alveoli passes into the air sacs, where it is expelled.* ***B****, Normally, this cycle is repeated 18 to 20 times every minute. Normal respiration is automatic, effortless and quiet. (Courtesy of Mallinckrodt Medical TPI, Inc. Irvine, CA. Shiley* Tracheostomy Care *Figure 2-A and 2-B, p. 5.)*

PULMONARY COMPLIANCE

The term *compliance* is used to describe the measure of ease at which the lungs expand. Compliance reflects elasticity of the lung tissue and alveolar surface tension.

$$\text{Compliance} = \frac{1}{\text{Elasticity}} \qquad \text{or } C = \frac{1}{E}$$

Compliance can also be described as the volume change per pressure change causing the lungs to inflate and deflate. Compliance equals the change in volume during inflation and deflation of the lungs divided by the change in pressure during inflation and deflation within the thoracic cavity.

$$\text{Compliance} = \frac{\text{Change in volume}}{\text{Change in pressure}} \qquad \text{or } C = \frac{V}{P}$$

V or P equals the final pressure or volume minus the initial pressure or volume:

$$V = V\ \text{final} - V\ \text{initial}$$
$$P = P\ \text{final} - P\ \text{initial}$$

Compliance is important because it reflects pathological conditions, assisting in the diagnosis of disease processes; for example, compliance thus decreases with pulmonary fibrosis or edema but increases with emphysema.

VENTILATION

Ventilation is achieved by the interaction of the pressures inside the lungs and the air pressure in the environment, also termed external gas exchange. The pressure of the air that surrounds us is referred to as the atmospheric pressure. The pressure inside the lungs is referred to as intrapleural pressure and changes throughout the respiratory cycle. For example, we are able to inspire air by increasing the volume of the thoracic cavity. This increase in volume causes the pressure inside the lungs (intrapleural pressure) to momentarily become negative relative to the outside. Air always flows from a region of higher pressure to a region of lower pressure. Therefore, air flows from the outside to the inside of the lungs, where the pressure is lower. Expiration is achieved in the opposite manner. The intrapleural pressure becomes positive relative to the pressure outside, resulting in air flow outward.

The process of inspiration is an active process, requiring muscle activity from the inspiratory muscles. In other words, the inspiratory muscles are responsible for increasing the volume of the thoracic cavity by raising the rib cage and lowering the diaphragm. As mentioned previously, this increase in volume results in the negative intrapleural pressure needed for inspiration.

Quiet expiration is normally a passive process and is achieved by a relaxation of the inspiratory muscles. The elasticity of the chest wall and lungs forces the structures to return to their rest position. In this process, the volume of the thoracic cavity is reduced and the pressure is momentarily increased, producing the pressure differential needed for expiration. During forced expiration (example - when exercising) the expiratory muscles actively aid in reducing the volume of the thoracic cavity. This increases the intrapleural pressure and results in a more rapid flow of air to the outside.

MUSCLES OF VENTILATION

Muscles of inspiration:

Diaphragm
External intercostal muscles
Pectoralis major
Serratus posterior superior
Levator scapulae
Sternocleidomastoid
Levatores costarum
Pectoralis minor
Trapezius
Rhomboid major
Rhomboid minor
Serratus anterior muscle
Scalene muscles

Muscles of expiration:

Abdominal muscles:
External oblique
Internal oblique
Transverse Abdominous
Internal intercostal muscles
Quadratus lumborum
Serratus posterior inferior

Muscles of Inspiration

The Diaphragm

The diaphragm is the most important inspiratory muscle (Figure 1-30) and can account for 70% of the tidal volume during normal breathing (eupena). It is a thin muscle that separates the bottom of the chest cavity from the abdominal cavity. It is dome-shaped, with the dome sticking up into the chest. The diaphragm is located completely within the thoracic cavity and cannot be felt from the outside.

The diaphragm attaches to the lower perimeter of the deep surface of the thoracic wall. The muscle fibers rise vertically upward and then turn centrally to insert into an elevated central tendon. Several structures pass through this tendon to supply the lower body (i.e., descending aorta, inferior vena cava, esophagus, and nerves). The diaphragm is controlled by the phrenic nerve, which is located at the C3 to C5 level of the spinal column.

The central part of the diaphragm is higher than the attachments to the inside of the rib cage. When the diaphragm contracts, the central part of the diaphragm lowers and is very effective in increasing the volume of the thoracic cavity. For example, if the diaphragm descends only 1 cm, it could increase thoracic volume 270 ml and a movement of 2.5 cm may increase the volume 700 ml. As mentioned previously, this increase in volume results in a decrease in intrapleural pressure, producing inspiration.

Quiet expiration is normally a passive process, or the relaxation of the inspiratory muscles. During expiration, the diaphragm stops contracting and the diaphragm returns to its relaxed elevated state. This is due to the elasticity of the lung tissue and the upward forces of the abdominal viscera.

When an individual primarily uses the diaphragm for respiration, it is referred to as diaphragmatic breathing. External signs will be little movement of the rib cage during respiration and a slight bulging outward of the abdomen, due to the forces of the compressed viscera that may be apparent.

Inspiratory Muscles That Affect the Rib Cage

There are a number of inspiratory muscles that enhance inspiration by lifting the rib cage up and out. This also increases the volume of the thoracic cavity, resulting in inspiration. This type of breathing is called costal breathing.

The external intercostal muscle (Figure 1-31) is one of the primary muscles for deep inspiration. It attaches from the lower portion of each rib above it and to the upper portion of the rib below it. These muscle fibers extend forward and downward. The action of the external intercostal muscle is to lift the ribs up and outward, increasing chest diameter. The external intercostal muscle is innervated by the intercostal nerve.

The pectoralis major (Figure 1-31) assists in raising the chest for deep inspiration. It begins from the medial clavicle and lateral sternum to the seventh costal cartilage and inserts at the greater tubercle of the humerus crest.

The serratus posterior superior (Figure 1-32) is another assistive muscle for deep inspiration. It acts to further raise the ribs for chest expansion during inspiration. The serratus posterior superior is located at the cranial and dorsal part of the thorax and originates from the spinal vertebrae C7 to T3 superior to the serratus posterior inferior muscle and the caudal portion of the nuchae ligament. This muscle inserts through the upper portion of the second through fifth ribs.

The levator scapulae (Figure 1-32) also can assist with deep inspiration and is located at the lateral and dorsal portion of the neck. It begins at the transverse processes of the axis and atlas and

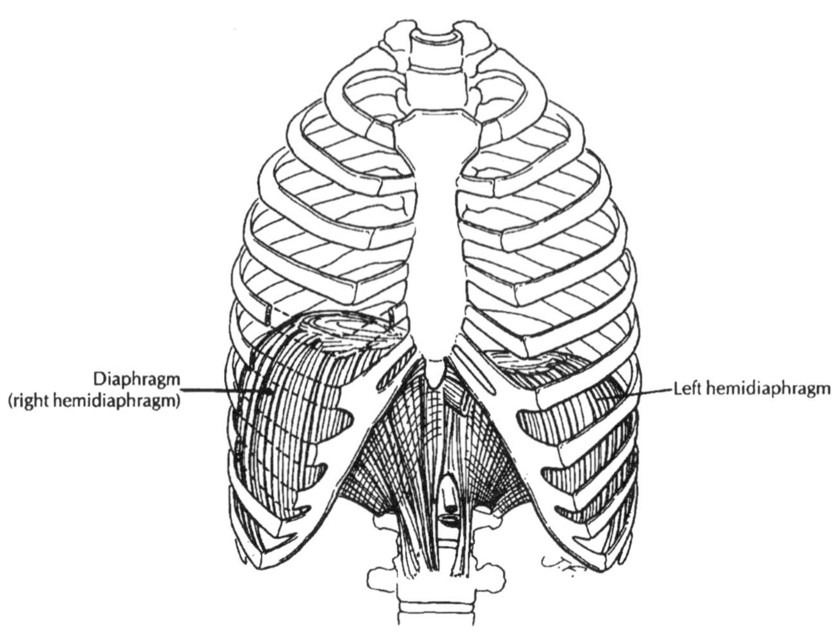

Figure 1-30 The diaphragm. (From Eubanks, D., and Bone, R.C., Comprehensive Respiratory Care: A Learning System, *2nd Edition, St. Louis; The C.V. Mosby Company, 1990.)*

from the transverse process of the level of C3 and C4 of the spinal column. It then attaches to the vertebral border of the scapula, fixing it in position. It causes the chest to rise during deep inspiratory efforts.

Inspiratory Muscles that Assist in Labored Respiration

Sternocleidomastoid

Sternocleidomastoid muscles (Figure 1-31) extend from the mastoid process behind the ear to the upper sternum and proximal part of the clavicle. These muscles turn the head and can be utilized to lift the chest during labored inspiration.

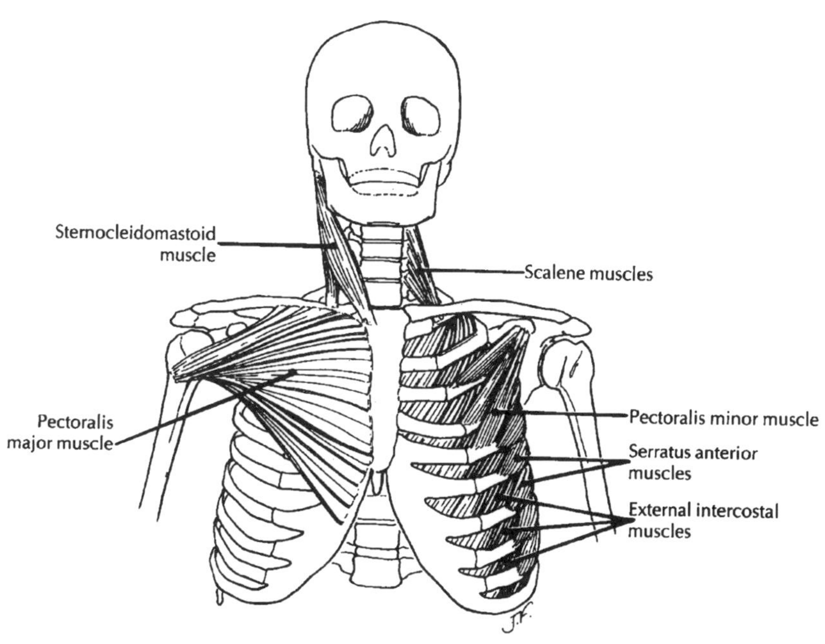

Figure 1-31 Muscles of inspiration, showing pectoralis major, sternocleidomastoid, and external intercostals. (From Eubanks, D., and Bone, R.C., Comprehensive Respiratory Care: A Learning System, *2nd Edition, St. Louis; The C.V. Mosby Company, 1990.)*

Levatores Costarum

The levatores costarum muscles (Figure 1-32) have twelve small tendons that originate from the C7 through T1 transverse processes. They extend laterally and obliquely downward and attach to the outer surfaces of the ribs directly adjacent to their vertebrae of origin. The action of these muscles causes the ribs to rise, increasing the amount of air within the thoracic cavity and allowing for increased lung volume.

Pectoralis Minor

The pectoralis minor (Figure 1-31) begins at the surface of the third to fifth ribs and attaches to the scapula coracoid process. It contributes to lifting the ribs.

Trapezius

The trapezius (Figure 1-32) is a triangular, flat muscle covering the upper neck and back. It begins from the skull's occipital bone, extending to the seventh cervical vertebra, clavicle, scapular spine, and all thoracic vertebrae. The primary use of the trapezius is to lift the upper chest (which can be used to assist inspiration), moving the head from side to side, lifting the shoulders and pulling the scapula down.

Rhomboid Major

The rhomboid major (Figure 1-32) begins at the inferior portion of the supraspinal ligament and spinous processes of T2 to T5 and attaches to the root of the scapular spine. As it contracts, it lifts and fixes the scapula, allowing the pectoral and serratus muscles to raise the ribs during labored inspiration.

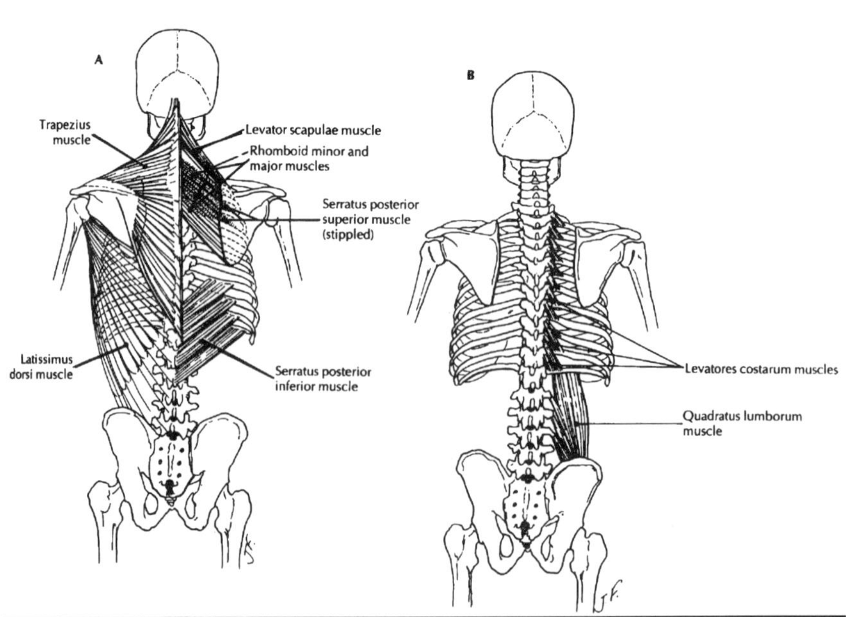

Figure 1-32 Muscles of breathing, including serratus posterior superior and levator scapulae, trapezius, rhomboid major, rhomboid minor, quadratum lumborum, and serratus posterior inferior. (From Eubanks, D., and Bone, R.C., Comprehensive Respiratory Care: A Learning System, *2nd Edition, St. Louis; The C.V. Mosby Company, 1990.)*

Rhomboid Minor

The rhomboid minor (Figure 1-32) begins at the spinous processes of C7 to T1 and the ligamentum nuchae. It then attaches to the root of the spinal scapula. This fixes the scapula to that pectoralis, and the serratus muscles can lift the ribs.

Serratus Anterior

The serratus anterior muscle (Figure 1-31) begins at the superior and outer surfaces of the eighth and ninth ribs and attaches to the anterior surface of the scapular ventricle border. Its primary function is to pull the shoulder forward and upward, causing the chest and ribs to rise.

Scalene Muscles: Anterior, Medial, and Posterior

The scalene muscles (Figure 1-31) begin at the second through seventh cervical transverse processes and attach to the first two ribs. These muscles raise the ribs during inspiration.

Muscles of Expiration

Abdominal muscles are the primary muscles of forced exhalation and include the external oblique, internal oblique, and transversus abdominis. Oblique contraction causes abdominal pressure increases that force the diaphragm upward to assist in forced exhalation. The external oblique muscles begin at the eighth rib and are attached to the crest of the iliac and the pubis bones. The internal obliques begin at the third rib and attach to the crest of the iliac and inguinal ligament.

Intercostal Muscles

There are eleven pairs of intercostal muscles that begin at the inner surface of the ribs and attach to the upper portion of the rib below (Figure 1-31). They extend from the sternum to the angle of each rib and cause the lower ribs to compress the chest wall, forcing expiration.

Quadratus Lumborum

The quadratus lumborum (Figure 1-32) begins at the iliolumbar ligament and associated part of the iliac crest and attaches to the last rib and apices of the L1 to L5 transverse processes. Its contraction fixes the eleventh and twelfth ribs during forced exhalation.

Serratus Posterior Inferior

The serratus posterior inferior muscle (Figure 1-32) is a thin muscle on the dorsum of the thorax. It begins from the supraspinal ligament spines of vertebrae T11 to L3 and attaches laterally to the lower angle portion of the ninth and twelfth ribs. Its contraction lowers the ribs during forced exhalation.

In summary, during quiet inspiration the diaphragm contracts, increasing the anteroposterior size of the chest and decreasing intrathoracic pressure, causing the inspiratory flow of air. Exhalation is a passive process. During labored respiration, all muscles are used for deep respiration. In addition, the scapulae are fixed in position by the contractions of the levator scapulae, trapezius, and rhomboids so that the pectoralis muscles will lift the ribs further. In labored respiration exhalation is forced with the use of the quadratus, lumborum, internal intercostals, subcostals, transverse thoracic, and serratus posterior inferior muscles. In addition, the contraction of the abdominal muscles increases pressure under the diaphragm, forcing it upward and decreasing thoracic cavity size, forcing expiration.

Central Nervous System Control of Ventilation

Body systems are controlled autonomically and volitionally by the cerebral and brain stem complexes (Figure 1-33 and 1-34). Although breathing is autonomic, it can be consciously controlled at any time because it is under the control of voluntary skeletal muscles.

Ventilation rate and depth will automatically adjust to the body's needs. Throughout the medulla oblongata and pons of the brain are clusters of neurons or nerve cells that work together directly to control and direct the muscles of ventilation. These groups of neurons are called the *respiratory centers*. Normally, these groups of neurons automatically discharge impulses to control muscles to meet body demand. This autonomic process can be voluntarily overridden at any time by cortical control. Several neural reflex mechanisms exist to ensure automatic changes in ventilation. The Hering Breuer reflex is composed of neural stretch receptors in the walls of the lungs and chest. As the walls of the lungs stretch, these receptors also stretch, sending the message to the brain to end inspiration. This is thought to provide a switching mechanism and may prevent over stretching during extreme inspiration.

Neural receptors called *chemoreceptors* play a much more important role in the regulation of breathing. Chemoreceptors are sensitive to changes in the partial pressure of carbon dioxide (PCO_2), partial pressure of oxygen (PO_2), and hydrogen ion concentration

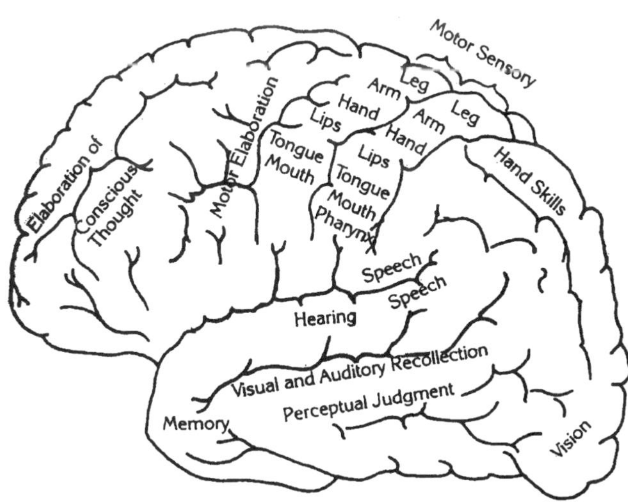

Figure 1-33 Diagrammatic cerebral functions. Some are well established; others are speculative or hypothetical. (From Shames, G.H., and Wiig, E.H., Human Communication Disorders: An Introduction, *Columbus, OH: Charles Merrill Publishing Co., 1982.)*

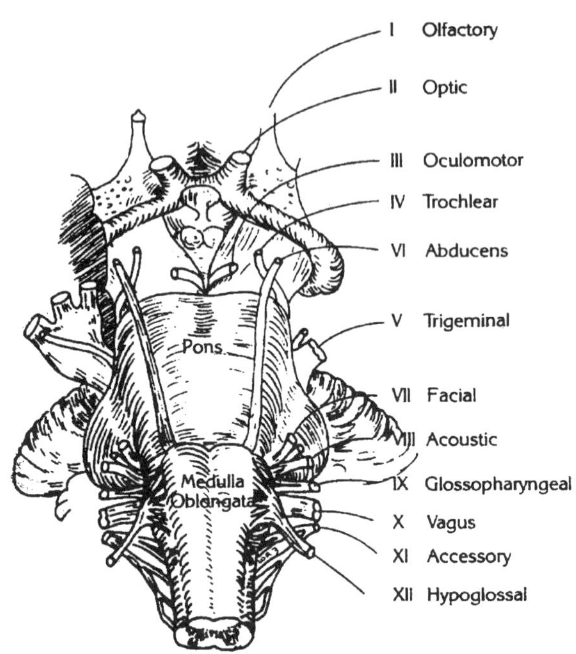

Figure 1-34 Emergence of the cranial nerves from the base of the brain. The nerves are numbered in the order they emerge. (From Shames, G.H., and Wiig, E.H., Human Communication Disorders: An Introduction, *Columbus, OH: Charles Merrill Publishing Co., 1982.)*

(pH) in the blood. Carotid bodies are special chemoreceptors located in the aortic arch. Carotid bodies are chemoreceptors especially sensitive to drops in partial pressure of oxygen (PO_2) . These carotid bodies are located in the carotid sinuses in the neck. If the PO_2 of blood falls below 65 mm Hg, the chemoreceptors will activate impulses to the brain's respiratory center, which will stimulate an increase in breath rate and depth to increase ventilation and the presence of oxygen. Carotid bodies activate this mechanism, referred to as the *hypoxic drive*. Another type of chemoreceptor resides in the fourth ventricle of the brain, located within the medulla oblongata. These are called *medullary chemoreceptors* and they detect the level of pH of fluid. If the pH of cerebrospinal fluid drops (becomes more acidic), medullary chemoreceptors will send impulses to stimulate the rate of ventilation. This decreases the level of carbon dioxide in the blood, which in turn lowers the amount of carbon dioxide entering cerebrospinal fluid. In cerebrospinal fluid, carbon dioxide combines with water to form carbonic acid and releases a hydrogen ion in this process, increasing the acidity of cerebrospinal fluid.

Reaction: $CO_2 + H_2O = H_2CO_3 = H + HCO_3$

Carbonic Anhydrase

This reaction can be increased 13,000 times by the enzyme catalyst of carbonic anhydrase, which is found in red blood cells and kidneys. Reducing carbon dioxide in the blood ultimately will reduce carbon dioxide entering the cerebrospinal fluid, thus raising the pH of this fluid.

PATTERNS OF BREATHING

Normal breathing, or eupnea, is rhythmic. Each breath should be approximately equal in depth and duration. A breath in the normal adult should be approximately 3 to 4 seconds in duration, with an average tidal volume (depth) of 500 ml. Tidal volume refers to the volume of air moved with each breath.

With disease, abnormal patterns of breathing may develop. Diagnostically, it is important to be familiar with these patterns as they will indicate distress. In this chapter, several abnormal breathing patterns will be discussed. The first type is Kussmaul's breathing. This is an extremely deep but steady and rhythmic pattern. The hyperventilation pattern of Kussmaul's breaths usually is indicative of metabolic acidosis as a result of overstimulation of the carotid bodies of the aortic arch. For example, Kussmaul's type breathing could indicate diabetic ketoacidosis.

The Cheyne-Stokes pattern of breathing is the most commonly encountered abnormal pattern of breathing. It involves periods of rhythmic breathing where the depth of the breath first becomes more shallow, then deepens to a maximum level, and then reduces again. The Cheyne-Stokes pattern of breathing is commonly seen in association with congestive heart failure conditions. It can also be seen in persons after long periods of hyperventilation or at high altitudes in individuals not accustomed to these altitudes.

Apena is a condition in which no breathing occurs for an extended period of time. This cessation of breathing often occurs during sleep and is referred to as sleep apena. If the cessation of breathing is prolonged, it can severely disrupt sleep. Apena may also be responsible for some occurences of sudden infant death syndrome (SIDS).

Respiratory Quotient

The respiratory quotient is a means of determining gas exchange. It is equal to the ratio of the volume of carbon dioxide produced to the volume of oxygen consumed:

$$\text{Respiratory quotient} = \frac{\text{Volume of carbon dioxide produced}}{\text{Volume of oxygen consumed}}$$

Stated as a formula, the respiratory quotient is RQ, the volume of carbon dioxide produced per minute is VCO_2, and the volume of oxygen consumed per minute is VO_2; thus:

$$RQ = \frac{VCO_2}{VO_2}$$

In a normal fasted adult the RQ would be determined as follows:

$$RQ = \frac{200\text{ ml}}{250\text{ml}} = 0.08$$

This quotient will actually range from 0.7 to 1.0, depending upon what the individual ate prior to the test.

BLOOD

Blood Types

Antigens are found in red blood cell membranes and are designated as A and B. Blood types can have either A or B antigens or both A and B antigens. Cell membranes without either A or B antigens are classified as type O blood. Blood type is determined by the type of antigen that results in development of antibodies to this antigen. For example, type A blood would not have antibodies to type A antigens but would to type B antigens. Type B blood would have antibodies to type A antigens but not to type B antigens.

Type AB blood would not have antibodies to either A or B antigens. Consequently, AB blood is the universal recipient to AB, A, or B type blood. Type O blood contains no A or B antigens or antibodies. It can be used as the universal donor. However, type O blood can only receive type O blood because of this lack of antigens and antibodies.

RH Factor

If the Rh antigen is present in the blood cell membrane, a person is considered to be Rh positive. If the blood cell membrane is without an Rh antigen, one is considered to be Rh negative. Rh factor can be critical during pregnancy if the mother has developed antibodies to a differing fetal Rh factor from a previous pregnancy. Blood type is vital when determining whole blood transfusion compatibility.

Immune Reaction

Antibodies and antigens involve the body's defense mechanisms against foreign matter. An antigen is a foreign or invading protein entering the body. An antibody is a protein substance found in plasma; it is produced by plasma cells and inactivates antigens. A specific antigen response is made by a specific antibody. Lymphocytes are formed when an antigen invades the plasma cells. This causes antibodies to be produced against this antigen. Antibodies chemically surround the antigen, sealing it off, and preventing its further interaction with body substances. This is referred to as the *antigen-antibody response*. It provides immunity to some diseases and is the basis of vaccination. Vaccination involves the introduction of a small amount of antigen into the body to initiate development of an antibody. As a result, a natural immunity to a specific disease is provided (e.g., measles, rubella, polio, and flu strain). This antigen-antibody response is also responsible for blood typing, allergic reactions, and organ transplant rejection.

The Circulatory System

Blood is the transport system of the body. Each cell in the body is dependent on blood supply. Blood brings oxygen and nutrients to tissues and filters out waste products through other body systems such as the lymphatic system, kidneys, spleen, liver, and lungs. There are three major types of blood cells (Figure 1-35): red blood cells (erythrocytes), white blood cells (leukocytes), and platelets.

Erythrocytes (Figure 1-35) (red blood cells or RBCs) are the most common blood cells and are simple in structure, appearing as small biconcave discs that are approximately 7 microns in diameter. Lacking a nucleus, mature cells are unable to reproduce or perform more complicated metabolic processes. There are approximately 5,000,000 RBCs in one milliliter of blood. Every second, 2 to 3 million new erythrocytes are formed. These cells are formed in the red bone marrow located in the diploe of the ribs, sternum, vertebrae, pelvis, and skull. This process is called hematopoiesis or erythropoiesis. During development the erythrocytes have a nucleus but this is lost at maturity.

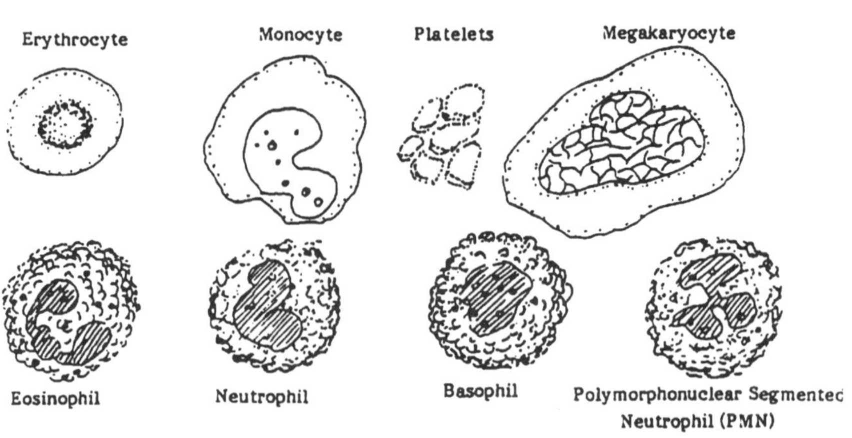

Figure 1-35 Types of blood cells. (From California College for Health Sciences, Entry Level Respiratory Therapy Program, Vol. 1, *Figure 1-2, p. [RTT 102] 1-5. National City, CA, 1985.)*

An erythrocyte circulates and functions in the blood for approximately 120 days and travels 700 miles through the body. During this travel, the cell comes in constant contact and collision with vessel walls and other cells. As the cell ages, it becomes fragile, and eventually the cell membrane ruptures and the cell dies. This cellular debris is removed by the macrophage activity of the reticuloendothelial systems of bone marrow, spleen, and liver. Part of the cellular debris of dead erythrocytes is hemoglobin. This could be harmful if left in the system so it is reduced to pigment called bilirubin and transported via plasma to the liver, which excretes it in bile.

A hemoglobin molecule takes up one third of the volume of the red blood cell. The molecular compound hemoglobin carries oxygen in blood. This molecule contains globin and four molecules of the pigment heme. A heme molecule contains one atom of iron. Heme molecules are binding sites for oxygen. Hemoglobin contains four heme sites and carries four molecules of oxygen. The carrying of oxygen is the most important function of red blood cells. Hemoglobin ensures the transport of 97% of the oxygen in blood. Its ability to transport oxygen is much greater than that of plasma, which carries the small percent of oxygen remaining.

Once oxygen is bound to hemoglobin it becomes oxyhemoglobin. The pulmonary vein carries the majority of the oxyhemoglobin from the lungs to the heart, but most oxyhemoglobin is carried in arterial blood vessels. Carboxyhemoglobin is formed when oxyhemoglobin binds to carbon dioxide instead of to oxygen. This waste product is carried in veins back to the lungs for gas exchange and exhalation. Carbon dioxide is the result of metabolism at a cellular level and is a waste product. Hemoglobin levels in males are 13 to 16 grams per 100 ml; for females the levels are 12 to 14 grams per 100 ml. Counts of less than 11 grams represent anemia and indicate that the ability of the blood to carry oxygen is greatly reduced. In contrast, a condition called polycythemia occurs when the hemoglobin level is more than 17 grams. Polycythemia may occur in chronic obstructive pulmonary disease as the body produces more hemoglobin to compensate for a lack of oxygen. Hematocrit is the volume of red blood cells in 100 cubic cm of whole blood, which is approximately 45 to 47%.

White blood cells (WBCs) combat infection and inflammation. The ratio of RBCs to WBCs is 700 to 1. WBCs are also referred to as leukocytes. WBCs are measured by diluting a blood sample and physically counting leukocytes. A CBC is a complete blood count. It reflects hemoglobin, white blood cells, red blood cells, and differential. Leukocytes have a nucleus unlike RBCs (erythrocytes) and do not contain hemoglobin. Leukocytes fall into two groups: granular and nongranular. This grouping is based on the cell cytoplasm type. Granular cells have a grainy appearance in cytoplasm. Nongranular cells have normal cytoplasm. Granular leukocyte types are neutrophils, eosinophils, and basophils, with mostly irregularly shaped and lobed nuclei, also called polymorphonuclear neutrophils (PMN). Red bone marrow is the manufacturing site of granular leukocytes. Basophils and eosinophils (Figure 1-35) combat allergies, basophils secrete the anticoagulant heparin, eosinophils destroy foreign material, and neutrophils are phagocytic.

Leukocytes that are nongranular are lymphocytes and monocytes with nuclei that are normally shaped. Lymphocytes and monocytes are produced in lymphatic tissue. The function of lymphocytes is antibody production. Phagocytic function is also provided by monocytes, and these cells can change into macrophage cells. Lymphocytes also have the ability to change into new cells that are phagocytic.

Platelets or thrombocytes are small cells (Figure 1-35). They do not have nuclei and are manufactured in red bone marrow. The main function of platelets is blood clotting. Blood clotting is vital to prevent excessive loss of body fluid by plugging cut or torn vessels. Platelets circulate normally in the blood and have the tendency to attach to any rough surface and then rupture as a result. Upon platelet rupture, platelet factor 3 is released causing calcium and proteins to join and form thromboplastin. Thrombin is formed when thromboplastin and protein globulin in blood (prothrombin) combine with platelets. Thrombin forms with fibrin to produce fibrinogen, creating a sticky fiber network at the cut site. As cells are caught in this network, a blood clot is formed. The liver synthesizes the active proteins fibrinogen and prothrombin. Increasing the production of prothrombin requires vitamin K. Until it joins with thrombin as a catalyst to clot formation, fibrinogen is not active. Blood vessels normally have a smooth surface, allowing for rapid flow.

Branches of the thyroid arteries (inferior) and venous drainage ends in the thyroid venus plexus supply blood to the trachea. The vagus and recurrent nerve branches innervate the trachea with the sympathetic system. The thyroid ima artery commonly arises on the right from the innominate and descends on the anterior tracheal wall in the midline. Its position can present a problem during tracheostomy. On the anterior wall of the midline trachea is the thyroid ima vein, which drains the anastomosed right and left inferior thyroid veins into the right or left brachiocephalic vein.

CARDIAC PHYSIOLOGY

The heart is a muscular organ roughly the size of a fist (Figure 1-36). It is roughly located in the center of the chest with two-thirds of the heart mass to the left of the medial line, and the remainder to the right. The bluntly pointed end, or apex is the left ventrical, and it points to the left. The heart consists of four chambers (Figure 1-36). The superior and bilateral left and right atria receive blood into the heart from the veins. The atria are separated by the interatrial septum, a muscular wall. Inferiorly and bilaterally are the right and left ventricles with the interventricular septum muscular wall separating them. The ventricles send blood from the heart via arteries. The thickness of the walls in the heart chambers relates to the difference in the amount of work performed by the chambers. The atria have thinner walls than the ventricles. The left ventricle wall is thicker due to the blood being pumped into the higher resistance pressures of the systemic circulation. The slightly thinner wall of the right ventricle reflects the lowest resistance of the pulmonary circulation.

The right side of the heart receives blood that has circulated throughout the body and is depleted of oxygen and contains high amounts of carbon dioxide (the waste product of metabolism). Blood is carried to the right side of the heart by the largest veins of the body, the superior and inferior venae cavae. Lower systemic system blood is carried by the inferior venae cavae. Blood from the head is carried by the superior venae cavae. From the venae cavae, blood flows into

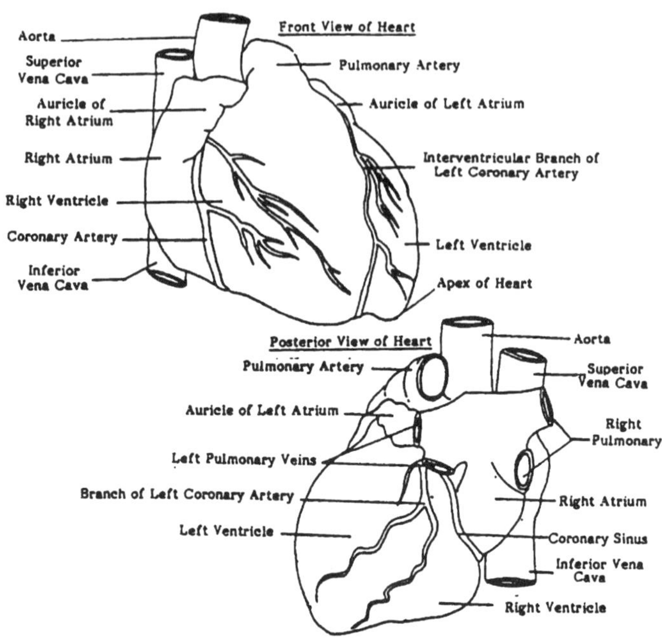

Figure 1-36 Frontal and posterior views of the heart. (From California College for Health Sciences, Entry Level Respiratory Therapy Program, Vol. 1, Figure 1-3, p. [RTT 102] 1-9. National City, CA, 1985.)

the right atrium, through the tricuspid valve, and into the right ventricle. The role of the tricuspid valve is to prevent blood from returning to the right atrium during right ventricle contraction. The tricuspid valve (Figure 1-37) withstands a great deal of pressure. It is able to remain closed and is prevented from inverting into the atria by the chordae tendineae. These cords are attached to the conical muscles (papillary muscles) in the ventricles. This is also true for the bicuspid valve. With right ventricle contraction, blood flows through the semilunar valve and directly into the pulmonary artery. This blood flow results in the pulmonary artery being the only artery with high carbon dioxide content. To supply the right and left lungs, the pulmonary artery splits into the left and right pulmonary arteries. This process allows the lungs to re-oxygenate blood and relieve the blood

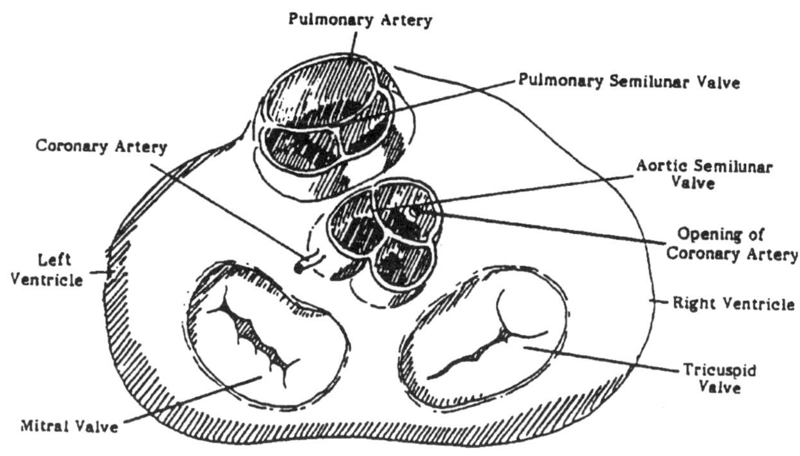

Figure 1-37 Heart with atria removed. (From California College for Health Sciences, Entry Level Respiratory Therapy Program, Vol. 1, *Figure 1-4, p. [RTT 102] 1-9. National City, CA, 1985.)*

of carbon dioxide waste. Re-oxygenated blood enters the pulmonary vein (the only vein in the body carrying highly oxygenated blood), which connects to the left side of the heart. Blood entering the left atrium travels through the mitral or bicuspid valve and enters the left ventricle. When contraction of the left ventricle occurs, oxygen-rich blood is pumped into the aortic arch and the descending aorta to the systemic system, beginning the circulatory process.

The layers of the heart include the pericardium, which forms a loose sac containing the heart. The two layers within the pericardium are (1) the parietal pericardium, which is the outer layer of fibrous tissue that attaches to the sternum and diaphragm, and (2) the visceral pericardium, which attaches directly to the heart. The space between these two pericardium layers is the pericardial cavity, which contains pericardial fluid to provide viscosity and reduce friction between the two pericardial layers. The third layer of the heart is the myocardial muscle itself, and the fourth layer of the heart is the endocardium on the inside of the thin smooth tissue lining of the cavities of the heart.

Heart Beat

The normal heart beat for an adult is 60 to 80 times per minute. The normal heart beat is 120 times for a child, and up to 140 to 160 beats a minute for a neonate.

Cycle of the Heart Beat

Systole is contraction of the ventricles, and diastole is relaxation of the ventricles. As the heart muscle acts as a pump, a pattern of four phases results. This pattern involves the atria acting primarily as reservoirs and the ventricles acting as pumps for blood flow.

The four phases of the heart beat are as follows:

1. The first phase occurs with contraction of both atria: the cuspid valves are open (two), and the semilunar valves are closed (two). Closing of the semilunar valves creates the diastolic sound "dubb."
2. The second phase begins with the relaxation of the atria and with the cuspid valves in the closed position, allowing blood to again fill the atria. Closing of the cuspid valves results in the systolic sound of "lubb."
3. The third phase occurs when the cuspid valves are closed, the ventricles contract, and the semilunar valves are in the open position, allowing for the emptying of blood from the ventricles.
4. The fourth phase involves relaxation of the ventricles, with the semilunar valves closed and the cuspid valves open. This marks the initiation of the first phase, again with the atria starting to contract.

Heart Beat Conduction

Conduction of the heart beat involves four separate structures (Figure 1-38). The first structure is the sinoatrial node (S-A node), in which the heart beat begins. The S-A node is located near the opening of the superior venae cavae of the right atrium. Nerve fibers from both divisions of the autonomic nervous system are contained in the S-A node. These nerve fibers that originate and influence heart rate are both parasympathetic and sympathetic. The impulse that fires the S-A node travels through other fibers in both the right and left atria.

Blood concentration of hormones can affect heart rate (i.e., epinephrine and thyroxine can both increase the heart rate).

The atrioventricular node (Figure 1-38)(A-V node) is the second structure of heart beat conduction. Directly next to the atrial septum is the small mass of the A-V node. Impulses from the S-A node cross the atrium where the A-V node picks up this impulse for a brief time. This delay allows the ventricles to fill and the atria to contract. Continuing from the A-V node, the impulse travels through the network of fibers of the bundle of His, the third structure of heart beat conduction, down to the ventricular septum and into the Purkinje fibers, the fourth structure of heart beat conduction, thus causing the contraction of the ventricles.

The inherent rhythm of the heart muscle varies throughout the structure of the heart. The fastest rate originates in the S-A node.

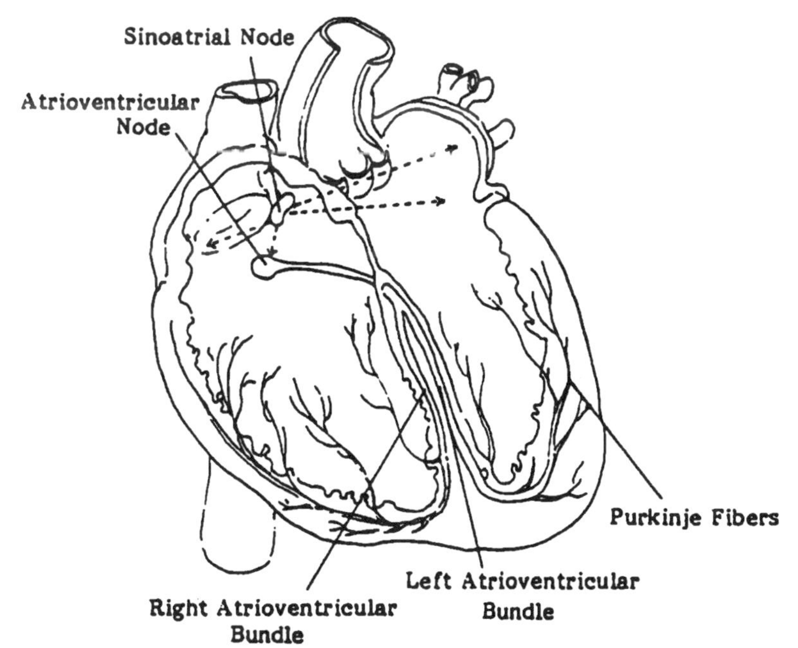

Figure 1-38 Conducting system of the heart. (From California College for Health Sciences, Entry Level Respiratory Therapy Program, Vol. 1, *Figure 1-6, p. [RTT 102] 1-12. National City, CA, 1985.)*

Impulses spread from the S-A node so fast that they depolarize other adjacent heart muscles covering the other inherent rhythms. The A-V node with the next highest rate of 40 to 60 beats per minutes can pace the heart rate if the S-A node is not functioning. Other parts of the heart muscle may have an inherent heart rate. A heart beat is considered an ectopic beat if it does not originate within the S-A node (i.e., the Purkinje fibers have an inherent rate [15-40] but impulse firing is usually disorganized). The term for an excessive heart rate of 100 to 120 beats per minute is *tachycardia*. The term for an excessively slow heart rate of less than 40 to 50 beats per minute is *bradycardia*.

Electrolyte function can affect heart beat rate. An excess of calcium can affect myoneural junction blocking (the release of troponin), causing the heart to become spastic. Calcium deficit can cause cardiac weakness. This occurrence should be rare as the body will pull calcium from the bones as it is required. Also, high levels of potassium can cause heart muscle to dilate and become flaccid, reducing heart rate. In contrast, a reduction in potassium can lead to fibrillation from heart irritability.

Heart rate is also affected by high sodium levels because this affects calcium absorption. Temperature increase also increases heart rate as the body tries to bring heat to the skin surface to be cooled. Effects on the heart can be described in several terms, including strength or inotropic effect, rate of conduction or dromotropic effect, and heart beat rate or chronotropic effect.

Blood supply to the heart comes from the right and left coronary arteries originating from the ascending aorta (Figure 1-39). The right coronary artery has two branches: (1) the posterior descending branch supplying blood to the right and left ventricles, and (2) the marginal branch supplying blood to the right ventricle. The anterior descending branch and the circumflex are contained in the left coronary artery. The circumflex supplies blood to the left ventricle and the left atrium. The anterior descending branch supplies blood to the right and left ventricles. It may be observed that the left ventricle receives more blood supply due to stress of workload.

Venous drainage from the heart occurs through several routes: (1) the anterior cardiac veins draining from all of the chambers of the heart; (2) the thebesian vein draining both right and left atria; and (3)

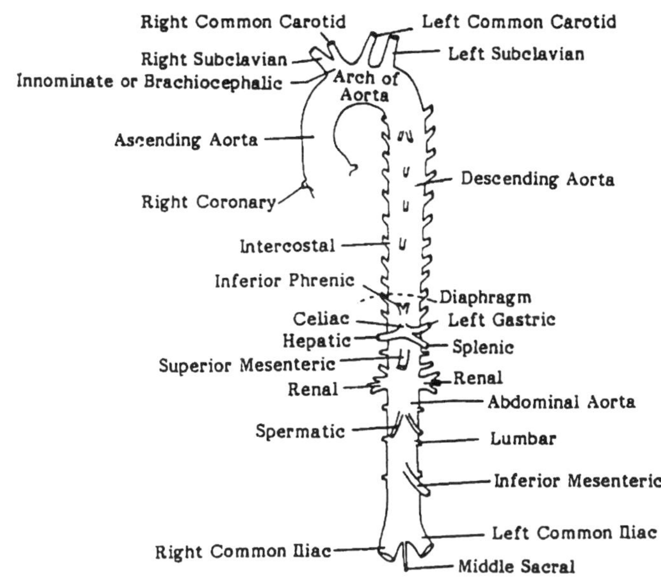

Figure 1-39 The aorta. (From California College for Health Sciences, Entry Level Respiratory Therapy Program, Vol. 1, *Figure 1-5, p. [RTT 102] 1-10. National City, CA, 1985.)*

the coronary sinus, which acts as a final point that mainly drains into the left ventricle and then empties into the right atrium.

Blood Vessels

Arteries carry blood away from the heart. As they become smaller in size they are termed *arterioles*. As blood leaves arterioles it enters smaller capillaries, which directly service the cell metabolism. Arteries have several layers, the tunica intima, the tunica media, and the tunica adventitia (Figure 1-40). The smooth inner wall of endothelial tissue surrounded by fibrous elastic material is the tunica intima. Two thick bands of fibers and smooth muscle make up the tunica media. The tunica media allows the artery to change size, increasing or decreasing as needed to regulate the pressure of the blood. The tunica adventitia is fibrous and primarily collagenous. It

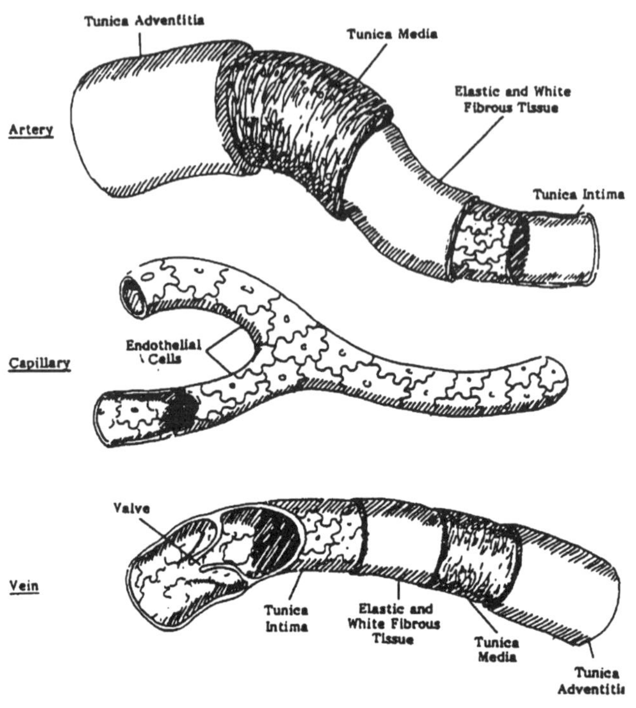

Figure 1-40 Artery, capillary, and vein structure. (From California College for Health Sciences, Entry Level Respiratory Therapy Program, Vol. 1, *Figure 1-7, p. [RTT 102] 1-14. National City, CA, 1985.)*

is the outer layer and acts as protection against excessive stretching. The vasa vasorum of vessels supplies nutrients to the artery muscles.

The basic structure of veins (Figure 1-40) is similar to that of arteries. However, the difference between arteries and veins is related to hydrostatic pressure. The chordae tendineae are attached to the conical musculature and elasticity aids in the ability to withhold the pressure of pulsing blood flow. In contrast, veins do not contract and have less elasticity as they do not withstand such pressures. Instead, they contain semilunar valves that act within the vein to prevent blood backflow.

Blood flows through the capillaries and enters the smallest of veins (venules) and is then carried through the veins back to the heart. Capillaries are made up of a single layer of endothelial cells (Figure 1-40) to allow for the easy diffusion of gases, waste products, and nutrients in and out of the cell. Capillaries contain sphincters (smooth circular rings of muscles), which are vital to the maintenance of blood pressure as is their small size. Capillaries carry blood directly to the cell site. Their diameter is approximately 1 mm. One and a half million capillaries are contained in a cubic inch of muscle.

Blood Pressure

Blood flow is due to an inherent pressure gradient within the circulatory system. Fluid flows from a higher pressure source to a lower pressure gradient. Systolic pressure normal in the adult are 120 mm Hg. Diastolic pressures normal to adults are between 60 and 80 mm Hg on the average.

Cardiac output and peripheral resistance combine to determine arterial blood pressure. The amount of blood pumped in one minute equals cardiac output. (The amount of blood pumped in one heart beat is called the stroke volume. Stroke volume times the rate equals cardiac output.)

According to Starling's law, the strength of heart muscle contraction is dependent on how stretched or lengthened the heart fibers were at the beginning of the contraction. The heart can lose its natural elasticity if it is stretched too long, as occurs in congestive heart failure.

Peripheral resistance determines blood pressure. The size of the venous or arterial lumen will affect the pressure of the blood being pumped through it. For example, in sclerotic heart disease, a residual build up of fatty materials deposits on the interior of the lumen, inhibiting blood flow and increasing blood pressure. In contrast, blood pressure will drop when resistance within the lumen lessens as with extreme blood loss.

As mentioned previously, veins do not have the elasticity of the arteries; thus blood flow is assisted by other factors. Breathing and skeletal and muscle movement help to reduce pressure in the veins. Movement of the muscles and supportive skeletal structures increases pressures on the veins to help push blood toward the heart. Abdominal pressure builds with the distention of the diaphragm and assists in moving blood to the heart. Thus, the act of breathing assists blood flow through the veins.

LYMPHATIC SYSTEM

The lymphatic system is anatomically associated with the circulatory system (Figure 1-41). Lymphatic vessels move fluid to and from the circulatory system. The lymphatic system has four functions. The first function is to return important proteins and fluids from interstitial spaces to the circulatory system after it has cleansed the fluids of harmful substances and accumulated waste. The lymphatic system acts as a bridge that nutrients and waste products pass between the body capillaries and cells. It also removes proteins or other foreign substances. The second function is that of fat absorption through central lacteal vessels in the small intestine villi. The third function is that of defense system. With use of the immune system and phagocytosis the body is able to fight microorganisms. The fourth function is the hematopoiesis of lymphocytes.

The lymph capillaries are vessels with a thickness of a single layer of cells. The ends of these vessels have a perforated, rounded hub that allows lymphatic fluid to move through these spaces easily. Internally, the lymph capillary contains numerous valves formed by overlapping edges of endothelial cells. Lymph capillaries are most easily found in loose portions of connective tissue or in the submucosal layers of organs.

Rising from the smaller lymph capillaries are lymph vessels. Larger lymph vessels are thinner and have many more valves than veins but still have layers of cells similar to those of blood vessels.

Drainage in the body occurs through two major lymphatic systems: the right lymphatic duct and the thoracic duct. Anterior to the second lumbar vertebra is the large sac of the chyle cistern, which is the origin of the thoracic duct. The thoracic duct receives lymph from the majority of the lymph vessel system. The exception to this is the upper right quadrant, which contains vessels for the right side of the head and the right side of the chest. Of the 120 ml of fluid moved every hour in the lymphatic system, the thoracic duct is responsible for 100 ml, with the right lymphatic duct handling the remaining 20 ml of

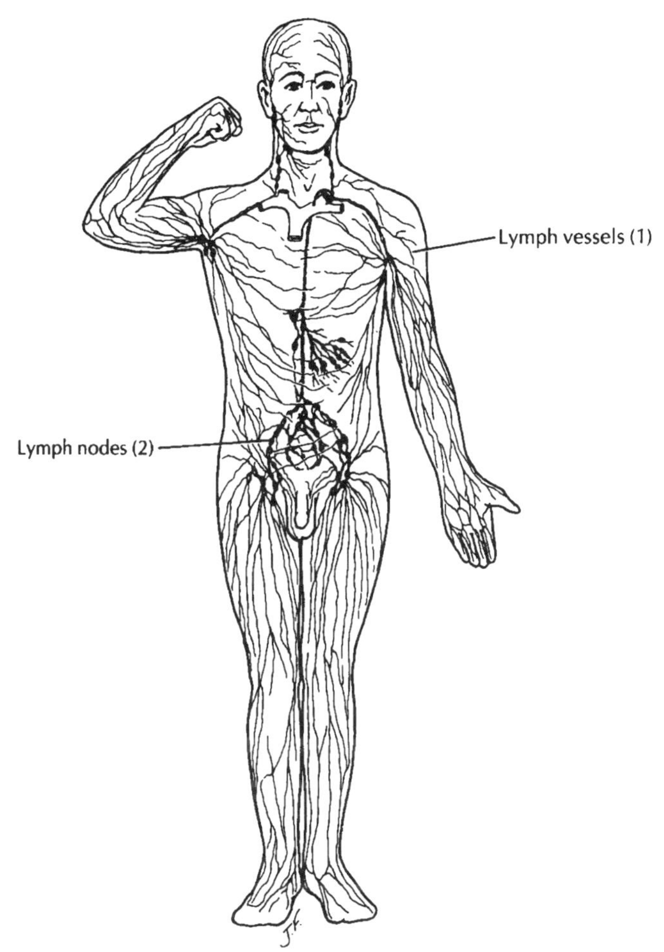

Figure 1-41 Lymphatic system showing lymph vessels and lymph nodes. (From Eubanks, D., and Bone, R.C., Comprehensive Respiratory Care: A Learning System, *2nd Edition, St. Louis: The C.V. Mosby Company, 1990.)*

fluid. This distribution is due to the larger area of the body covered by the thoracic duct. The thoracic duct drains lymph into the left subclavian and jugular vein junction. The upper right quadrant lymph drains into the right lymphatic duct and returns to the venous system at the junction of the right subclavian and jugular veins.

The entire pathway of the lymphatic system is lined with lymph nodes. Lymphatic fluid must pass through a series of nodes before it can be returned to the general circulatory system. Nodes contain larger portions of lymphatic tissue with a fibrous covering. Lymphatic fluid can enter nodes from a variety of directions through small afferent vessels and then exit through only one large efferent vessel. Internally, the node contains a medulla and a cortex. The medulla of the lymph node serves as an area of sinuses in a structure suspended for support in a trabecular framework. The medulla serves the function of filtration of lymphatic fluid with the assistance of large numbers of macrophages to remove substances by phagocytosis. Macrophages within the medulla can be wandering and capable of amoeboid type movement to pursue particles, or may be fixed with no movement. (The cortex layer is the outer layer of the lymph node wherein germinal center dense patches of lymphatic tissue are located.) Germinal centers are the active production sites of lymphocytes. Once manufactured in the germinal centers, lymphocytes find their way to the circulatory system.

The major groups of lymph nodes are axillary (under the arm), submaxillary (under the neck), and inguinal (in the groin). The tonsils, adenoids, and lingual tonsils also contain lymphatic tissues, which filter fluid and produce lymphocytes. This group of nodes surrounds the pharynx, protecting the throat (airway) from infections.

Located below the left diaphragm, above the kidneys, and behind the stomach is the spleen. This oval-shaped structure can act as a blood reservoir as it stores up to 350 ml of blood and can hold up to 500 ml. If necessary, the spleen can release up to 150 ml per minute. It also holds onto erythrocytes, giving it the ability to contract and release blood with a high hematocrit to help in the event of blood loss. The spleen also serves in the role of destroying old red blood cells. In a fetus, the spleen is a site for red blood cell production. The spleen also serves as a site of lymph filtering and lymphocyte production. Despite its many functions, a person can survive with no obvious disability if the spleen is removed.

Lymphatic tissue is also in the thymus. The thyroid serves in the manufacturing of lymphocytes to stimulate lymphocyte production in other lymphatic tissues as these cells migrate to other parts of the body. However, the thyroid cannot filter lymph. The thymus serves an important role in the development of the immune system as the lymphocytes it produces travel throughout the lymphatic system.

BLOOD PRESSURE

Highly sensitive specialized cells called *cardiac baroreceptors* are located in the carotid sinus and the aortic arch. These cells send a message via sensory fibers from the aortic baroreceptors from the vagus nerve directly to the medulla. Carotid sinus baroreceptors send impulses along fibers to the glossopharyngeal nerve, sending them to the medulla. The cardiac center within the medulla generates parasympathetic and sympathetic impulses to regulate heart beat. Increases in pressure in the carotid sinus or aortic arch are detected by the medulla, which in turn activates the parasympathetic system. This action slows the heart rate and lowers the blood pressure. A drop in blood pressure will signal the medulla to activate the sympathetic system to increase the heart rate and to raise the blood pressure to normal levels.

The tracheobronchial tree has its own arterial and venous systems for blood flow and nutrients. These consist of the large pulmonary veins and arteries. In addition to the pulmonary vein and arteries, the tracheobronchial tree is supplied by the bronchial arteries all the way through to the level of the bronchioles. Blood returns from bronchial veins to the right atrium via the azygos system (the system of the spinal column veins). Hypertrophy of bronchial collateral circulation compensates for blockage of the pulmonary artery and any areas of the lung that are under perfused during disease processes.

RENAL SYSTEM

The renal system, or excretory system, includes the kidneys urinary bladder, ureters, and urethra (Figure 1-42). The kidneys are located at the level T11 to L2 of the spinal column, high in the posterior of the abdomen. They are situated close to the liver, spleen, and diaphragm. The kidney's structures include the nephron, which filters toxic wastes from the blood. the primary function of the kidneys is to regulate the composition and volume of extracellular fluid. They

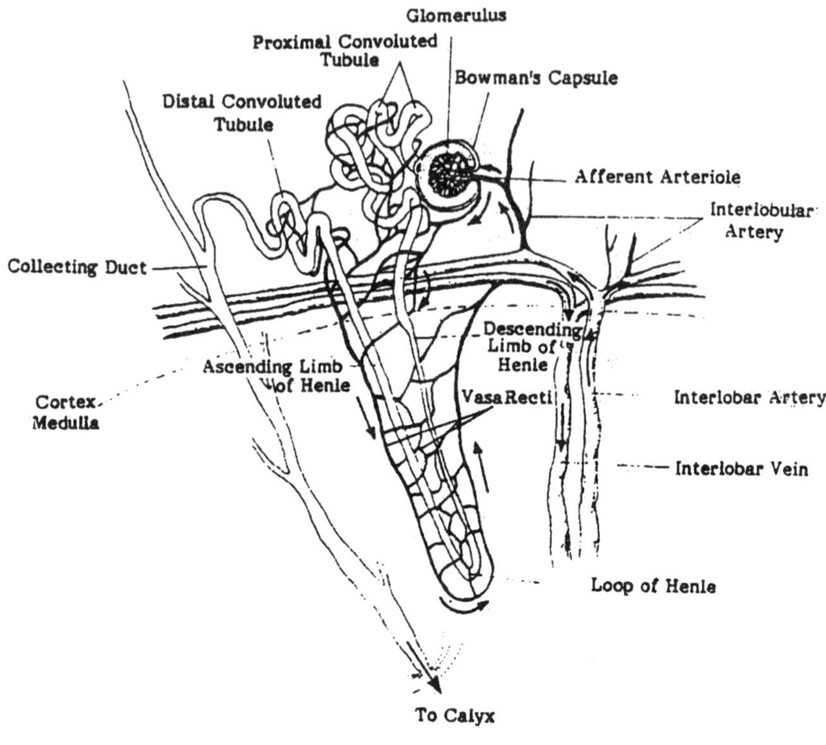

Figure 1-42 The renal system. (From California College for Health Sciences, Entry Level Respiratory Therapy Program, *Vol. 1, Figure 7-4 p. [RTT 7-5]. National City, CA, 1985.)*

are vital for the homeostasis of the body. For respiratory patients the kidneys serve a major role by regulating arterial blood pH (acid or base content). This is accomplished by the retention or excretion of acid and bicarbonate (base). The kidney structures are efficient enough to support the body even if only 25% of the renal mass remains.

The actual structures within the nephron where filtration takes place include the glomerulus, Bowman's capsule, proximal tubule, convoluted loop of Henle, and distal tubule. The filtration of blood takes place within the renal corpuscle, which is the combination of Bowman's capsule and the glomerulus. Blood flows through the glomerulus to the tubules, where high capillary pressure drives plasma fluid out of the blood across the capillary membrane and into the Bowman's capsule. The tubules filter out useful materials such as sugars and salt and send them into the blood via active transport and osmosis. Waste products are excreted from the tubules into the ureter and to the bladder. Blood flows at approximately 1,200 ml per minute. Of this volume, 125 ml is filtered into Bowman's capsule. Approximately 124 ml per minute is reabsorbed via the vasa recti in the kidney's tubular system, a net of about 1 ml of urine produced each minute. Most of the material that is reabsorbed is water. Eliminated material contains waste, toxins, urea, creatinine, uric acid, ammonia, phosphates, sodium potassium, chloride, magnesium, sulfates, and some hormones. Normal adult production of urine is 1500 ml per day.

Reabsorption of water from the renal system is essential to the body. Thus, if this function is ineffective, it can have deadly consequences. The body produces two substances that affect the amount of water absorbed. The first substance is antidiuretic hormone (ADH), which is manufactured by the pituitary gland and regulated by the hypothalamus. In response to low blood pressure, ADH is produced to ensure osmotic pressure. ADH increases the size of the pores in the membranes of the cells so that water is reabsorbed at a faster rate into the blood. For an unknown reason, mechanical ventilation may stimulate the hypothalamus, increasing water reabsorption and leading to renal shutdown. The substance that signals reabsorption of water is aldosterone, a hormone and a type of mineralocorticoid. It stimulates the tubular reabsorption of sodium. Low levels of sodium can cause an increase in levels of aldosterone. Renal tubules reabsorb more sodium along with water. The volume of blood may need to be reduced in some situations, such as in congestive heart failure, due to circulatory overload. Urine production may need to increase. This can be done by reducing water reabsorption into the blood by use of a diuretic.

The kidneys perform the metabolic function of maintaining the acid-base balance (pH) of the blood. Normal pH levels are maintained by regulation of hydrogen ions (H^+) and bicarbonate ions (HCO_3). Kidney function includes the excretion of hydrogen ions or reabsorption of bicarbonate ions if the blood is too acidic. If the blood is too alkaline, the kidneys will excrete bicarbonate ions and reabsorb hydrogen ions.

In the case of alkalosis, the body will attempt to restore homeostasis (normal pH) by increasing the acid condition of the blood. The kidneys will excrete bicarbonate ions, increasing the level of hydrogen ions in the blood and correcting the pH. The excretion of hydrogen ions is more difficult. To decrease acid as the result of acidosis, hydrogen ion levels must be reduced and reabsorbed. This is done through urine when hydrogen ions combine with bicarbonate ions to form carbonic acid, which dissociates into water and carbon dioxide. Carbon dioxide diffuses easily across cell membranes into the blood where it recombines with water to form carbonic acid, which then dissociates into hydrogen ions and bicarbonate ions. New hydrogen ions combine with ammonium ions (NH_3) to form ammonia ions (NH_4) which diffuse back into the renal tubules for excretion. This is the reabsorption of bicarbonate ions, which corrects acidosis.

CENTRAL NERVOUS SYSTEM

The central nervous system plays the primary role of receiving and transmitting stimuli and coordinating body activity. The nervous system is responsible for body reaction to all external and internal stimuli.

Neurons

The basic unit of the nervous system is the neuron. The cell body of the neuron contains similar structures as other cells (Figure1-43), including a nucleus, mitochondria, and ribosomes. They have the capacity to synthesize proteins and ATP (adenosine5'- triphosphate). Neurons differ from other cells in that they have specialized membranes that are capable of conducting electrochemical impulses called action potentials.

The typical neuron contains relatively short processes that extend from the cell called dendrites. These are the input side of the cell and transmit information to the cell body. In the Central Nervous System (CNS) there are many neurons that may converge on one neuron by attaching to the dendrites. The axon is typically a long, thin projection that transmits information from the cell body to another neuron, a muscle, or organ.

Neurons in the Peripheral Nervous System (PNS) are often divided into afferent and efferent neurons. The afferent neurons convey sensory information (from sensory receptors in the body) to the CNS. These sensory neurons have a different structure form the typical neuron described above (e.g., the "dendrite" can be very long and has the same structure as an axon). Efferent neurons are often referred to as motor neurons and convey information from the CNS to the muscles and organs of the body. An example of a motor neuron attached to a muscle is in Figure 1-43. These motor neurons are

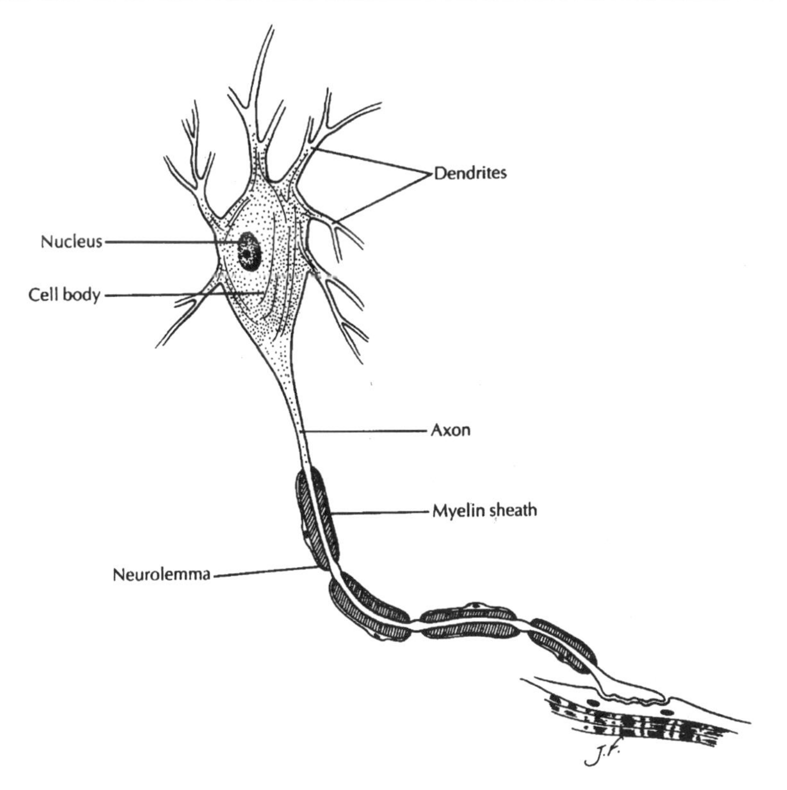

Figure 1-43 Structures of a neuron. (From Eubanks, D., and Bone, R.C., Comprehensive Respiratory Care: A Learning System, *2nd Edition, St. Louis: The C.V. Mosby Company, 1990.)*

responsible for informing all of the muscles when to contract, how long to contract, and how strong to contract.

In order to speed up the transmission of the action potentials, many neurons are myelinated. Schwann cells attach to the axons of neurons and surround the axon with its cell membrane. This is called a neurilemma or myelin sheath. In between each myelin sheath is a node (nodes of Ranvier) where the naked membrane is exposed. Action potentials travel faster down myelinated axons because the action potential jumps from node to node. Myelinated fibers are important to the nervous system because they are able to convey information at a much faster rate. The synaptic junction is a gap at the end of one axon and the point of impulse transmission at the site of a dendrite from another neuron. The neurotransmitter acetylcholine is released at the synaptic junction eliciting muscle contraction. It is deactivated by the chemical cholinesterase.

There are times when it is advantageous to have reactions to external stimuli which are extremely rapid. The nervous system accomplishes many of these tasks by forming reflex arcs. Sensory information is passed to the spinal cord, (or brain stem for structures of the head) where it directly affects the motor neurons. The motor neurons produce the muscle contractions needed in order to achieve the desired affect. An example of this is the removal of a limb in response to a pain stimuli. If an individual steps on a nail, the reflex arc is used to remove the foot from the stimuli. Before the individual is even aware of what has happened (e.g., the information has not made it to the cortex) the reflex arc has already initiated the process of removing the leg from the pain stimuli. There are many reflexes that range from this simple example to extremely complex reflex responses.

The Brain

The central nervous system comprises of the brain and spinal cord (Figure 1-44). The brain contains three major divisions: forebrain, midbrain, and hindbrain. The structures of the brain are primarily responsible as the body's controlling organ. The forebrain contains the cerebrum and thalamus. The midbrain contains the corpora

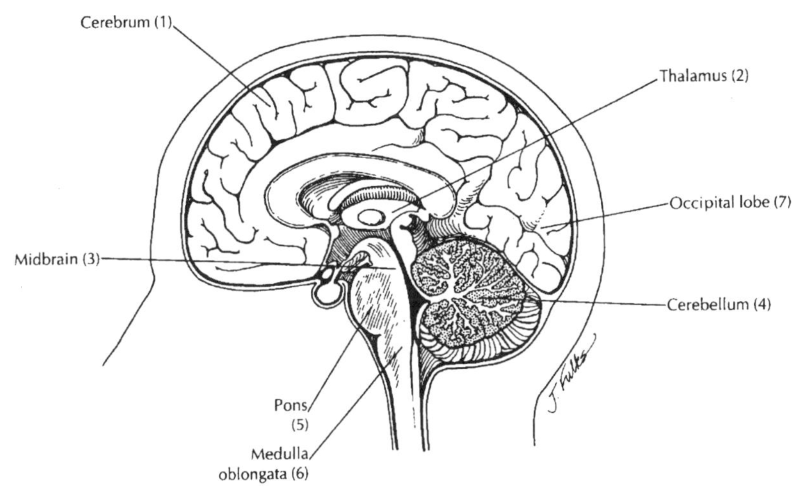

Figure 1-44 Structures of the brain. (From Eubanks, D., and Bone, R.C., Comprehensive Respiratory Care: A Learning System, *2nd Edition, St. Louis: The C.V. Mosby Company, 1990.)*

quadrigemina and cerebral peduncle located directly below the thalamus. The hindbrain contains the medulla oblongata, pons, and cerebellum.

The Cerebrum

The cerebrum is the largest area of the brain and makes up seven-eighths the total weight of the brain. The cortex is divided down the center by a long fissure, producing two hemispheres. The left hemisphere, in most individuals, is the primary hemisphere involved with language production and reception.

The cerebrum is composed of gray and white neuron matter mainly composed of myelinated axons. Each of the two hemispheres divide into the frontal, parietal, temporal, and occipital lobes. Although cortical function is highly integrated, we can make some general assumptions concerning the main functions of the lobes. The frontal lobes contain the motor cortex and associated motor areas. These areas are responsible for planning an executing movements. The parietal lobes contain the primary sensory cortex, where sensations from the body are received and analyzed. The temporal lobe contains the primary auditory cortex, where sound information is received and analyzed, and the occipital lobe receives visual information from the receptors in the retina of the eyes.

The Cerebellum

The cerebellum is located in the posterior part of the skull under the occipital lobe. It is part of the hindbrain and the second largest portion of the brain. The interior of the cerebellum is white matter with an exterior or cortex of mainly gray matter. The cerebellum is responsible for the coordination of body positioning and maintenance of posture.

The Medulla Oblongata

Also part of the hindbrain is the medulla oblongata, which forms the lowest portion of the brain. It begins in the central portion of the brain and extends to the spinal cord. It functions as the nerve center for most involuntary functions, including heart beat, respiratory rate, and control of vein and artery diameter.

The Pons

The pons is located in the hindbrain. It is between the midbrain and medulla and anterior to the cerebellum. The pons is composed of white matter and performs the linking of brain structures such as the medulla and higher cortical centers. The pons has a bridge-like structure and functions between these two cortical centers.

The Midbrain

Above the pons and inferior to the surface of the cerebrum is the midbrain. The midbrain is made up mostly of white matter with some gray matter located around the cerebral aqueduct. Connected to head movements, the midbrain serves as the center for visual reflexes. If the position of body has been dramatically disturbed, the midbrain is vital in maintaining upright posture.

SKELETAL SYSTEM

Because the skeletal system supports major organs and muscle function, we will briefly review basic bone structure and type. Bones also store minerals such as calcium and phosphorus. In addition, they are the site of red blood cell manufacturing.

The Spinal Cord

The spinal cord is in the canal of the spinal column and is approximately 46 cm long (Figure 1-45). Shaped like a cable with each end tapered, it extends from the occipital bone to the vertebral disc level between lumbar 1 (L1) and lumbar 2 (L2). From this area, the cord begins to taper to a pointed shape where it then extends branches into the nerves that extend into the lumbar and sacral areas.

The spinal cord is similar to the brain in that it contains white and gray matter. It is also covered with meninges, thin layers of tissue called pia mater, the arachnoid, and the dura mater. The subarachnoid space is located between the arachnoid mater and pia mater. Gray matter forms an "H" shape within the cord center (Figure 1-46); surrounding it are bundles of white matter myelinated fibers. The spinal nerves extend from the white matter myelinated fibers and form the pathways that coordinate and interconnect all body nervous functions. The ramus communicans, a branching of nerve fibers, connects the sympathetic ganglion to the spinal nerves. Thirty-one pairs of spinal nerves extend from the openings of the spinal vertebrae at each level. Each of these levels corresponds to body functions. For example, nerves from the top of the spinal cord branch and form trunks to control functions of the arms, hands, and upper torso (including the primary muscle of respiration, the diaphragm). Also, nerves from the lower cord extend to form trunks that control the legs, feet, thighs, and pelvis. Through the dorsal or sensory root, afferent

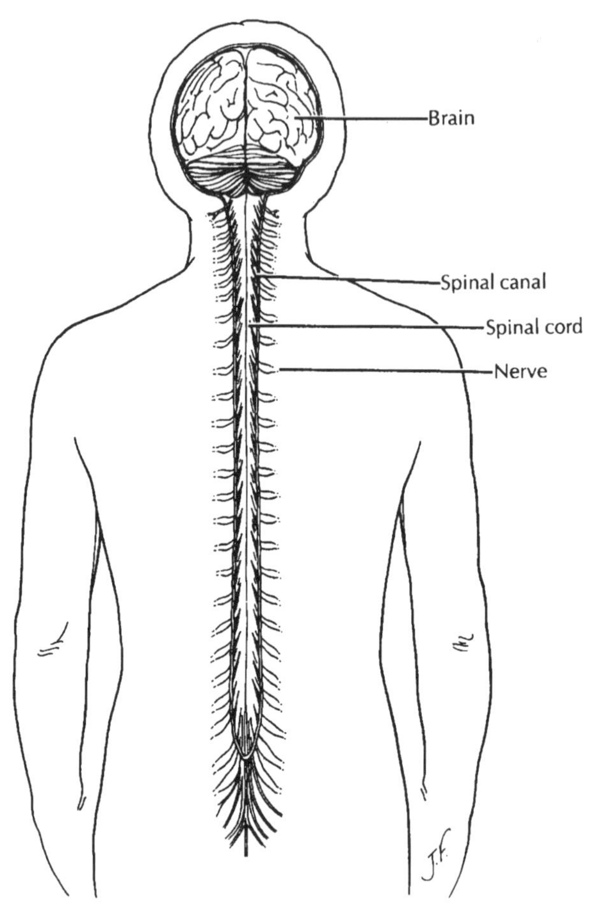

Figure 1-45 Central nervous system showing brain and spinal cord. (From Eubanks, D., and Bone, R.C., Comprehensive Respiratory Care: A Learning System, *2nd Edition, St. Louis: The C.V. Mosby Company, 1990.)*

signals are sent to the spinal cord and brain. The ventral or motor root sends efferent signals from the spinal cord.

Since each level of the spinal column holds the beginning of major innervation for the body, if nerves are severed or damaged beyond repair, paralysis or disfunction of remaining muscle groups and body structures results.

Bones of the Spinal Column

The spine contains three major groups of vertebrae: cervical, C1 to C7 (Figure 1-47), forming the bones of the neck; thoracic, T1 to T12, forming the bones of the upper back and attaching to the ribs of the thorax; and lumbar, L1 to L5, forming the bones of the lower back. The sacrum articulates with the sacroiliac in the pelvic girdle. The coccyx is fused into one structure in the adult and is formed by the smallest bones of the spine.

There are 26 irregularly shaped bones (Figures 1-46 and 1-48) of the spinal column that extend most of the length of the spine until the sacrum at the lower end of the spine. These irregularly shaped bones provide housing for the spinal cord. As this structure protects the spinal cord, it also becomes one of the body's major supportive

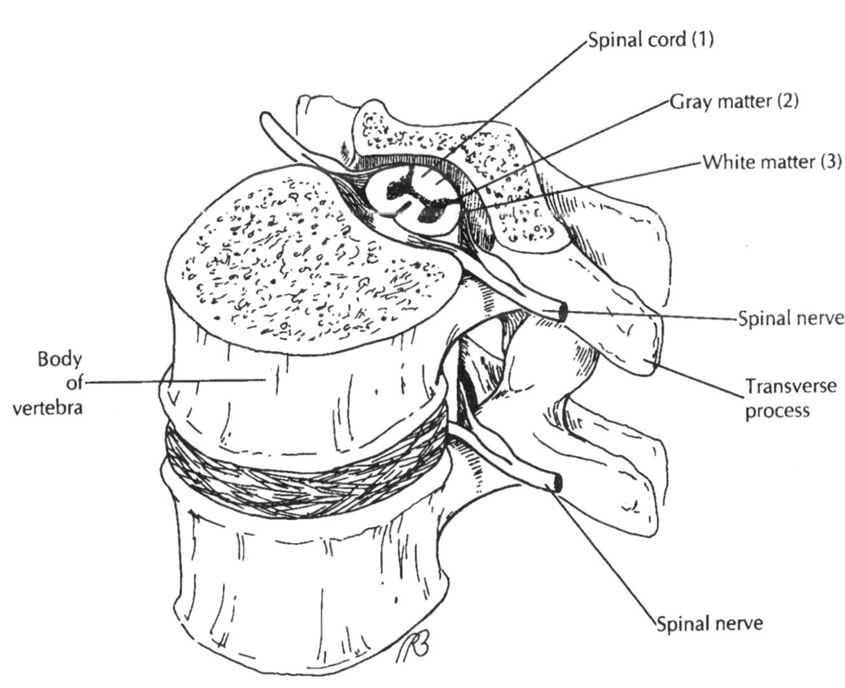

Figure 1-46 Spinal cord. (From Eubanks, D., and Bone, R.C., Comprehensive Respiratory Care: A Learning System, *2nd Edition, St. Louis: The C.V. Mosby Company, 1990.)*

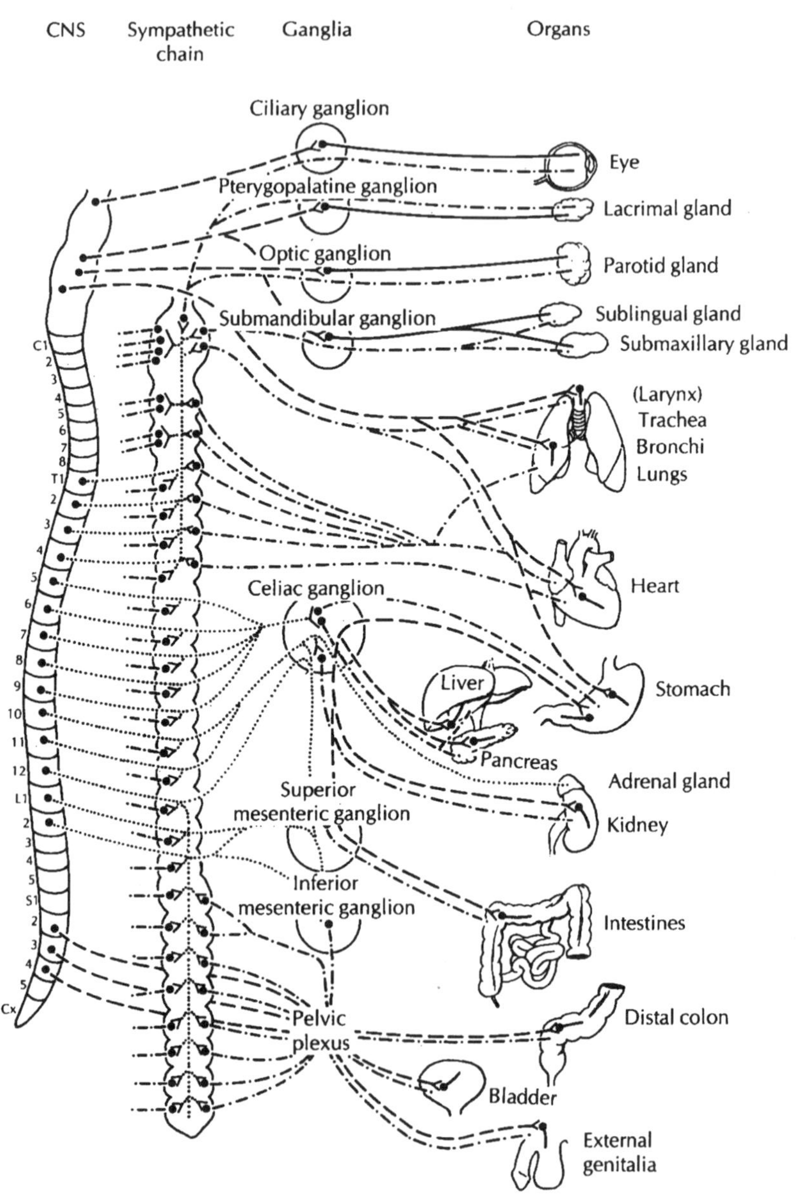

Figure 1-47 Routes and effector organs of sympathetic and parasympathetic nerves. (From Eubanks, D., and Bone, R.C., Comprehensive Respiratory Care: A Learning System, 2nd Edition, St. Louis: The C.V. Mosby Company, 1990.)

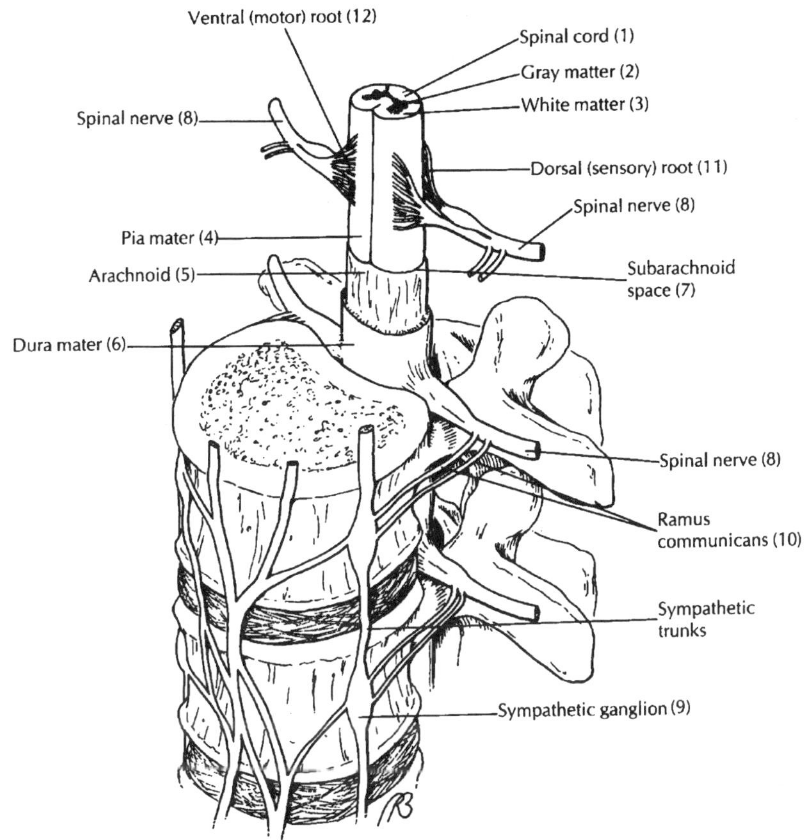

Figure 1-48 Cross section of spinal cord showing its structures. (From Eubanks, D., and Bone, R.C., Comprehensive Respiratory Care: A Learning System, *2nd Edition, St. Louis: The C.V. Mosby Company, 1990.)*

structures. By affording muscles attachment to the spinous process and transverse process, the spinal column becomes the major structural support. The spinous process is located on the posterior aspect of the spinal column or dorsal spine. The transverse process is located on the lateral aspect of the spinal column. In addition, the spinal column allows for the attachment of ribs of the thorax, forming the posterior boundary of the thorax. The sacrum is the lowest portion of the spine, formed by its smallest bones, and it articulates with the pelvic girdle.

Cerebrospinal Fluid

Spinal fluid and the cushion of tissue covering, the meninges, protect the brain and spinal cord. As mentioned earlier, the subarachnoid space is located between the pia mater and dura mater of the meninges, and it is here where the spinal fluid resides. The subarachnoid space is continuous, surrounding the length of the spinal and cranial space, and contains the protective cerebrospinal fluid. Cerebrospinal fluid is clear and cushions the brain by absorbing shock during trauma. High filtration pressure forces cerebrospinal fluid from the choroid plexus into the four brain ventricles and circulates it until it returns to venous circulation. Cerebrospinal fluid is thought to play a major role in the control of ventilation because it has a pH of 7.32 as does blood. The pH will change when there are changes in arterial carbon dioxide levels, effecting changes in respiration sent by the spinal cord.

Bones of the Thorax

The thorax is commonly referred to as the rib cage. It contains 12 pairs of ribs with cartilages, 12 vertebrae, and the sternum.

The Sternum

The beginning of the sternum is located at the suprasternal notch (Figure 1-49). The sternum forms the medial portion of the thorax or chest. It is the anterior attachment point for the majority of the ribs directly (seven upper pairs) or indirectly (eighth to tenth ribs). The sternum has three major parts, consisting of the manubrium, body, and xiphoid. The manubrium is the sternum's thickest portion and is located between clavicle notches and first ribs. The body of the sternum is where most ribs attach anteriorly, beginning with the second rib. The xiphoid process is the very tip of the sternum. It may easily be broken in cardiopulmonary resuscitation attempts when compression of the chest is extreme. When broken, the xiphoid can injure underlying organs or tissue such as the liver and diaphragm. It also becomes brittle as most adults age.

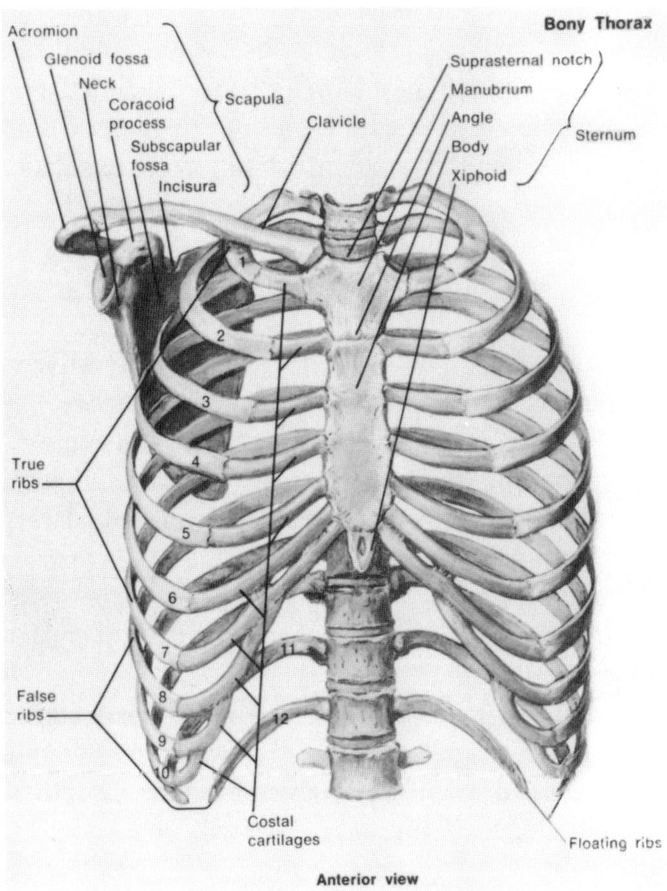

Fig. 1-49 Bony thorax. (Copyright 1988 CIBA-GEIGY Corporation. Reproduced with permission from the CIBA COLLECTION OF MEDICAL ILLUSTRATIONS *by Frank H. Netter, M.D., West Caldwell, NJ, All rights reserved.)*

Each rib is shaped so that it curves more than the rib above it. The first and second ribs are in a fixed position and provide stability (fulcrum) with the sternum for the movement of the ribs below during breathing excursions. When the ribs rise upward with muscle contraction, thoracic diameter increases, allowing for decreased pressure in the lungs that demands inspiratory flow. Anteriorly, ribs one through seven articulate directly to the sternum. These attaching or articulating ribs are termed *true ribs*. The seventh to tenth ribs fuse together and attach below the sixth rib. The remaining eleventh and twelfth ribs do not attach and are called floating ribs. As the ribs reach forward, downward, and outward, they form a structure that in the process of breathing excursion acts as a lid to raise the chest, becoming larger during inspiration and then smaller during passive exhalation. Posteriorly each rib attaches to the spinal column vertebrae.

GASTROINTESTINAL TRACT

The gastrointestinal tract, also known as the digestive system or alimentary canal, serves a primary function to change foods from complex substances into materials that can be utilized by cells. Its secondary function is to eliminate material that is unprocessed or toxic from the body. Components of the gastrointestinal tract include the mouth, pharynx, esophagus, stomach, small intestine, large intestine, and rectum (Figure 1-50). Many of these structures or organs have been discussed earlier in this chapter so we will concentrate on those remaining.

Additional organs that assist the gastrointestinal tract include the salivary glands, liver, gallbladder, pancreas, spleen, vermiform appendix, and teeth. To go into detail about the function of these organs is beyond the scope of this text. We will concentrate on those structures that immediately affect respiration and swallowing, primarily the esophagus and stomach.

A primary structure of importance is the esophagus (Figure 1-50). Dysfunctions and deviations of the esophagus and stomach structure or sphincters contribute dramatically to the management problems of gastric reflux and may prohibit feeding and cause chronic aspiration pneumonia. Structurally, the esophagus is a muscular tube approximately 25 cm long, depending on individual anatomy, that extends from the larynx to below the diaphragm to the stomach. There is some controversy as to the mechanism of esophageal function. Traditionally, it has been thought that peristalsis, or the contraction of the muscular esophageal walls, causes the transport of material to the stomach. Recent studies have indicated that airway pressure may contribute to swallowing and that pressures generated within the

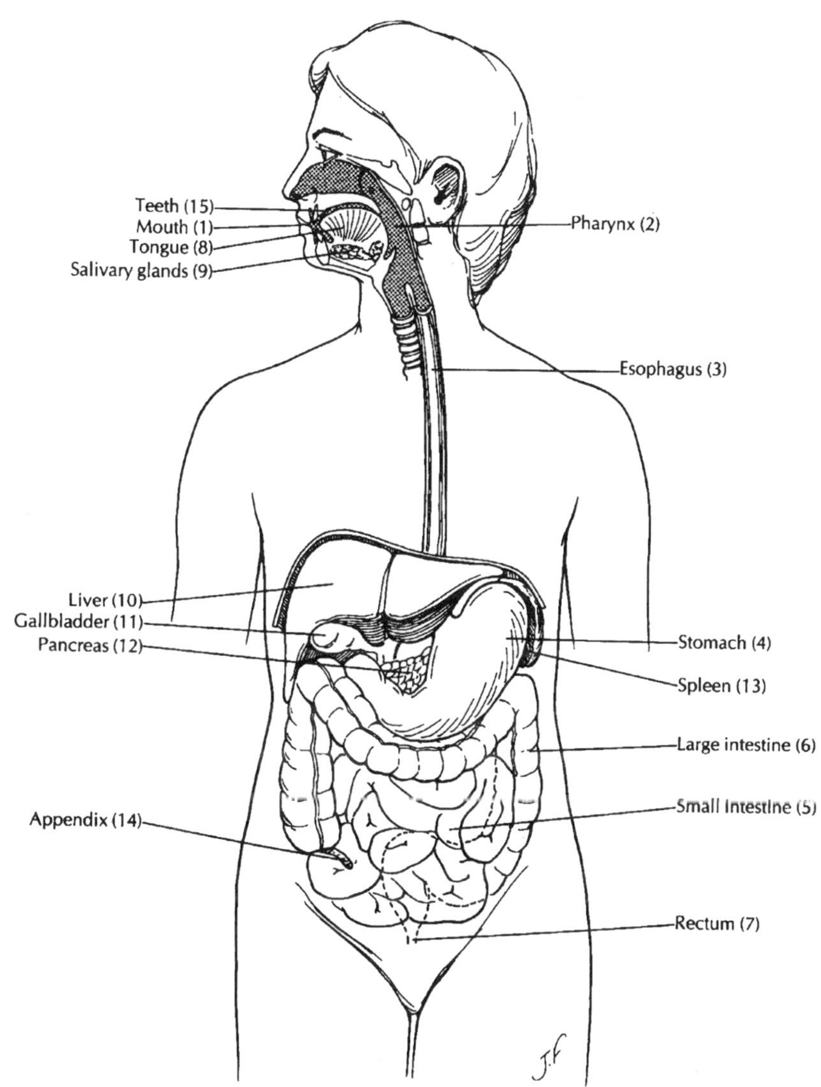

Figure 1-50 Organs of the digestive system. (From Eubanks, D., and Bone, R.C., Comprehensive Respiratory Care: A Learning System, *2nd Edition, St. Louis: The C.V. Mosby Company, 1990.)*

esophagus itself may propel the food bolus downward. It can be measured readily with manometry that there is a pressure wave created in the esophagus during swallowing. The origin of this pressure still remains unclear. It is generally agreed that gravity plays little or no role in food bolus transport.

The stomach (Figure 1-50) is a bladder-shaped organ residing in the upper left quadrant of the abdomen below the diaphragm. The stomach has three smooth layers of muscle fiber that continue lengthwise around and obliquely to the stomach wall. Peristaltic contractions mix food with the stomach enzymes pepsin and hydrochloric acid. This mixture exits the stomach via the sphincter into the duodenum. The duodenum is the first portion of the small intestine. In the small intestine this food, enzyme, and acid mixture comes in contact with villi. The villi are responsible for transferring the nutrients of the food into the blood and lymph systems. Food that is not used is propelled to the large intestine. In the large intestine water is absorbed from the material and bacterial action begins to take place. Within 10 to 12 hours feces is formed and expelled via the rectum from the body.

ENDOCRINE SYSTEM

The endocrine system (Figure 1-51) includes glands that secrete hormones into the blood system. Glandular function is to secrete some substance. The body has two types of glands: endocrine and exocrine. Endocrine glands regulate chemicals in the body. These chemicals readily move into the bloodstream. The secretions of exocrine glands move on an outward path via a system of ducts to the surface of the body. Typical areas to find exocrine glands include the respiratory system, gastrointestinal tract lining, and skin. These glands excrete sweat, mucus, saliva, and milk.

Endocrine glands adjust the body's internal processes slowly. This is in contrast to the almost instant response time of the nervous system. The major glands of the endocrine system are as follows: the pituitary gland at the base of the brain; the thyroid gland in the neck on either side of the trachea; the four parathyroid glands located behind the thyroid; the adrenal glands atop the kidney; the islets of Langerhans located in the pancreas (responsible for insulin); and the ovaries located in the female abdomen and the testes located in the male scrotum. The brain, liver, and placenta in the fetus can act as endocrine glands as they can excrete special substances.

The islets of Langerhans in the pancreas control sugar balance as

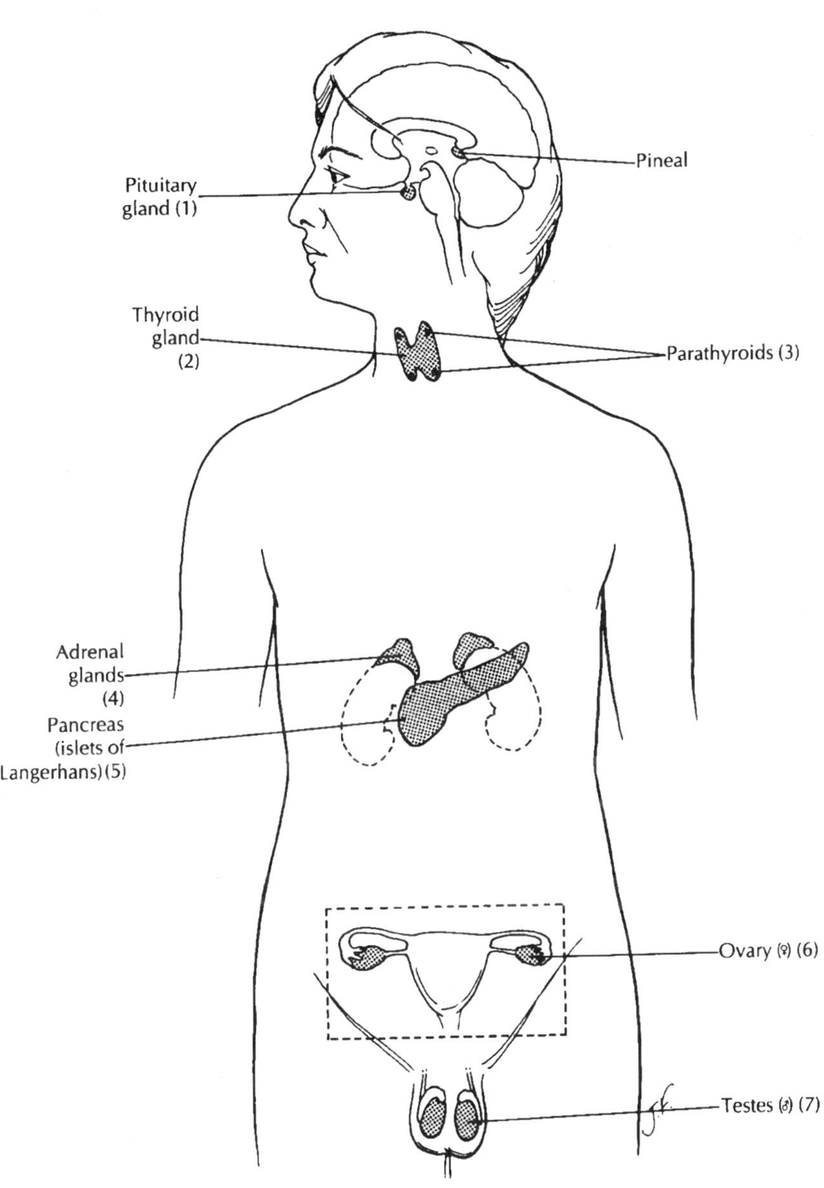

Figure 1-51 The endocrine system. (From Eubanks, D., and Bone, R.C., Comprehensive Respiratory Care: A Learning System, *2nd Edition, St. Louis: The C.V. Mosby Company, 1990.)*

they secrete insulin. The adrenal cortex in the brain can produce steroids such as cortisone and aldosterone, which also regulate sugar and salt balance. Steroids can be very helpful in the reduction of inflammation. Each endocrine gland can produce at least one hormone to regulate the body; some, for example the pituitary gland, can produce up to nine hormones.

All glands play a role in the homeostasis of the body. The adrenal glands excrete epinephrine (adrenaline) and norepinephrine, hormones that in a time of severe stress speed the respiratory rate, raise the blood pressure, and prepare the body for fight or flight. In contrast, in response to hypertension, norepinephrine causes the amount of blood flow to the heart to be reduced by constricting capillaries and causing the blood to be forced to other major body organs.

BIBLIOGRAPHY

California College for Health Sciences, *Entry Level Respiratory Therapy Program* Vol. I and Vol. II, National City, CA, 1983.

Chernick, V., and Kendig, E.L., Jr., *Kendig's Disorders of the Respiratory Tract in Children,* 5th Edition, Philadelphia: W.B. Saunders Co., 1990.

Clemente, C.D., *Gray's Anatomy,* 30th Edition, Philadelphia: Lea & Febiger, 1985.

Dickson, D.R., and Dickson, W.M., *Anatomical and Physiological Bases of Speech,* Boston: Little, Brown & Co., 1982.

Eubanks, D.H., and Bone, R.C., *Comprehensive Respiratory Care,* St. Louis: The C.V. Mosby Company, 1990.

Gates, G.A., "Biochemistry of the salivary glands and saliva." In Paparella, M.M., and Shumrick, D.A. (Eds.)., *Otolaryngology,* 1, Philadelphia: W.B. Saunders Co., 1973: 401-407.

Mason, M., & Watkins, C., *Communication Approaches for Tracheostomized and Ventilator Dependent Patients*, Newport Beach, CA: Voicing! Inc., 1993.

Meyers, E.N., Stool, S.E. and Johnson, J.T., *Tracheostomy*, New York: Churchill-Livingstone, Inc., 1985.

Netter, F.A., *The CIBA Collection of Medical Illustrations,* Vol. 7 *Respiratory System,* West Caldwell, NJ: CIBA, 1988.

Netter, F.A., *The CIBA Collection of Medical Illustrations,* Vol. 3 *Digestive System,* West Caldwell, NJ: CIBA, 1989.

Shames, G.H., and Wigg E.H., *Human Communication Disorders: An Introduction,* Columbus, OH: Charles Merrill Publishing Co., 1982.

Shapiro, B.A., *Clinical Application of Respiratory Care* (Fourth Edition), St. Louis, MO: Mosby-Year Book, 1991.

Van Riper, C. and Emerick, L., "An Introduction to Speech Pathology and Audiology." *Speech Correction*:, Englewood Cliffs, NJ: Prentice Hall, 1990.

Welsh, M.H., "Ventilatory function of the lungs." In Guenter, C.A., and Welch, M.H., (Eds.), *Pulmonary Medicine* (2nd Ed.), Philadelphia: J.B. Lippincott Company, 1982.

Yokachi, C., Rohen, J.W. and Weinreb, E.L., *Photographic Anatomy of the Human Body,* 3rd Edition, Tokyo: Igaku-Shoin, Ltd., 1989.

Zemlin, W.R., *Speech and Hearing Science,* 2nd Edition, Englewood Cliffs, NJ: Prentice Hall, 1981.

CHAPTER II

AIRWAY ISSUES

Mary F. Mason, *M.S., C.C.C.-SLP*

Edited by:

Barbara M. Baker, *Ph.D.*
Associate Professor of Surgery
Division of Communicative Disorders
University of Louisville School of Medicine
Private Practice
University Speech Pathology Associates
Louisville, Kentucky

Lauren D. Holinger, *M.D., F.A.C.S.*
Head, Division Pediatric Otolaryngology
The Children's Memorial Hospital
Professor
Department of Otolaryngology-Head and Neck Surgery
Northwestern University Medical School
Chicago, Illinois

OBSTRUCTED AIRWAY

There is a need for an airway alternative when a definitive airway cannot be established by the usual oral and/or nasal means. Anatomically speaking, there is great potential for an airway obstruction to occur due to the delicate makeup of the upper airway. When the patency of the upper airway is compromised in any way, the amount of air entering and leaving the lungs, the lower airway is consequently affected. There can be an obstruction due to neurological occurrences that diminish tone in the oral and nasal cavity, causing airway obstruction by the tongue. In this case the tongue gravitates toward the pharynx, blocking the passage of air to the lower airway. There may also be peripheral obstruction in the upper airway. This blocks the passage of air to the lower airway for proper ventilation. This category may include a foreign body, tumor, infection, and so forth. An upper airway obstruction can occur at any level of the upper airway from the oral cavity down to the larynx where the lower airway begins. "The most common cause of an airway obstruction is the tongue."[1] When a seizure, stroke, or heart attack occurs, the tongue, which normally stays on the floor of the oral cavity, may fall backward in the throat, blocking free air exchange into the trachea. When rescue methods are attempted, the rescuer must properly align the tongue to prevent any airway obstruction.

Airway obstructions occur in both acute and chronic forms. The acute obstruction is most recognizable because the patient demonstrates overt signs of respiratory distress. The chronic form is more subtle and can easily go undetected and become an acute obstruction, which could be total airway occlusion. Any obstruction, whether acute or chronic, is very serious. In infants and children, because pediatric anatomy is so much smaller than that of adults, a small narrowing or obstruction can seriously and quickly increase the work of breathing and compromise the airway, whereas in the adult it may make very little or no difference in the breathing process.

UNIVERSAL DISTRESS SIGNS

There are recognizable distress signs that indicate either a partial or total airway obstruction. The procedure for assisting a person with either obstruction is the same. The partial obstruction is detected by a noticeable change in a person's breathing pattern. This can be recognized by a gasping-of-air sound, wheezing, coughing, vocal gurgle, or any noticeable struggle in breath attempts. The total obstruction is indicated with the well-known universal distress sign of the person's hand to the throat, indicating he or she is choking (Figure 2-1). Other noticeable signs of complete obstruction are when the person cannot speak at all or get any type of vocalization out, when there is no ability to cough, and when no breathing attempts are observed, such as chest movements or breath sounds heard or felt. There may also be marked chest wall retractions, cyanosis, or loss of consciousness.

MANAGING THE OBSTRUCTED AIRWAY

After determining that there is an airway obstruction, appropriate management to relieve the obstruction is initiated (Figure 2-2). In 1961, a team of researchers at Johns Hopkins Hospital[2] in Baltimore

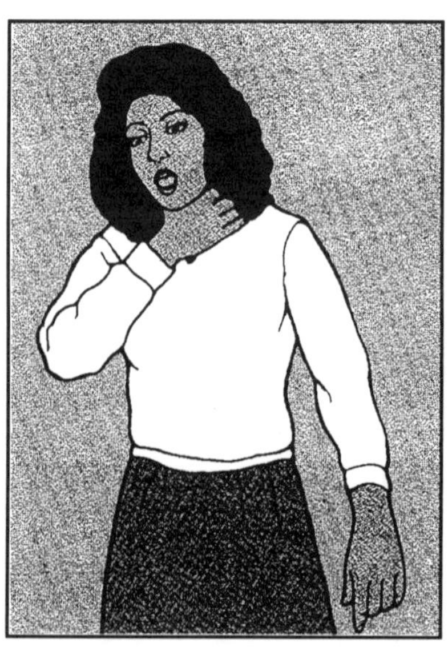

Figure 2-1 The universal distress signal for choking. (From American Red Cross Standard First Aid Workbook, *1991, Washington, D.C.: The American Red Cross, Figure 10, p. 29.)*

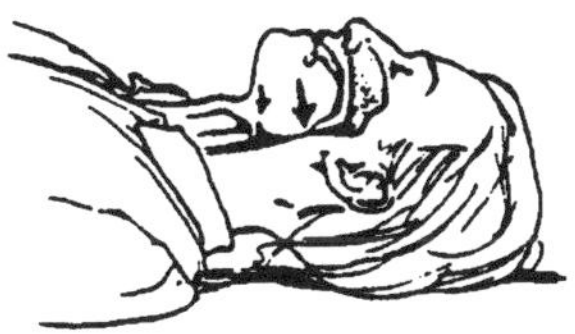

Figure 2-2 The obstructed airway. (From Entry-Level Respiratory Therapy Program Volume 1, *National City: California College for Health Sciences, 1985, Figure 1-1, p. (RTT 108) 1- 4.)*

outlined a technique for restoration of circulation when a person's heart has stopped. Ten years later, a group of health officials[2] in Seattle, Washington, started a public information campaign to teach the basics of CPR (cardiopulmonary resuscitation).

Cardio refers to the heart, *pulmonary* to the lungs, and *resuscitation* means to bring back to life. The American Heart Association[2] and the American Red Cross[2] have trained over a million people in these basic measures since CPR was first advocated. If breathing stops, the heart will continue to pump blood throughout the body for only a few minutes. Respiration and circulation are interrelated and interdependent on each other. It is therefore very important that an obstructed airway be relieved as soon as possible to prevent death. Lindsay Curtis, M.D.,[2] outlines in her CPR manual that artificial breathing and circulation will be effective only if there is an open airway. Airway, breathing, and circulation are essential to basic life support.[2] It is important to remember, that if a person is attempting to clear his or her airway by coughing not to interfere. The person is attempting to expel the object that is blocking the airway. Interference may further obstruct the airway. If the airway becomes completely obstructed, there are several methods that can be used to clear the airway. These include the Heimlich maneuver, abdominal or chest thrusts, finger sweeps, and back blows.

The Heimlich Maneuver

In 1974, Dr. Henry Heimlich[3] of Cincinnati, Ohio, first initiated the now well- known Heimlich maneuver.[3] He first attempted this procedure on beagles. This maneuver is now widely used in emergency medical situations and has decreased the need to perform an emergency tracheotomy or cricothyroidotomy to open an airway. When food or foreign objects are aspirated during inspiration, the lungs of the individual are expanded and "pressing one's fist upward in the abdomen above the navel, but below the rib cage, elevates the diaphragm. Sudden elevation of the diaphragm compresses the lungs within the boundaries of the rib cage increasing the air pressure, forcing it through the wind pipe. Along with the air, the food or foreign object will be ejected, thus alleviating the obstructed airway"[3] (Figure 2-3).

Abdominal/Chest Thrust

The abdominal thrust is done with the rescuer's arms around the victim's stomach with the fist and thumb toward the victim. The other hand grabs the fisted hand between the navel and the sternum. Four

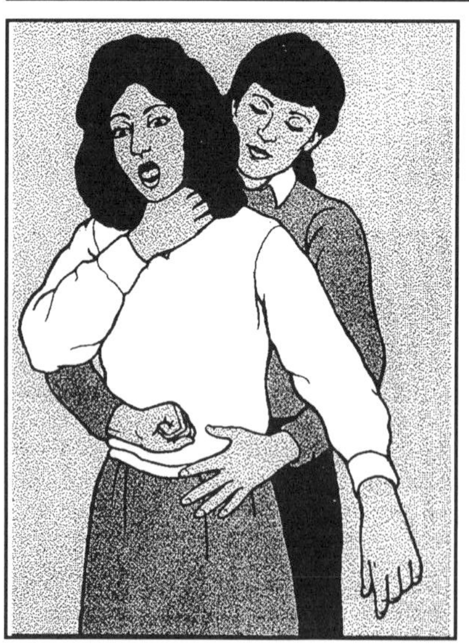

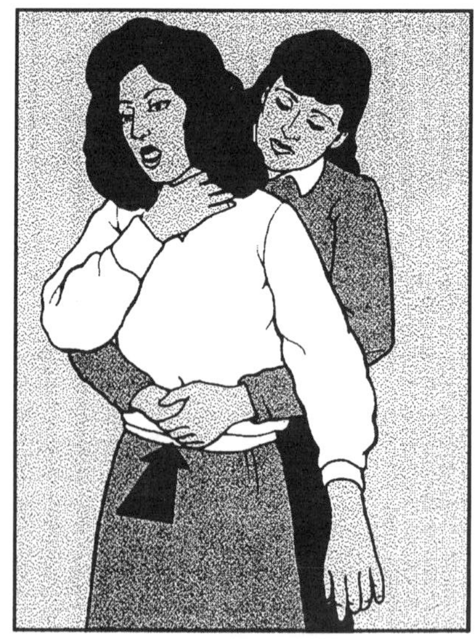

Figure 2-3 The Heimlich maneuver. Stand behind the victim. Wrap your arms around the victim's waist. Make a fist with one hand and place the thumb side of your fist against the middle of the victim's abdomen just above the navel and well below the lower tip of the breast bone. Grasp your fist with your other hand. Keeping elbows out, press your fist into the victim's abdomen with a quick upward thrust. Each thrust should be a separate and distinct attempt to dislodge the object. Repeat thrusts until the airway obstruction is cleared or the victim becomes unconscious. (From American Red Cross Standard First Aid Workbook, *1991, Washington, D.C.: The American Red Cross, p. 32.)*

quick thrusts are given to dislodge the object causing the obstruction.

The chest is utilized with the obese or the pregnant individual. The objective is the same as with the abdominal thrust. The rescuer puts his arms around the victim's chest with one hand above the tip of the sternum and with the other hand over this hand. Four quick thrusts are given, compressing the ribs with the arms of the rescuer while using the hands to compress the lower sternum (Figure 2-4).

Finger Sweeps

To finger sweep inside the victim's mouth, the rescuer must stabilize the victim's tongue and lower jaw with one hand and insert a forefinger of the other hand deep into the victim's mouth. The key is to push the foreign object to one side, dislodging it and hooking the finger underneath it to lift it out (Figure 2-5).

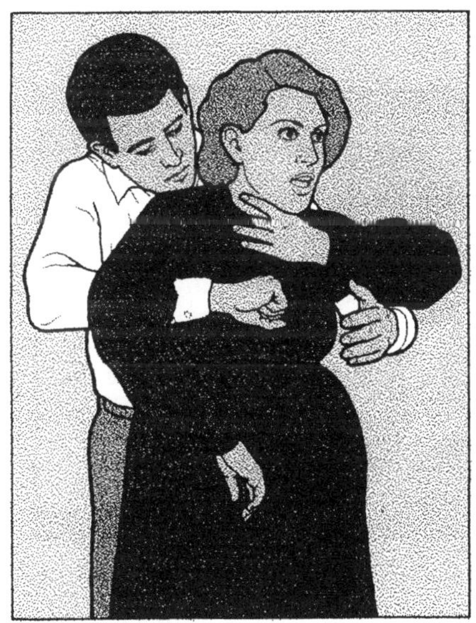

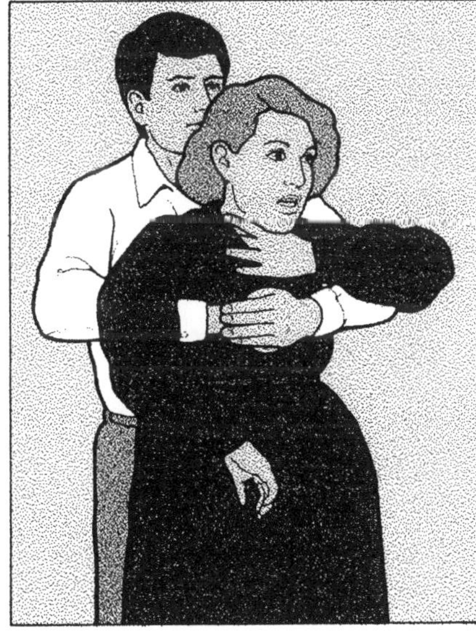

Figure 2-4 Chest thrust. With the person either standing or sitting: (1) Stand behind the victim and place your arms under the victim's armpits and around the chest. (2) Place the thumb side of your fist on the middle of the breast bone. (3) Grasp your fist with your other hand. (4) Give thrusts against the chest until the obstruction is cleared or until the person loses consciousness. (From American Red Cross Standard First Aid Workbook, *1991, Washington, D.C.: The American Red Cross, Figures 11 and 12, p. 38.)*

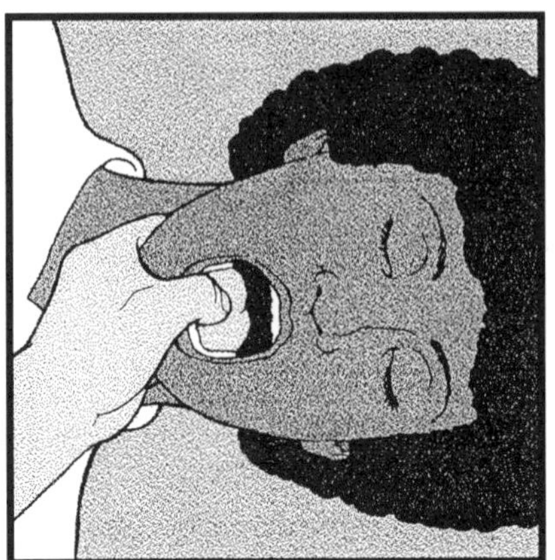

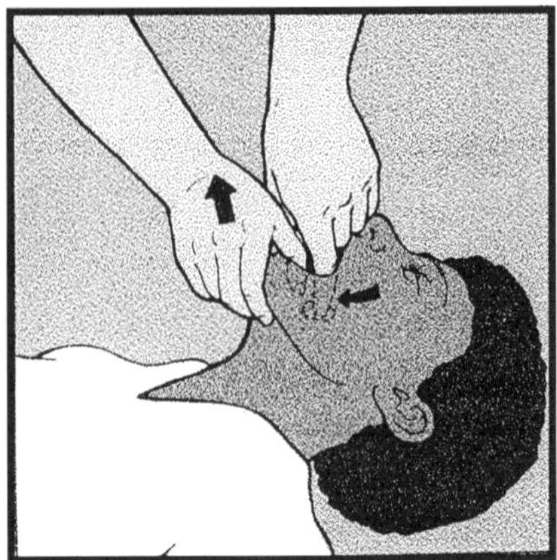

Figure 2-5 Finger sweep. Kneel beside the victim's head. With the victim's face up, open the mouth and grasp both the tongue and the lower jaw between the thumb and fingers of your hand nearer the victim's legs; lift jaw. Insert your index finger into the victim's mouth along the inside of the cheek and deep into the throat to the base of the tongue. Use a "hooking" action to dislodge any object that might be there and move it into the mouth for removal. (From American Red Cross Standard First Aid Workbook, *1991, Washington, D.C.: The American Red Cross, p. 36.)*

ALTERNATIVE AIRWAYS

When it has been determined that the patient cannot oxygenate and ventilate adequately, alternative airways are considered to maintain appropriate airway patency. The following will address oropharyngeal airways, nasopharyngeal airways, esophageal obturator airway, manual resuscitation bags, and endotracheal tubes.

Oropharyngeal Airways

These are curved rubber or plastic tubes that are shaped to follow the natural curvature of the tongue and soft palate. Oropharyngeal airways extend past the base of the tongue to hold the tongue away from the pharynx, maintaining a route around the tube for airway patency to the lower airway. This procedure should be used with caution, as the placement of this tube may elicit the gag or vomiting reflex. These airways are often used with seizure patients to keep the tongue clear from the hypopharynx. Oropharyngeal airways are easily dislodged (Figure 2-6).

Nasopharyngeal Airways

These are soft rubber or latex tubes. The tube is inserted into one of the nares and follows the posterior nasopharyngeal and oropharyngeal walls to the base of the tongue. This airway is very similar to the oral airway, as the concept remains to maintain airway patency. This airway is preferred over the oral airway as it can be tolerated for longer periods of time. The airway remains more stable in the nares (providing the ring is attached to the proximal end to prevent slipping). Although there is a decreased tendency for the initiation of the gag reflex as well as vomiting, the risk for tissue necrosis and laryngospasm exists with this airway; it is therefore temporary (Figure 2-7).

Esophageal Airways

There are special circumstances where this unusual artificial airway is utilized. The esophageal obturator is used when the risk of aspirating gastric contents is great. The purpose of this tube is to

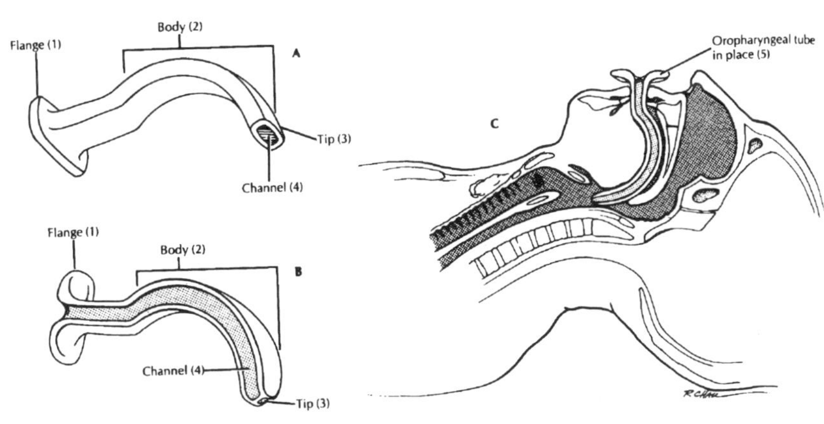

Figure 2-6 Oropharyngeal airways. ***A****, Guedel airway.* ***B****, Berman airway.* ***C****, Airway in place. (From Eubanks, D., and Bone, R.C.,* Comprehensive Respiratory Care: A Learning System, *2nd Edition, St. Louis: The C.V. Mosby Company, 1990, Figure 20-25, p. 548.)*

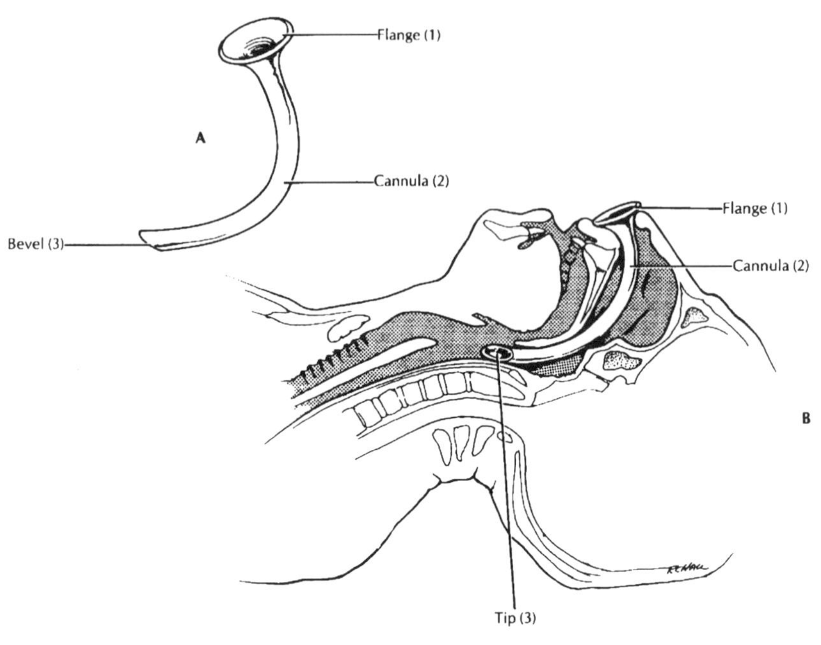

*Figure 2-7 Nasopharyngeal airways. **A**, Parts of airway. **B**, Airway in place. (From Eubanks, D., and Bone, R.C.,* Comprehensive Respiratory Care: A Learning System, *2nd Edition, St. Louis: The C.V. Mosby Company, 1990, Figure 20-26, p. 548.)*

prevent aspiration of the stomach contents. It is recommended for use with the unconscious patient only. Risks include pharyngeal trauma, accidental entrance into the trachea, total obstruction of the airway, gastric distention, and impaired ventilation with an improperly inflated cuff. There is also a great risk of aspiration with this tube, as the patient may vomit when it is removed. The placement of an endotracheal tube is possible (if needed) in conjunction with this tube (Figure 2-8).

Manual Resuscitation Bags/Masks

Adequate ventilation and oxygenation can be maintained with a manual bag or mask connected to an oxygen source. These methods are often utilized until another source of ventilation can be established, such as endotracheal tube placement. When utilizing a mask,

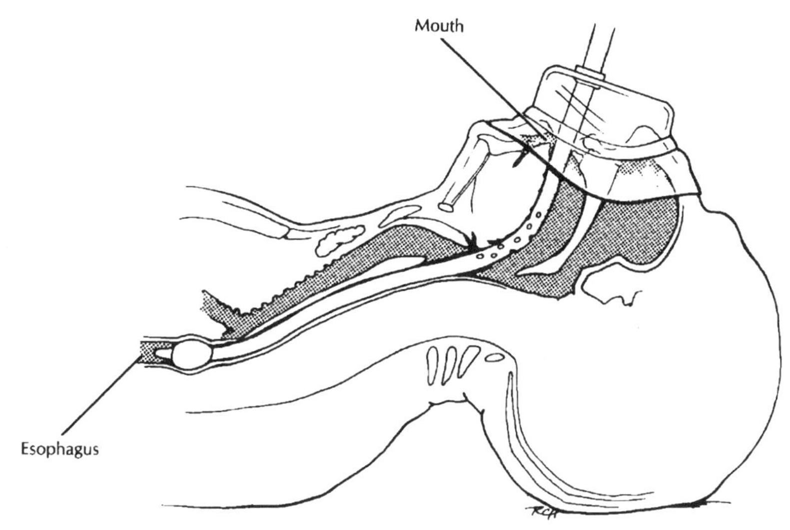

Figure 2-8 Esophageal obturator airway in place. (From Eubanks, D., and Bone, R.C., Comprehensive Respiratory Care: A Learning System, *2nd Edition, St. Louis: The C.V. Mosby Company, 1990, Figure 20-19, p. 549.)*

it is important to angle the patient's mandible upward to maintain a patent airway. The resuscitation bag delivers room air or may be connected to an oxygen source for an oxygen mixture necessary for ventilation.

Endotracheal Tubes

The purpose of endotracheal intubation is to provide an artificial airway into the trachea for maintenance of airway patency. The reasons for endotracheal tube placement may include:

1. Upper airway obstruction
2. Impending airway obstruction (due to infections, trauma, allergic reactions, etc.)
3. Airway protection against aspiration
4. A means to remove secretions retained in the central airway
5. To provide a means for short-term mechanical ventilation

The most effective method used to intubate a patient is with an instrument known as the laryngoscope. The laryngoscope helps to ensure that the tube is properly placed between the vocal cords. The patient is positioned flat on his back with his or head hyperextended and airway opened, with the mouth, larynx, and trachea properly aligned. The laryngoscope blade is placed in the mouth and positioned over the tongue into the posterior pharynx, and depending on the type of blade, it is either placed into the vallecula or under the epiglottis. The endotracheal tube itself is then placed alongside the laryngoscope blade, past the glottis, into the larynx, and down the trachea. Sometimes there are wire stylets in the tube to stiffen it, thus further assisting the physician in its placement.

There are orotracheal tubes as well as nasal endotracheal tubes. Tracheal intubation can be accomplished most expediently through the oral route as the vocal cords are usually visualized during orotracheal intubation; thus the tube can be placed with greater assurance.[4] This method of intubation is the most widely utilized when a person undergoes general anesthesia for surgical

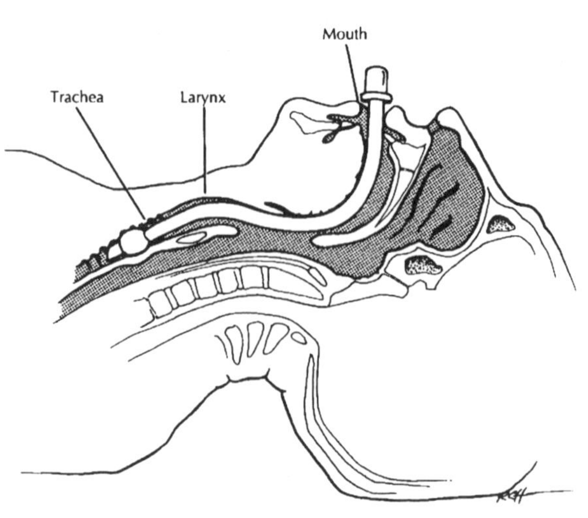

Figure 2-9 Orotracheal tube in place. (From Eubanks, D., and Bone, R.C., Comprehensive Respiratory Care: A Learning System, *2nd Edition, St. Louis: The C.V. Mosby Company, 1990, Figure 20-17, p. 549.)*

purposes. The tube is placed in the oral cavity and down between the vocal cords of the larynx and is maintained in the trachea. The tube remains in place with an air-inflated tracheal cuff (Figure 2-9).

The nasotracheal intubation method is preferred to orotracheal intubation in some situations. These may include surgery in the oral cavity, poor oral access, and prolonged ventilation. "The nasal tracheal route is usually better tolerated by the patient, especially those who require tracheal intubation for extended periods. The nasotracheal tube is easier to stabilize after its placement and does not run the risk of being occluded by the patient biting on the tube."[4] The complications with use of this tube are nasal tissue destruction, hemorrhage, and the potential for the development of sinusitis after a patient has been intubated for several days. The nasotracheal tube is inserted through the nares, runs down through the pharynx, and is maintained between the vocal cords of the larynx. This tube is also kept in place by an air-inflated tracheal cuff (Figure 2-10).

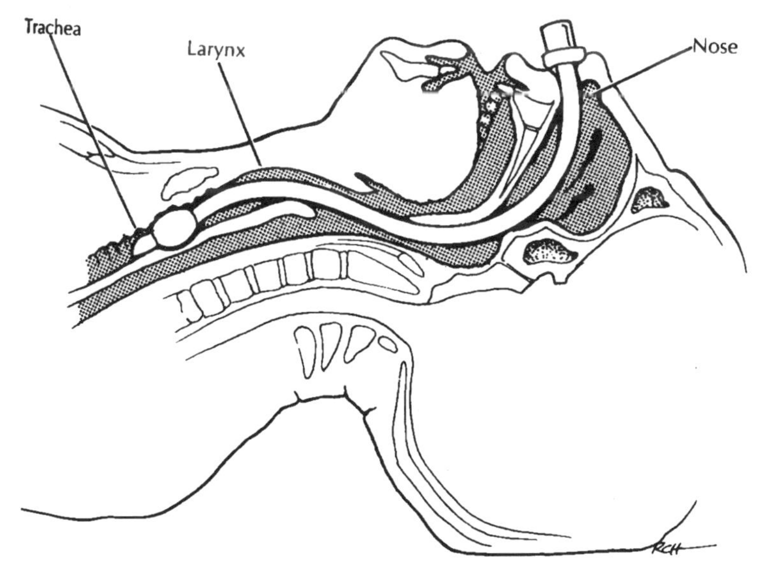

Figure 2-10 Nasotracheal tube in place. (From Eubanks, D., and Bone, R.C., Comprehensive Respiratory Care: A Learning System, *2nd Edition, St. Louis: The C.V. Mosby Company, 1990, Figure 20-18, p. 549.)*

Tracheal Cuffs

There are many complications with the use of the cuff, including laryngeal lesions and tracheal stenosis. The newer design of cuffs developed in the 1970s caused the patient and practitioner fewer problems. These cuffs are low-pressure designs, which are made differently from the old low-volume/high-pressure cuffs used previously. However, these newly designed cuffs still may cause problems if the tube size is inappropriate and the cuff needs to be stretched to fill the tracheal space or if any pressure points exist between the cuff and the tracheal wall. There are measuring devices that can be utilized to determine if the pressures in the cuff are great enough to cause any ischemia. These devices are pressure manometers. The purpose of the cuff is to provide a seal in the airway below the point of airway pressures. There are also pressure-relief valves to prevent any tracheal trauma. The respiratory therapist can use different techniques to evaluate cuff pressures. One technique is called the *minimal leak technique,* which involves auscultation of the area above the tracheal cuff for sounds of air movement around the cuff. A small amount of air is permitted to leak during inhalation. Another technique, known as *minimal occluding volume*, is utilized when there is just enough volume injected into the cuff to occlude the airway. A method utilized to prevent mucosal damage from the cuff is to adjust the cuff position. This is done by actually moving the endotracheal tube up or down at least 2 cm on a daily basis. High-frequency ventilation does not require a cuff and therefore changing to this mode will also help with this complication. Cuffs are also used during the placement of tracheostomy tubes, also known as *translaryngeal* or *transtracheal tube placement*. There are similar complications with these tubes. These are discussed in Chapter 3.

Complications With Intubation

There are several complications with orotracheal and nasotracheal intubation tubes. The patient cannot communicate because the oral articulators are blocked as is the airflow for vocal production. Oral nutrition is affected, and therefore the patient may need a nasogastric or gastric tube. The placement of this tube along with the intubation tube may cause complications for the patient. Sometimes, the endotracheal tube may be inadvertently placed into the right mainstem bronchus. The result of this complication is that only one lung will ventilate. It is important to always check the tube placement so that the tube can be repositioned if needed.

An improperly positioned tube can also cause either partial or total airway obstruction. Sometimes during an emergency intubation, teeth fractures may occur and damage to the vocal cords (due to the tube being placed right between the cords). After the intubation tube is removed, many patients have hoarseness of the voice, laryngeal/tracheal edema, compromised cough reflex, as well as all the complications mentioned previously regarding cuffs, such as tracheal stenosis.

INTUBATION VS. TRACHEOTOMY

The issue of whether to perform a tracheotomy or intubation has always presented much controversy. There are many situations where the decision is obvious, such as when oral or transnasal intubation is difficult due to an obstruction. In this case the need for a tracheotomy procedure would be obvious. The controversy involves the time frame that a person should remain intubated before a tracheostomy should be performed. An endotracheal tube is placed when a patient undergoes general anesthesia for a surgical procedure that requires short-term mechanical ventilation. Finucane and Santora[1] outlined two philosophies relating to the decision of how long a patient can be intubated before a tracheotomy should be considered. The more traditional and widely followed guideline is to perform a tracheotomy after two weeks of endotracheal intubation. Watson[5] conducted a survey in 1983 of critical care professionals concerning the recommended length of intubation. The average acceptable duration of prolonged intubation among 280 responders was two weeks, with many practitioners electing to perform tracheotomy only for specific indications such as patient comfort and to avoid chronic ventilatory care.

Establishment of a secure airway is the main goal in the event of respiratory insufficiency. The means to obtaining this goal is often a crucial and quick decision made by the physician. Each method involves complications.

CRICOTHYROIDOTOMY

Cricothyroidotomy is believed to be the fastest way to open and maintain an airway when there is a severe upper airway obstruction. Many medical professionals advocate this as an alternative to a tracheotomy procedure. "The procedure itself is very simple: an incision is made through the skin directly overlying the thin and relatively avascular membrane which joins the thyroid cartilage to the cricoid cartilage. This incision can be enlarged horizontally and then spread vertically to allow insertion of a standard tracheostomy tube."[6] The advantage given by medical professionals who support this procedure is that it can be performed faster than a tracheotomy and by a non-surgeon. There is much controversy over the safety of this procedure, and more studies need to be conducted to further examine this procedure. Brantigan and Grow[7] in 1976 reviewed the experiences of 655 patients who underwent a cricothyroidotomy instead of a tracheostomy procedure. In each case the cricothyroidotomy was done preoperatively by a thoracic surgeon. None of the patients had laryngeal infections, neoplasms, pneumothorax, or hemorrhage, as are often seen with a tracheostomy procedure. Both Nelson[8] in 1957 and Koopmann and Feld[9] in 1981 studied the effects of this procedure on dogs. Nelson found marked stenosis with dogs who had severed cricoid cartilages. The average time of intubation was 20 days. Koopmann and Feld performed cricothyroidotomies in 40 dogs. They found no stenosis or cricoid cartilage necrosis, but granulation tissue development was noted. Standard tracheostomy tubes are used for this procedure because cricothyroidotomy tubes have not been developed. "Standard tracheostomy tubes are not anatomically suited for use in cricothyroidotomy. The normal cricothyroid membrane measures 9 mm in height, with a range of 5 to 12 mm. The outside diameter of a Shiley No. 4 tracheostomy tube is 8.5 mm, while that of a No. 6 measures 10 mm. Similarly, the shape of a tube designed to traverse the soft tissues of the neck before curving gently into the trachea at the level of the second or third tracheal ring is different from that required for cricothyroidotomy intubation."[6] There appears to be a need for further studies to support the safe use of a cricothyroidotomy over a tracheotomy. It is important to keep in mind that this procedure is faster than the tracheotomy procedure for emergency purposes. A tracheotomy procedure can always be done after the cricothyroidotomy is established to open an airway (Figure 2-11).

TRACHEOSTOMY

Some patients will require a tracheostomy procedure as an alternative for ventilation. Severe upper airway obstruction, necrosis

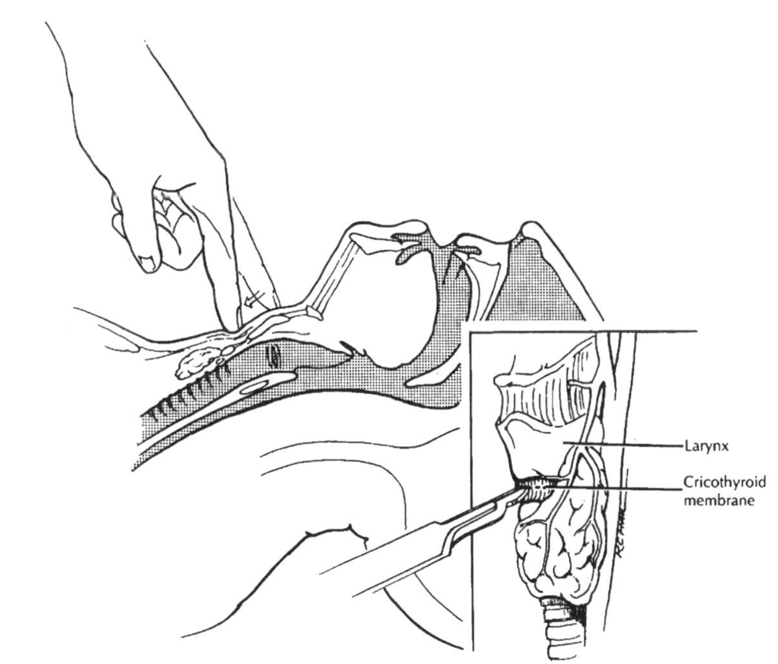

Figure 2-11 Cricothyroidotomy. (From Eubanks, D., and Bone, R.C., Comprehensive Respiratory Care: A Learning System, *2nd Edition, St. Louis: The C.V. Mosby Company, 1990, Figure 20-25, p. 555.)*

of tissue that prevents the passage of an intubation tube, the need for long-term mechanical ventilation, a predisposition to pulmonary aspiration, and retention of bronchopulmonary secretions are some of the indications for tracheostomy. "It should suffice, however, to emphasize that tracheotomy is the operation that opens the door to breath because of its value in the management of many diseases and conditions."[10] The decision to perform a tracheostomy procedure is a very complex one and has risks that should be compared to other airway methods previously described.

A tracheostomy procedure is usually performed under a general anesthetic in an operating room. The procedure creates a hole in the trachea through which a tube can be placed for air exchange. Air bypasses the upper airway to provide adequate ventilation (Figure 2-12).

There has been confusion between the terms *tracheotomy* and *tracheostomy*. "The surgical procedure is a *tracheotomy*; the surgical opening into a patient's trachea is the tracheostomy. The procedure takes place with the patient positioned with the neck hyperextended. A horizontal skin incision is made about one finger in breadth below the level of the cartilage. When the trachea is located, the surgeon

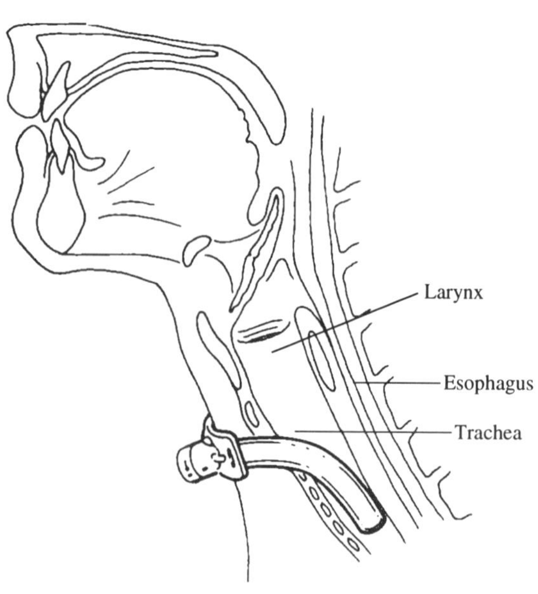

Figure 2-12 Tracheostomy tube placement.

makes a vertical incision through the second, third, and fourth tracheal rings."[10] The trachea is then widened and the tracheostomy tube is inserted. After the retractors are removed, the pretracheal fascia approximate spontaneously to the midline. Sutures are normally unnecessary. Complications can include laryngeal lesions, ischemia, hemorrhage, ulceration, tracheoesophageal fistula, and tracheal stenosis. Cuff overinflation creates pressure against the tracheal mucosa, creating complications as discussed in Chapter 3. As with the placement of an endotracheal tube, a tracheostomy tube can also create many complications.

TRACHEOSTOMY COMPLICATIONS

The patient's history should be reviewed in regard to any predisposition to excessive bleeding because hemorrhage is an obvious complication of any surgical procedure. It is also important to note that the area of the neck in which this procedure is done is extremely venous. Diligence on the part of the surgeon is critical due to the risk of creating a tracheoesophageal fistula. "In order to avoid creating a fistula between the posterior wall of the trachea and the anterior wall of the esophagus, the surgeon must be careful not to penetrate the tracheal wall. Opening the trachea over a bronchoscope or endotracheal tube and then enlarging the incision with scissors will help to avoid injuring the trachea in this way."[6] A diminished airway can occur when the tracheostomy tube is incorrectly inserted into soft tissue, missing the trachea altogether. Injury of the recurrent laryngeal nerve can be caused by a knick or cut during the tracheostomy procedure, resulting in vocal cord paralysis. Infections, swallowing problems, granuloma tissue formation, and laryngotracheal stenosis are frequent and serious complications. "Jackson accurately analyzed the factors leading to complications of tracheotomy. He pointed out that making the incision high in the neck, dividing the cricoid cartilage, performing the operation hastily, using an improper cannula, and poor postoperative care were the most frequent causes of complications."[11]

Jackson further describes tracheotomy: "It is one of the oldest operations in the history of surgery, yet it is probably more often improperly performed today, and more often followed by needless mortality and needless crippling, than any other operation."[12]

There are also many secondary anatomical and physiological changes that occur due to the placement of the tracheostomy tube. One of the most significant complications is the inability to naturally phonate or vocalize for speech production. This complication along with other physiological changes are described in Chapter 3.

REFERENCES

1. Finucane, B.T., and Santora, A. H., *Principles of Airway Management*. Philadelphia: F.A. Davis Company, 1988.

2. Lindsey, C.R., *How to Save a Life Using CPR* (Cardiopulmonary Resuscitation). Tucson, Arizona, HP Books 1981.

3. Armellino, D., *C.P.R. It Could Save Your Life.* Chicago: Contemporary Books, 1979.

4. Burton, G.G., Hodgkin, J.E., and Ward, J.J., *Respiratory Care, A Guide to Clinical Practice.* 3rd Edition, Philadelphia: J.B. Lippincott Co., 1991.

5. Watson, C.B., *ENT Journal.* Cleveland: International Publishing Group, 1983.

6. Myers, E.N., *Tracheotomy.* New York: Churchill Livingston, 1985.

7. Brantigan, C.O., and Grow J.B., "Cricothyroidotomy: Elective use in respiratory problems requiring tracheotomy." *J Thorac Cardiovasc Surg*, 1976; 71-72.

8. Nelson, T.G., "Tracheotomy: A clincial and experimental study." *Am Surg*,1957; 23:660, 750, 841.

9. Koopmann C.F., Feld, R.A., and Coulthard, S.W., "The effects of cricoid cartilage injury and antibiotics in cricothyroidolomy." *Am J Otolaryngol*, 1981; 2:123.

10. Beatrous, W.P., "Tracheostomy; Its expanded indications and its present status." *Laryngoscope*, 1968; 78:16.

11. Jackson, C., and Jackson, C.L., *The Larynx and Its Diseases.* Philadelphia: W.B. Saunders, 1937.

12. Jackson, C., "High Tracheotomy and other errors: The chief causes of chronic laryngeal stenosis." *Surg Gynecol Obstet,* 1923; 32:392.

BIBLIOGRAPHY

Eubanks, D.H., and Bone, R.C., *Comprehensive Respiratory Care,* St. Louis: The C.V. Mosby Company, 1990.

Kirby, R.R., Smith, R.A., and Desautels, D.A. (Eds.), *Mechanical Ventilation*, New York: Churchill Livingstone, 1985.

CHAPTER III

TRACHEOSTOMY AND TRACHEOSTOMY TUBES

Mary F. Mason, *M.S., C.C.C.-SLP*

Kaye Meehan, *R.N.C.S., A.N.P., C.O.R.L.N.*
Certified Adult Nurse Practitioner
Department of Otolaryngology-Head and Neck Surgery
Carle Clinic Association
Urbana, Illinois

Edited by:

Lauren D. Holinger, *M.D., F.A.C.S.*
Head, Division Pediatric Otolaryngology
The Children's Memorial Hospital
Chicago, Illinois
Professor
Department of Otolaryngology-Head and Neck Surgery
Northwestern University Medical School
Chicago, Illinois

HISTORY

Tracheostomy has been performed for over 3500 years and is described by Elizabeth Frost as originating from the Greek words meaning "I cut the trachea."[1]

One of the earliest references to tracheostomy is found in the sacred book of Hindu medicine, the Rig Veda,[2] which was written around 2000 B.C. and refers to "the bountiful one who, without a ligature, can cause the windpipe to unite when the cervical cartilages are cut across, provided they are not entirely severed." Eber's Papyrus, another historical medical text published around 1550 B.C., and translated by Joachimo, delineates a tracheostomy procedure as "incision of a fatty tumor in the throat, taking care of the vessels."[3] The early history of tracheostomy, 1500 B.C. to 1500 A.D., is recorded more as opinion and perhaps even rumor than published writings of documented procedures, as in the tracheostomy allegedly performed by Alexander the Great on the battlefield around the fourth century, B.C. As a soldier was choking on a bone, Alexander was said to have punctured his trachea with his sword and inserted a reed.[4] We do not know, however, if this was a successful procedure.

Robert Eavey describes the evolution of tracheostomy through early history as performed by physicians only in life-threatening situations as it was met with skepticism and disapproval by the medical profession.[5] The Greeks and Romans during this time had a very limited knowledge of anatomy and physiology, and the basic principles of medicine evolved around the four humors of the body. These were thought to be blood, phlegm, yellow bile, and black bile. People in good health were considered to have harmony of the four humors, and people who were unhealthy or ill were regarded as having an imbalance of their four humors. It was believed that the carotid artery in the neck carried both air and blood, and therefore the concept of cutting into the carotid and allowing these "vital forces" to escape was unthinkable as it would leave the patient unconscious or dead.[6] Goodall[7] describes the reluctance of physicians to perform such a "scandalous surgery" as tracheostomy as it was reasoned to be irresponsible and futile. Because of a lack of knowledge of anatomy and physiology and fear of compromising their reputations, few physicians would perform the procedure. About 100 B.C. Galen[8] described the first elective tracheostomy performed by Asclepiode of Bithynia. Aretaeus, in his textbook *The Therapeutics of Acute Diseases,*[9] discusses and condemns Asclepiodes' tracheostomy surgery based on his theory that cartilage could not heal.

Paulus Aegineta performed several tracheostomies in the 7th century and wrote of the work of the Greek surgeon, Antyllus (A.D. 340).[10] His operation was described as making a transverse incision into the trachea between the third and fourth rings, drawing the cartilages apart with hoods, and sewing the edges of the wound together when the patient could breathe more freely.

The wars, conflicts, and religious persecutions of the Dark Ages repressed literature, scientific exploration, and medicine, and little was written of surgeries of any kind until after the 15th century.[1]

In 1546, Andreas Visalius described in *De Humani Corporis Fabrica,*[11] his comprehensive text on anatomy, an operation performed on a newborn lamb that was cyanotic, bradycardic, and gasping as a result of the clamping of the umbilical cord. A tracheostomy was performed and the lamb's lungs were ventilated with bellows through the tracheostomy, which successfully restored the lamb's breathing and heart rate. Also, in 1546, Musa Brassarolo published his description of the first successful tracheostomy on a patient near death from "an abscess in the windpipe."[5] Though the procedure was still quite controversial, Brassarolo's reputation apparently was not jeopardized as he, over the years, provided medical care to several sovereigns, including Henry VIII of England and several royal popes.

From the 16th century to the mid 19th century tracheostomy was considered dangerous and futile. Although many modifications were developed for the operation, they were immediately criticized and abandoned.[1] Physicians were fearful and skeptical of this procedure, and the literature reveals only 28 successful tracheostomies performed during this 300-year period.[7]

The first book on tracheostomy was published in 1620 in Paris by Nicholas Habicot, in which he described four successful tracheostomies.[7] One patient was a young boy thought to be dead from knife wounds to the neck. Habicot saved the boy's life by performing a tracheostomy and removing a blood clot from the boy's larynx.

Another young boy's airway was obstructed by a bag of gold coins stuck in his esophagus after he swallowed it to keep from being robbed. Habicot performed a tracheostomy to provide an airway while manipulating the bag of coins down the esophagus. Several days later the coins were excreted and recovered. Another adventurous procedure was performed on a highwayman who was scheduled to be hanged. A surgeon was paid to perform a tracheostomy and place a tube in his neck for airway prior to the scheduled hanging. The hangman saw blood on the highwayman's neck and became suspicious. However, he was advised that the highwayman had tried to commit suicide. He proceeded with the hanging. The tracheostomy was not effective, and the highwayman died.[7]

In the early 1600s, Fabricius acknowledged that surgeons were terrified to perform a tracheostomy because it was labeled a "scandalous operation."[12] Fabricius successfully performed a tracheostomy procedure on several patients with airway obstruction from foreign bodies in the larynx. At the same time, Cosserius, one of Fabricius' students developed a curved tracheostomy cannula and neck tapes to tie the cannula into position. Although an improvement, this advancement was ignored, and the straight tube was used instead of the curved tube for many years to come.[12]

In 1650, the report of the tragic death of a 7-year-old boy was published by Thraphilus Bonetus,[13] a pathological anatomist. He had recommended a tracheostomy for the child, who had an upper airway obstruction from a bone he had aspirated. The internist overruled the recommendation and the child died.

In 1739, Heister[14] used a straight tube and trocar in the procedure he actually named "tracheotomy." He chastised his contemporaries for neglecting to utilize this valuable procedure. At the Royal Academy of Surgery of Paris, in 1759, M. Louis[15] presented a memoir on bronchotomy and advocated tracheostomy in particular for removal of foreign bodies. Although he was most judicious in his recommendations on tracheostomy, Louis was vehemently criticized by celebrated surgeons Sharp[16] and Van Swieten.[17]

In 1770, the double cannula was developed by George Martin.[18] Although another important advance, it was discarded. Herholdt and Rafn,[19] in 1796, recommended orotracheal intubation and bellows ventilation for near-drowning patients.

P.J. Desault,[20] Surgeon in Chief of the Great Hospital of Humanity, Paris, described the procedure of passing a nasotracheal catheter into the larynx of a child with severe glottic edema. This procedure was considered an improvement over laryngotomy because it provided a secured airway while generating a cough reflex. The child recovered and the catheter was removed after 36 hours. Also in Paris, Favier[21] performed laryngotomies on dogs whose airways were obstructed by foreign bodies. He found in his research that the airway was cleared by the coughing that was created by making an incision. He concluded that this was not a difficult procedure and that his colleagues were merely timid.

Croup, an upper airway inflammation associated with harsh breathing and a sore throat, was so named by Francis Home,[22] a Scottish physician, in 1765. Home recommended tracheostomy for children in distress from croup symptoms. The treatment was still not enthusiastically embraced by the medical community at that time. The bias and fear of the tracheostomy procedure that permeated the medical profession in Europe soon traveled across the ocean to the United States. Even though croup was widespread in this country in the early 1800s, tracheostomy was not accepted as a treatment. When George Washington developed an upper airway obstruction, only one of his three physicians recommended tracheostomy. The surgery was not performed and Washington died on December 14, 1799.

Pierre Bretonneau published his description of symptoms of nonspecific swellings of the head and neck that had been historically referred to as abscesses, angina, or cyannache.[11,23] He defined these conditions as a disease, which he named *diphtheria*. Bretonneau was instrumental in changing the perspective of tracheostomy which he accomplished when he performed a lifesaving tracheostomy on a 5-year-old girl suffering from diphtheria.

Tracheostomy at this point had been a radical procedure performed in life and death situations by only the most aggressive surgeons. It was not an operation performed or recommended by conservative physicians. McKenzie's textbook, *Diseases of the Pharynx, Larynx, and Trachea*, refers to this critical issue as "the question always rises in the mind of the young surgeon whether the symptoms are sufficiently urgent to render the operation necessary."[10]

Following Bretonneau's experience, by 1833 Trousseau[24] had established diphtheria as an appropriate indication for tracheostomy. He cited 200 children with life-threatening diphtheria who had a tracheostomy, with successful results in one fourth of the cases.

By 1860, tracheostomy was becoming an acceptable procedure for treating upper airway obstruction caused by foreign bodies, diphtheria, croup, and trauma. For the first time in history, physicians began to focus on the issues of techniques, complications, and postoperative care. Over 38 papers on tracheostomy were published and the controversies were being reviewed in a text by Max Schuller[25] in 1880. With experience, physicians began to improve techniques and develop new instruments and cannulas.

Conway[26] also reported in the *Edinburgh Medical Journal* in 1860 that the mortality rate for croup and diphtheria patients in France was only 68% because of the use of tracheostomy for these patients, and he advocated more extensive use of the procedure in Scotland.

The British physician, Dr. Erichsen, in 1869, commented that tracheostomy was seldom successful because it was not usually done until it was a last resort for "hopeless" cases.[27] Erichsen acknowledged that the initial incision may cause death; however, resuscitation may be possible if a large silver tube were used after the surgery was completed. He recommended no anesthesia for adults and that chloroform be used as an anesthetic for children. He suggested that the critical issues of tracheostomy were the incision into the trachea, the opening of the airway, the risk of hemorrhage and the positioning of the tube. Tracheostomy was recommended by Sir William Jenner[27] for diphtheria patients because he felt patients might die anyway, but in a less painful manner than by asphyxiation.

In 1886, Norton described four different operations that relieved upper airway obstruction. "The incision could be made from the hyoid cartilage to the trachea and sponging the trachea with silver nitrate to enhance post operative recovery."[28] These procedures are illustrated in Figure 3-1.

By the early part of the 20th century, Chevalier Jackson [29,30] had extensive experience with tracheostomy procedures and took an analytical approach to the management of airway obstruction. Via

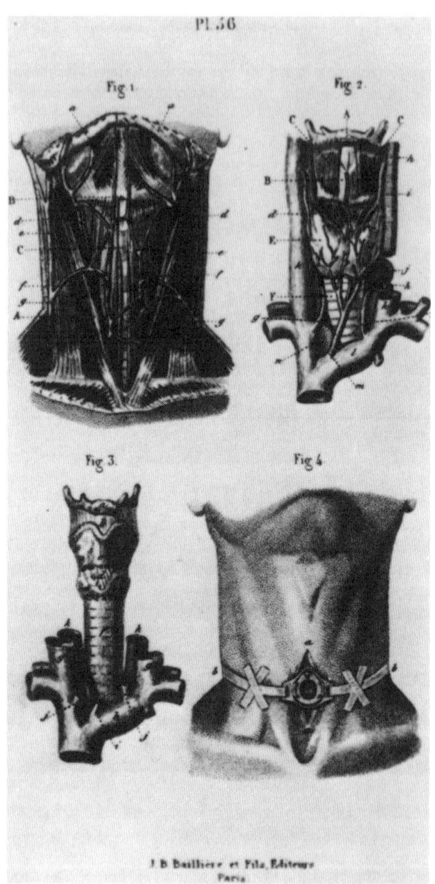

Figure 3-1 The illustration may appear contemporary, but the accompanying legend reveals that surgeons of the last century actually described four different procedures, only one of which is similar to what we term tracheotomy. *They described making incisions (1) into the larynx by the thyroid membrane (subhyoid bronchotomy); (2) through the hyoid cartilage (laryngotomy); (3) into the larynx and the upper rings of the trachea (laryngotomy); or (4) into the trachea (tracheotomy). (From Norton, A.H.:* A Text Book of Operative Surgery and Surgical Anatomy, *London: Long, Bailliere, Tindel and Cox, 1886.)*

bronchoscopy, tracheostomy, and direct laryngoscopy, he delineated a universally accepted tracheostomy procedure using a double-cannula silver tube for airway obstruction in pediatric and adult patients.

Jackson's published work[29,30] defined the critical issues of the tracheostomy operation such as positioning the incision too high, the choice of cannula used, hurried surgery, and inappropriate postoperative care. Jackson recommended avoidance of high cartilage dissection and careful methodical surgery using a long incision dividing the thyroid isthmus. Jackson's historical perspectives are as pertinent today as they were at the time:

> Tracheotomy is one of the oldest operations in the history of surgery, yet it is probably more often improperly performed today, and more often followed by needless mortality and needless crippling, than any other operation. The two chief preventable sequelae are death from improper routine surgical care and wrongly fitted tube and stenosis from too high an incision.[29, 30]

Jackson's recommendations on tracheostomy positioning:

> Every medical graduate has been taught that there are two kinds of tracheotomy, high and low, the low operation being very difficult, the high operation very easy. When he is suddenly called upon to do an emergency tracheotomy, this erroneous teaching is about all that remains in the dim recesses of his memory; consequently he makes sure of doing the operation high enough, and goes in through the larynx, usually dividing the cricoid cartilage, the only complete ring in the trachea. As originally made, the distinction between high and low as applied to tracheotomy referred to operations above and below the isthmus of the thyroid gland, in a day when primitive surgery attached too much importance to operations upon the thyroid gland. The isthmus is entitled to absolutely no consideration whatever in deciding the location at which to divide a structure as vital as the trachea.[29,30]

Jackson's comments regarding postoperative care:

> 1. Always bear in mind that the tracheotomy is not the ultimate object. The ultimate object is to pipe air down into the lungs. Tracheotomy is only a means to the end.

> 2. After-care in tracheotomy cases is one of good "plumbing," that is, keeping the "pipes," natural and artificial, clear of obstruction. Air must be piped not merely into the trachea, but also into the lungs, and it must be the constant duty of someone to know by seeing, feeling and hearing that it gets there.
> 3. [After tracheotomy] do not give cough sedatives or narcotics. The cough reflex is the watchdog of the lungs.[29,30]

With Jackson's work, the mortality of tracheostomy was reduced from 25% to 1 or 2% while also reducing the complication of laryngeal stenosis.

Diphtheria began to disappear with the advent of immunizations in the early 20th century. Sulfonamides were developed to treat upper respiratory infections, and the indications for tracheostomy began to change. Foreign body removal was performed via endoscopy, thus replacing tracheostomy as the preferred procedure. However, with the onset of poliomyelitis, physicians enthusiastically embraced Dr. Wilson's[31] recommendation of the use of tracheostomy as prophylactic treatment to reduce the incidence of pulmonary infections for these patients.

The medical community began to advocate tracheostomy for most major surgeries, drug overdoses, and head and chest trauma. During the mid 1900s, tracheostomy was recommended for the treatment of chronic lung diseases, emphysema, pneumonia, and chronic bronchitis. Galloway[32] defined the primary indications for tracheostomy to be pulmonary toilet and mechanical ventilation. The development of intermittent positive pressure ventilation after World War II via tracheostomy tubes revolutionized the management of patients with severe pulmonary disease.

By 1965, nasal and oral intubation, instead of tracheostomy, quickly became more popular as safer and faster procedures to provide an adequate airway with fewer complications. Tracheostomy has evolved from a scandalous procedure performed by only the most aggressive physician in life-threatening or hopeless case, to a procedure that had to be justified as more appropriate than oral/nasal intubation. Over a 3,000-year span, tracheostomy has developed from a straight reed thrust over the point of a sword into a choking soldier on the battlefield to the meticulous aseptic insertion of a curved, nonreactive tube with a low-pressure cuff into an anesthetized patient whose airway may have already been secured by endotracheal intubation.

Today tracheostomies are a routine procedure performed ideally in an operating room but sometimes performed in emergency situations by paramedics in the field and by emergency room staff in the trauma room. The debate is no longer whether a surgeon should intervene to secure the airway but rather when a tracheostomy should be performed and oral/nasal intubation discontinued. Many institutions and physicians discontinue intubation after 10 to 14 days. However, this is a very controversial issue and can vary from physician to physician even within the same institution. It is postulated that complications of oral/nasal intubation can be diminished by performing a tracheostomy. With today's ever-increasing number of high-risk pregnancies producing severely compromised neonates and a medical system that provides extensive treatment to prolong life, tracheostomy procedures are increasing. Tracheostomy tubes have improved and there are several designs that address some of the complication issues regarding cuff design and tube materials.

The conventional surgical procedure has not changed extensively in the past few years. However, in the late 1980s, the percutaneous dilation tracheostomy (PDT) method gained favor, specifically in emergency situations in the trauma rooms and intensive care units.[33,34,35]

The tracheostomy tube itself and the methods of care are continually being improved. Many devices and practices have been developed to assist the tracheostomized patient with the complications associated with having a tracheostomy. Today this procedure is a widely established lifesaving intervention routinely performed in all parts of the world.

TERMINOLOGY

Initially described by Galen[8] as a verb, "to cut the larynx," Aretaeus[9] used the description, "to make an incision in the artery" in the second century. The reference to trachea included artery, bronchus, and larynx. It wasn't until the 16th century that the term *artery* was replaced by the term *trachea.* In 1600 a procedure illustrated as a laryngotomia was actually an incision into the trachea (Figure 3-2).

It wasn't until 1649 that the term *tracheotomy* appeared. Heister campaigned for the use of this term in 1718. In 1762, Quincy insisted *tracheotomy* was an incorrect term for *bronchotomy.* Desault[20] defined the difference between laryngotomy and tracheotomy in the 18th century and described them as "subdivisions under bronchotomy."

Since Bretonneau and Trousseau in the 1820s, the procedure was described as the commonly known tracheotomy. The terms *tracheotomy* and *tracheostomy* are often used interchangeably today. The term *tracheotomy* is derived from the Greek words *trachea arteria* ("rough artery") and *tome* ("to cut"). Tracheostomy is derived from the Greek ending *stoma* ("to furnish with an opening"). Today we usually refer to the operation or the procedure as *tracheotomy* and the opening that remains after the procedure as *tracheostomy.*

SURGICAL TECHNIQUES

Conventional

The procedure is performed in an operating room using local, intravenous sedation or a general anesthetic, by a general surgeon, but more commonly by an otolaryngologist (ENT), an ear, nose, throat, head, and neck physician. A surgical opening is made in the trachea and a tube is placed for the exchange of air directly into the trachea. This air exchange bypasses the normal respiratory system, that is, oral/nasal respiration. The patient is positioned with the neck hyperextended, and a horizontal incision approximately 3 to 4 cm in length is made into the skin The sternohyoid and the sternothyroid muscles are separated. The thyroid gland, now exposed, is either raised or lowered. The isthmus may be divided. A vertical incision is made between the second and third tracheal rings, the trachea is widened, and a tracheostomy tube is inserted. When the retracting instruments are removed, the pretracheal fascia approximates to the midline and there is usually no need for sutures. A chest x-ray is usually recommended on a new tracheostomy to confirm correct position of the tracheostomy tube. This procedure has remained as one of the most widely performed and effective lifesaving procedures in the history of medicine (Figures 3-3 and 3-4).

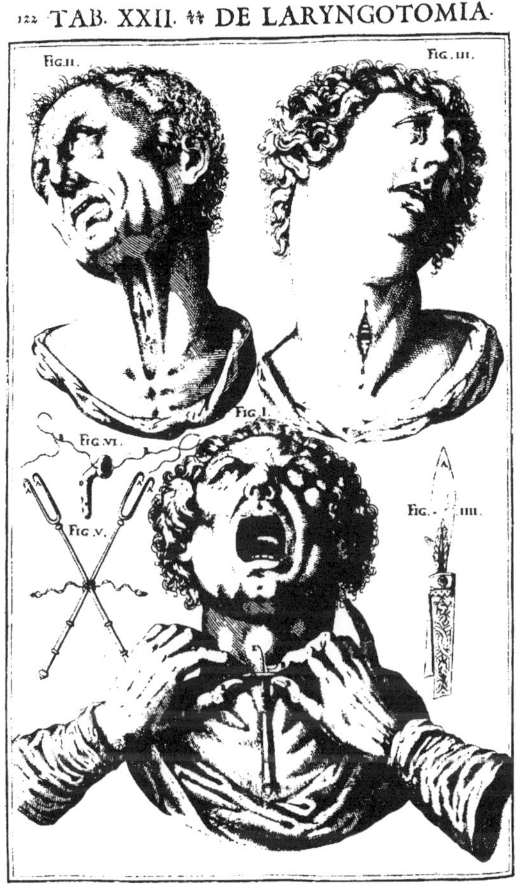

Figure 3-2 Note the name of the operation, although the incision appears to be in the trachea. Note also the curved tube. This design was forgotten and later rediscovered. (From Casserius, J:. De vocis auditusque organis historia singulari fide methodo ac industria concinnati tractatibus duobus explicata ac variis iconibus aere excusis illustrata . . . (Ferrariae, 122, 1600-1601.)

Percutaneous Tracheostomy

A percutaneous tracheostomy is described by Hazard[33] and colleagues as a "modification of Seldinger's technique for vascular cannulation, in which a flexible guidewire is inserted into the trachea

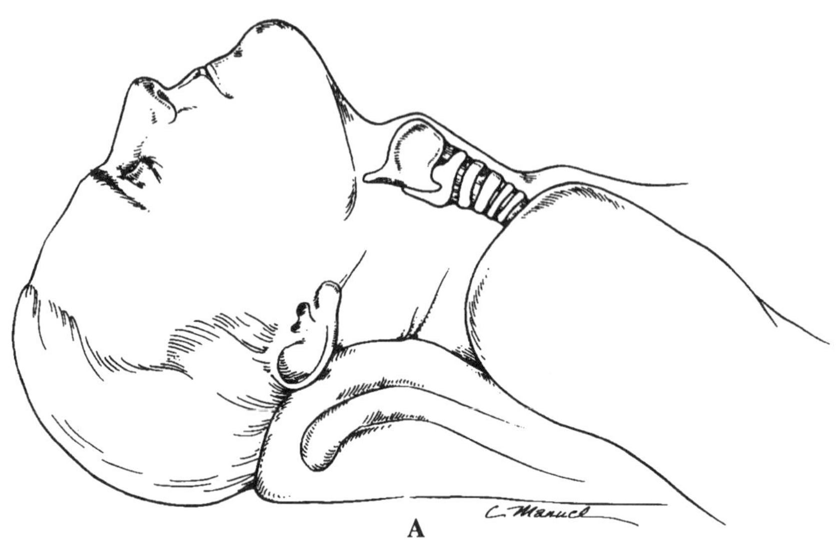

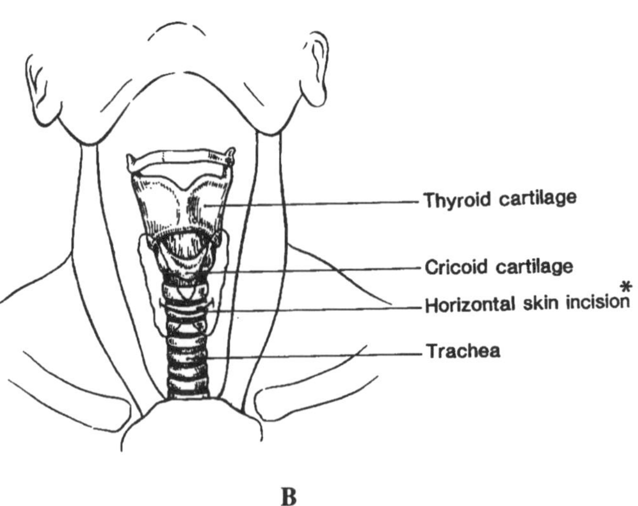

Figure 3-3 ***A****, Patient positioned with the neck hyperextended.* ***B****, Skin incision is made about one finger's breadth below the level of the cricoid cartilage. (Courtesy of Mallinckrodt Medical TPI, Inc. Irvine, CA.)*

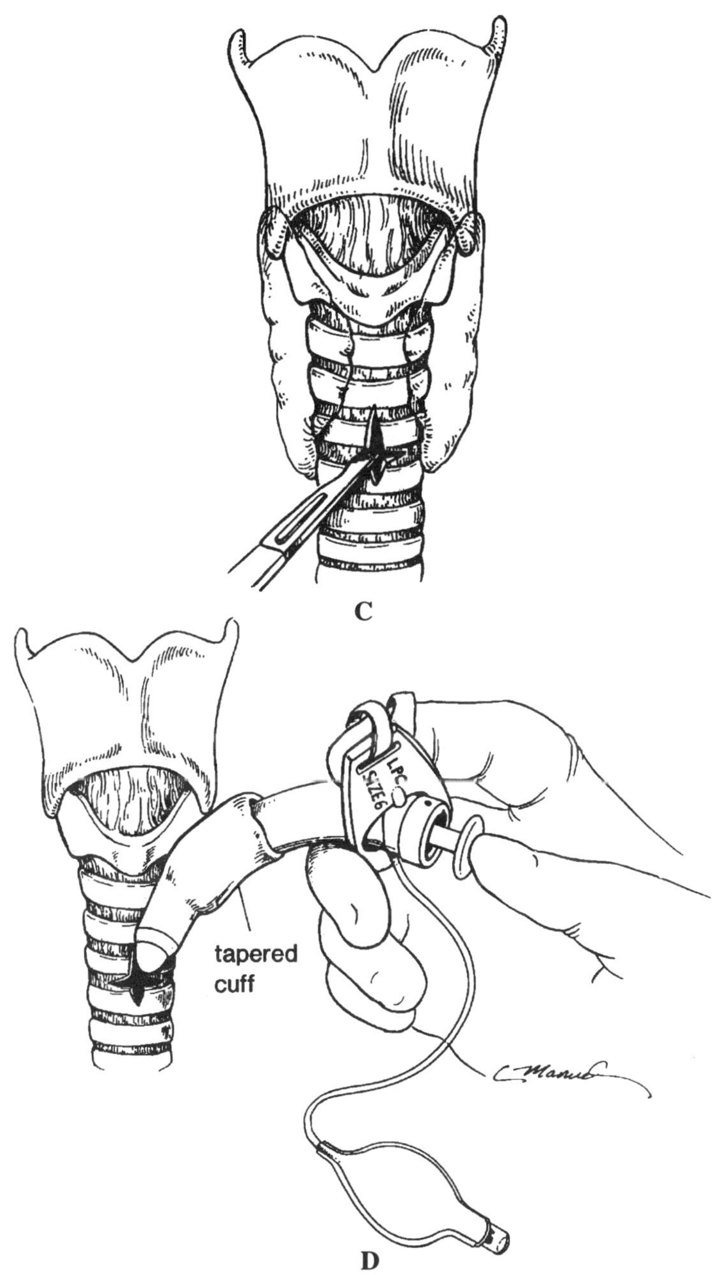

Figure 3-4 ***C****, The surgeon makes an incision through the second, third, and fourth tracheal rings.* ***D****, A cuffed tracheostomy tube is then placed carefully through the incision into the anterior tracheal wall. (Courtesy of Mallinckrodt Medical TPI, Inc. Irvine, CA.)*

through a percutaneously introduced needle."[34] After identifying the landmarks, a horizontal skin incision is made in the neck. A large-bore needle is inserted into the tracheal lumen through which a flexible metal guidewire is inserted. The needle is removed, the space is dilated, the wire is removed, and the tracheostomy cannula is inserted. The procedure is easily performed at the bedside, using prepackaged kits. The procedure takes about 10 minutes to complete. Emergency tracheostomies are often done in the traditional procedure, or possibly through the cricothyroid membrane, and then converted to the traditional location. This is still a controversial procedure and is not performed as routinely as is the conventional method.

INDICATIONS FOR TRACHEOSTOMY

The purpose of a tracheostomy is to bypass a compromised upper airway and to provide access to the lower airway for basic air exchange and ventilation. Some indications for this procedure are acute or chronic upper airway obstruction, such as a foreign body or retention of pulmonary secretions; prolonged mechanical ventilation; neoplasm; intolerance or long-term placement of an endotracheal tube; retention of bronchopulmonary secretions or glottic incompetence; trauma; or sleep apnea. It is important to consider that although the placement of the tracheostomy tube is important to establish a patent airway and is a life-sustaining procedure, it is also a foreign body. Significant complications as well as many physiological changes occur secondary to the placement of a tracheostomy tube, and complications may develop.

COMPLICATIONS OF TRACHEOSTOMY

As described in Chapter 2, immediate, intermediate and long-term complications can occur with this procedure.

Apnea and hemorrhage are the most dramatic complications. Apnea occurs when the increased flow of oxygen decreases the respiratory drive. Hemorrhage occurs when one of the major vessels is inadvertently cut. Other immediate complications could damage the recurrent laryngeal nerve, causing paralysis of the vocal cords; trauma to the esophagus, causing a fistula or swallowing dysfunction; subcutaneous or mediastinal emphysema (accumulated air) or pneumothorax; and collapse of a lung.

Intermediate difficulties include aspiration, lung abscess, or tracheitis, due to the bypass of the upper respiratory system.

Long-term complications include tracheal granulations or malacia (softening), persistent tracheoesophageal fistula, tracheal or stomal stenosis, or ulceration of the tracheal wall into the innominate artery. These conditions can develop as a result of excessive pressure in the tracheostomy tube cuff. Tracheostomy sites are colonized with bacteria within 24 hours; and nosocomial (hospital-acquired) infections are common.

Infection can occur and is noted by signs of purulent and foul-smelling drainage coming from the tracheostomy site, temperature increase, malaise, or pain. A displaced tube can be noted by an increase in work of breathing or an increase in pain associated with breathing. Increased bleeding around the stoma site from vessels or a major artery and other complications having to do with the direct access to the lower airway may include pneumonia, pulmonary aspiration, reduction of mucociliary transport, bacterial infections, tube and suctioning problems.

PHYSIOLOGICAL CHANGES SECONDARY TO TRACHEOSTOMY

Speech

The primary focus of a tracheostomy is to provide an adequate airway for the patient. Consequently, an important change that is often overlooked is the inability to phonate naturally. Because air enters and exits the lungs via the tracheostomy, the upper airway is bypassed, including the vocal cords. This could leave the patient virtually aphonic and unable to communicate. Frequently, a tracheotomy is performed as an emergency procedure to provide an airway to sustain life, and the patient is unable to receive the appropriate counseling needed to establish a system of communication that helps to relieve the postoperative frustration of the inability to communicate verbally. With ventilator dependent patients, lack of communication is one of the main instigators of fear, anxiety, agony, and panic, according to a survey by Berbom-Enberger and Haljamae.[36]

Secretions

Another physiological change is an increase of secretions and reduced ability to manage these secretions. Secretions become a problem for several reasons. The first, and most obvious, is the placement of the tracheostomy tube that generates the body's natural reaction to fight against a foreign body. The once closed pulmonary system is now compromised as well. Airflow now bypasses the upper airway, and respiration takes place through the tracheostomy tube rather than through the nasal cavity. Tissues in the nose provide humidification and warmth to the inspired air. Cilia (small hair-like structures), are present to filter particles and bacteria from the air. The change in the direction of airflow causes the inspired air to be dry and nonfiltered, increasing the viscosity of mucus and the possibility of infection. The intrathoracic pressure that is required to raise the mucus is decreased, and the secretions therefore accumulate, requiring suctioning. The suctioning procedure irritates the lower airway and in turn increases the amount of secretions produced. Increased secretions may also be the result of infection.

Olfaction and Gustation

A secondary effect of tracheal tube placement is the loss of the senses of smell and taste. Air must flow high in the nasal chamber to achieve olfaction. Tracheostomized patients report their ability to smell is affected by the change in the respiratory airflow through the tracheostomy tube. Tracheostomized patients comment that they cannot taste their food as well and experience diminished appetite. This loss of appetite is significant because good nutrition is vital to the process of healing.

Dysphagia

Dysphagia, known as a disorder in deglutition and swallowing, can be a secondary consequence of tracheostomy placement. It is known that the placement of the tracheostomy tube anchors the strap muscles and prevents elevation of the larynx. "The major effect of tracheotomy on deglutition occurs during the second stage of the swallow. At this time, as the bolus passes through the pharynx, the suprahyoid muscles elevate and move the larynx anteriorly under the tongue base, the epiglottis tilts backward, and the three-tiered laryngeal closure occurs. Tracheotomy causes fixation of the trachea to the anterior neck skin. This in turn causes reduced elevation and anterior movement of the larynx, allowing food and/or secretions to enter the partially unprotected airway."[37] It is also theorized that the pressures in the pharynx and the esophagus are altered with the placement of the tracheostomy tube, causing a swallowing dysfunction. Leverment, studying intraluminal esophageal pressure in dogs, felt that the swallowing dysfunction may be due to an increase of intraluminal pressure at the cuff level and 5 to 10 cm below the pharyngoesophageal junction, which can lead to the scenario just described.[38]

It is postulated that the presence of the tracheostomy tube reduces the ability of the vocal cords and larynx to close because of changes in stimulation of subglottic sensory receptors and reduced subglottic pressures. Sasaki and colleagues discussed the effects of tracheotomy in two studies. In the first study, they demonstrated in dogs that chronic upper airway bypass can lead to an uncoordinated laryngeal closure response, which may allow aspiration to occur; in the second, they discussed both this neurophysiological effect of the tracheotomy and the mechanical elevation of the larynx.[39] Currently there are studies being done on humans that may support these hypotheses on the effects of the tracheostomy tube on the pharynx and larynx during swallowing.[40] There is a need for increased research on the effects of tracheostomy on swallowing. Preliminary research indicates that use of finger occlusion over the tracheostomy tube opening or a one-way speaking valve such as the Passy-Muir may help restore pressures and pharyngeal sensation for swallowing purposes. This is discussed at length in Chapter 10 of this text.

Infection

With tracheostomy tube placement there is an increased chance of infection. This tube gives direct access to the lower airway, bypassing all the natural filtration protectors of the upper airway as previously noted. Bacteria breed in warm, moist, dark environments, and therefore the chances for an infection are increased with a tracheostomized patient. Strict, sterile technique and good hand-washing by the patient to prevent contamination from finger occlusion are necessary.

Energy and Well-Being

A physiological aspect that is often overlooked in the tracheostomized patient is the decrease in energy level. It is theorized that there is a less efficient gas exchange with a tracheostomy tube present, and therefore the patient feels less energetic. This feeling can influence the patient's ability to participate more fully in his recovery process and affect a patient's self-esteem and body image.

Airway Resistance

"Air flow resistance of the upper airway with nose breathing (including nose, pharynx, and larynx) is as much as 80 percent of the total airway resistance, and with mouth breathing it is 50 percent."[41] Therefore, the presence of a tracheostomy tube should significantly reduce the airway resistance. "In reality, however, flow resistance through the tracheostomy cannula may be as high as or even higher than that through the normal upper airways, because of the cannula's relatively small diameter [7 to 8 mm ID] for an adult-sized cannula."[5]

"A tracheostomy reduces the anatomical dead space by as much as 100 ml in adults. This may help patients who have diseases such as emphysema, whose tidal volume is decreased in relation to physiological dead space."[42]

Humidification

It is important to note that, during respiration, inspired air is warmed and humidified through the nasal passage. Since the normal airflow is bypassed, the air reaching the trachea through the tracheostomy tube is cold, dry air and it is usually necessary to have a humidification system available for the tracheostomized patient. It has been noted that the decrease in the humidity of inspired air causes drying in the tracheobronchial mucosa, as well as inflammatory changes in the mucosa. This is an important physiological change that could breed additional complications, such as bleeding tracheitis, thickened pulmonary secretions, poor air exchange in the alveoli and possible infections or atelectasis.

TRACHEOSTOMY TUBES

Once the surgical procedure is completed, the insertion of a tube is necessary to keep the tracheal stoma open. There are several tubes from which the surgeon can choose, and often the selection of a tube is relative to the specific reason the patient had the procedure. The various tubes have particular characteristics that distinguish them from one another.

The original tubes were made of hollow reeds and through the years have progressed from goose quills, lead, gold, silver, rubber, silicone, and nylon to stainless steel, polyvinylchloride (PVC), and other synthetic materials. Today, two common materials are the silver and polyvinylchloride tubes. "Silver has long been used to manufacture tracheostomy tubes because the metal walls of the tube can be kept very thin, which is especially advantageous when an inner cannula is used."[5]

Adult and pediatric metal or silver tubes are very rigid. The polyvinyl chloride and other synthetic products used today are much more flexible and provide varying degrees of rigidity.

SIZING THE TRACHEOSTOMY TUBE

The size of the tracheostomy tube as related to the patient's anatomy is controversial. There are no commonly accepted standards, and methods vary from physician to physician. It is important to provide air space around the tube for phonation and to reduce the possibility of complication (i.e., stenosis, granulomas, tracheoesophageal fistulas, trachea malacia, etc.). The tube should be no larger than necessary. Many physicians size the tube to accommodate two-thirds the size of the tracheal lumen. Usually, women are sized smaller than men because of their smaller anatomy. A bronchoscope is used to determine the diameter of the trachea for the pediatric patient, but usually this exam is not used for the adult. Careful sizing of the tracheostomy tube is necessary to prevent the risk of complications from an oversized tube. The length of the tube is also an important consideration. A chest x-ray is usually performed to confirm tube placement and position.

Adult tracheostomy tube sizes range from 4 to 10, and neonatal and pediatric sizes range from 000 to 4. The neonatal tracheostomy tubes are much shorter than the pediatric tubes.

Age	Laryngoscope Blade Size	Mask Size	ET tube I.D.(mm)	Suction Catheter (French)	Trach Tube Size
Premature	0	1, small	2.5	6	00
New born	1	1	3.0	6	00-0
6 months	2	1	3.5	8	0-1
1 year	2	2, med	4.0	8	1-2
2 years	2	3, med	4.5	8	2
4 years	2	3	5.0	10	3
6 years	2	3	5.5	10	4
8 years	3	3	6.0	10	4
10 years	3	3	6.5	10	4
12 years	3	4, large	7.0	12	5
14 years	3	4	7.5	12	5
Adult					
female	3	4	8.0-8.5	14	5
male	3-4	4	8.5-9.5	16	6

Table 3-1 Tracheostomy Equipment Sizes. (From Oakes, D., Clinical Practitioners Pocket Guide to Respiratory Care© *1984 and 1988 Health Educator Publications, Inc. Old Towne, ME.)*

TRACHEOSTOMY TUBE COMPONENTS

Tracheostomy tubes have several components. The outer cannula forms the primary structure of the tracheostomy tube.

Flange

The neck flange or plate, which is attached to the proximal end of the outer cannula, provides the collar of support and rests on the skin of the patient's neck (Figure 3-5). The flange is secured by various types of tracheostomy tube holders or "ties" that secure the outer cannula by tying around the neck. The tracheostomy "tie" prevents the tube from accidentally being dislodged, and the flange prevents the tube from slipping into the incision. The face plate is flat; some attach at an angle, some are made of very soft material, and many have the flexibility to move easily to adapt to the patient's neck anatomy. Secure ties help to prevent accidental dislodgment of the tube from the trachea.

For infants, an Aberdeen neck plate (Figure 3-6) is used because of its unique shape. The shape is similar to that of an airplane wing and can be more comfortable on the neck.

Inner Cannula

Some tubes have an inner cannula that may be inserted into the outer cannula. The purpose of the inner cannula is to have available

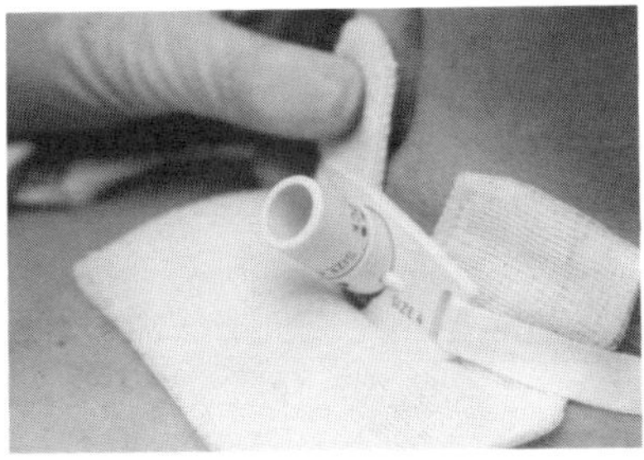

Figure 3-5 Neck flange. (Courtesy of Mallinckrodt Medical TPI, Inc. Irvine, CA.)

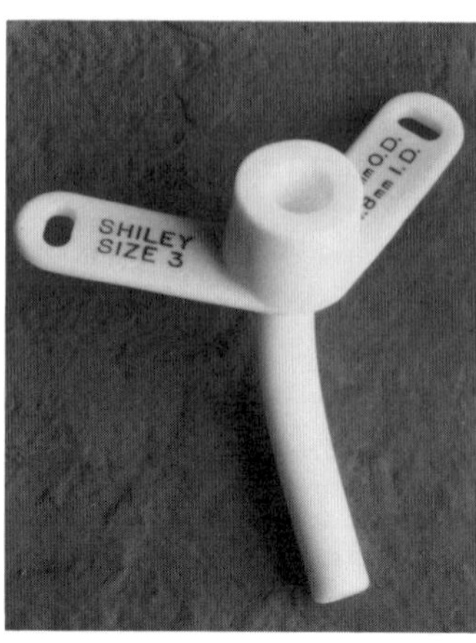

Figure 3-6 Shiley Aberdeen style neck plate. (Courtesy of Mallinckrodt Medical TPI, Inc., Irvine, CA.)

an insert that may be removed for cleaning. This allows the outer cannula to remain in place and prevents the outer cannula from becoming plugged, a distinct safety feature. The inner cannula takes up additional air space, decreasing the airflow. Inner cannulas are not used in pediatric tubes because the pediatric tube is already significantly smaller in internal diameter and an inner cannula would significantly impede airflow.

Inner cannula styles are generally slightly smaller in diameter than outer cannulas and may add to airway resistance for inspiratory/expiratory effort. Inner cannula styles vary and they attach by different methods. Some may lock into place (Shiley plastic [Figure 3-7]), or may be made of metal Figure 3-8), may clip on (Shiley disposable [Figure 3-9]) or may snap (coil) into place (Concord/Portex [Figure 3-10]). The Concord/Portex disposable tracheostomy tube utilizes an inner cannula that has a ring on the end to grasp for removal of the inner cannula. Although manufacturer recommendations are to always replace the inner cannula with a new inner cannula upon removal, if the inner cannula is reused the ring will protrude from the tracheostomy tube. Care should be taken to remove this type of inner cannula with speaking valves because the ring may obstruct the opening function of these valves. The Concord/Portex blue line tracheostomy tube design contains a corrugated inner cannula. The

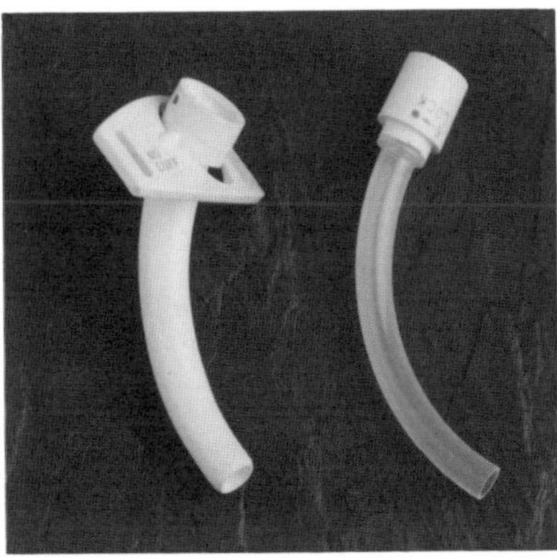

Figure 3-7 Shiley lock in inner cannula. (Courtesy of Mallinckrodt Medical TPI, Inc., Irvine, CA.)

need for this flexible inner cannula is due to the soft nature of the outer cannula and the necessity of the inner cannula to be able to move with the outer cannula.

Obturator

Each tube comes with an obturator. This is a solid component that has a rounded tip and protrudes beyond the end of the outer cannula. The rounded tip of the obturator facilitates insertion and prevents the tube from catching on tracheal mucosa. The obturator also provides some firmness to tracheostomy tubes that are made of less firm materials such as silicone. The obturator is removed immediately after insertion of the tube because it acts as a plug in the outer cannula, and it is kept at the patient's bedside in the event that a recannulation is needed if the tube is dislodged (Figure 3-11).

15 mm Hub

The tracheal hub refers to the proximal end of the inner cannula and is a standard 15 mm OD (outer diameter). This standard connector is necessary for all respiratory and anesthesia equipment adaptions. The 15 mm adapters are also manufactured separately and are used

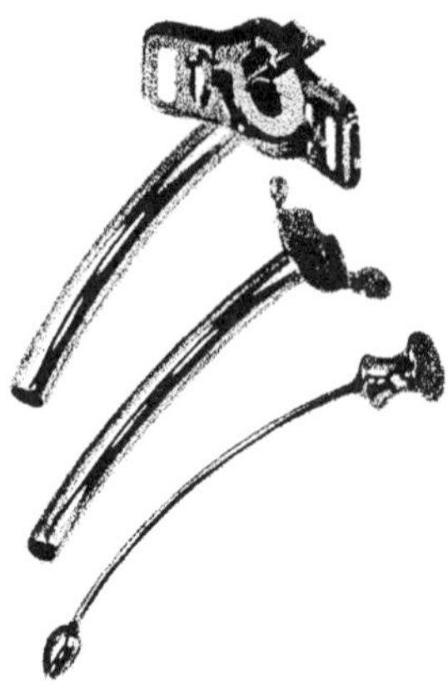

Figure 3-8 Jackson tracheostomy tube and inner cannula. (Courtesy of Pilling, Fort Washington, PA.)

with tracheostomy tubes that do not have hubs, for example, some metal tubes (Figures 3-12 and 3-13).

Cuff

The last component of some tracheostomy tubes is the cuff. The purpose of the tracheal cuff is to separate the upper from the lower airway for control of respiration, that is, to provide a closed ventilatory system and assist in directing air into the lungs. A large variety of cuffed tubes are available. The most widely used cuffed tubes have air-filled cuffs (Figure 3-14A).

Another variety, the silicone foam-filled cuff[†] permits the maintenance of low cuff pressures. The cuff is inflated by opening the inflating line to air. The purpose of this type of cuff is to reduce tracheal damage from high cuff-to-tracheal wall pressures and minimize tracheal dilation. The cuff increases and decreases in volume while continuously monitoring airway seal. Issues to consider with the foam cuff are possible foam hardening if the cuff develops a leak, thus making removal of this tube dangerous to the tracheal wall, and excessive bulk of the foam cuff, creating high pressure against the tracheal wall. However, proper monitoring of the cuff and following the manufacturer's directions may prevent these complications.

[†]This manufacturer refused permission to reference or to reprint photographs of these products.

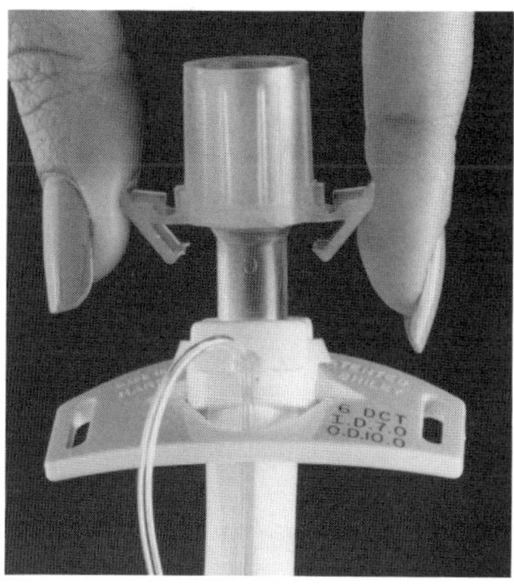

Figure 3-9 A Shiley 15 mm snap lock connector. (Courtesy of Mallinckrodt Medical TPI, Inc., Irvine, CA.)

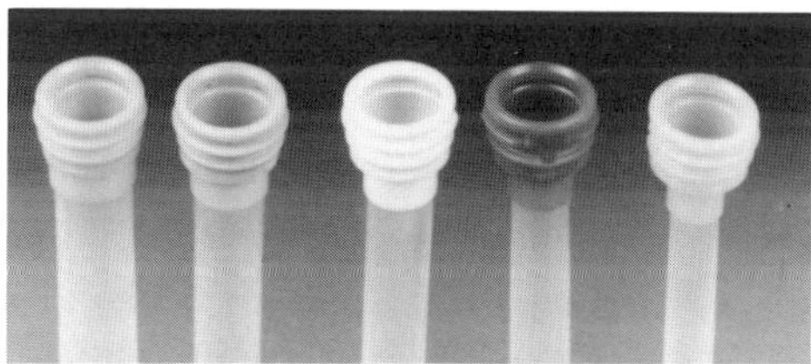

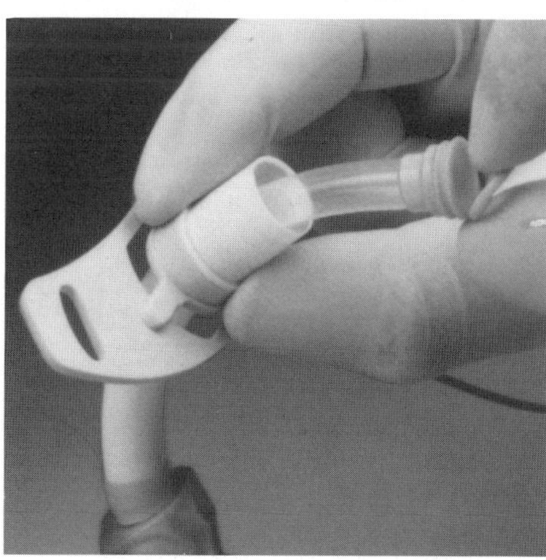

Figure 3-10 Inner cannula with "pull ring." (Courtesy of Concord/Portex, division of Smith's Industries Medical Systems, Keene, NH.)

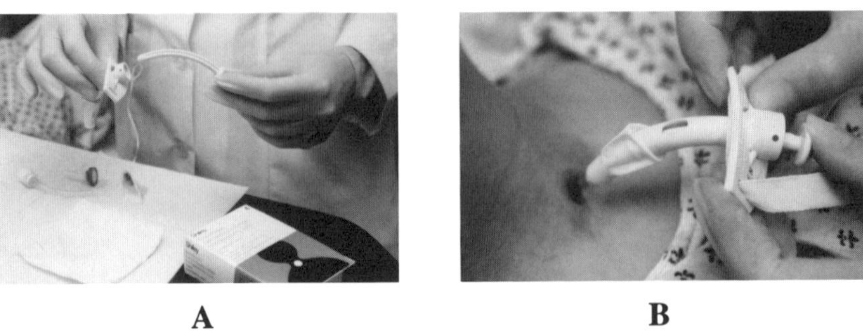

A B

Figure 3-11 ***A,*** *Shiley obturator insertion.* ***B,*** *Shiley tracheostomy tube insertion with use of obturator. (Courtesy of Mallinckrodt Medical TPI, Inc., Irvine, CA.)*

CUFF DEFLATION

There are two popular methods used for inflation of the air-filled cuff to ensure that appropriate pressures are present in the cuff:

Minimal Leak Technique (MLT)

MLT is achieved by inserting enough air into the cuff to maintain the necessary amount of ventilation pressures, allowing some air to pass around the cuff, thus protecting

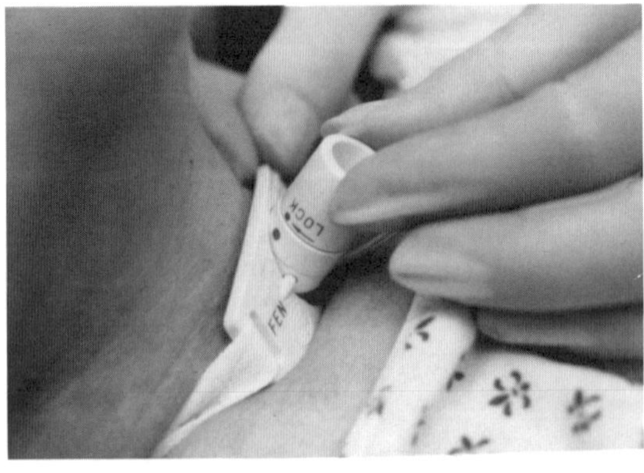

Figure 3-12 A 15 mm hub. (Courtesy of Mallinckrodt Medical TPI, Inc. Irvine, CA.)

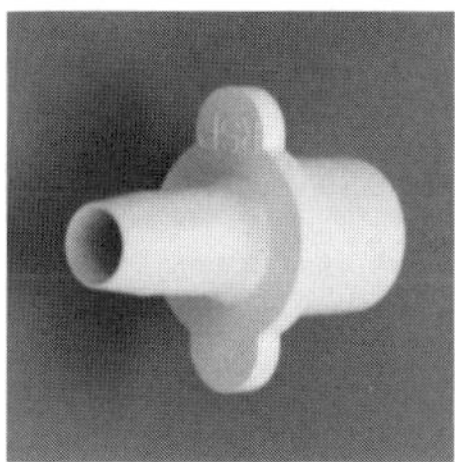

Figure 3-13 A 15 mm adapter. (Courtesy of Concord/Portex, division of Smith's Industries Medical Systems, Keene, NH.)

the tracheal mucosa from pressure from the air-filled cuff. MLT is verified by placing a stethoscope over the upper trachea and listening for air movement around the cuff during the last third of a positive inspiration.

Minimal Occlusal Volume (MOV)

MOV aims for the minimum amount of air in the cuff to prevent a leak around the tube, that is, a totally closed system. This method is required when the ventilatory pressures are high, for example when PEEP is required, and a leak around the cuff is not tolerated. This system is often used for aspiration as well, but can be very difficult to monitor by auscultation (listening).

The cuff pilot is used to instill air into the cuff and is attached via the connected tubing to the upper part of the cuff. Care must be taken to prevent leaks or kinks in the pilot tubing, which will allow air to leak from the cuff. Inflation of the cuff pilot does not indicate the amount of air in the cuff or the cuff pressure. It merely shows that air is present in the cuff (Figure 3-14).

CUFF MANOMETRY

Cuff pressure is best monitored by a cuff manometer and is the most appropriate technique to determine the tracheostomy tube cuff inflation point and the amount of pressure that will be exerted against the tracheal wall.

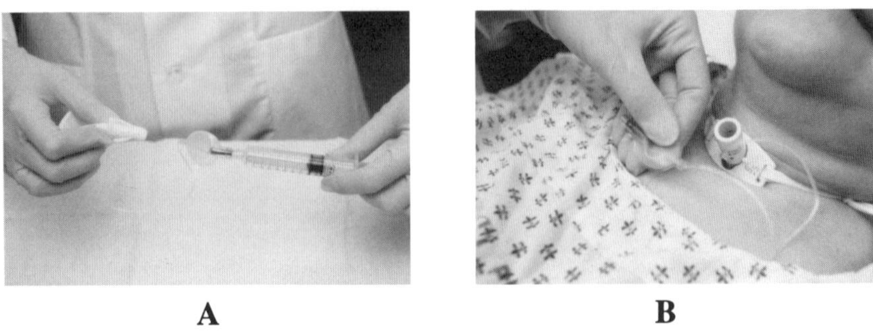

A B

Figure 3-14 **A**, *Air syringe insertion into Shiley cuff pilot.* **B**, *Exterior cuff pilot balloon confirms cuff inflation. (Courtesy of Mallinckrodt Medical TPI, Inc. Irvine, CA.)*

Typically, a tracheostomy tube cuff should not exceed pressures of 25 mm Hg against the tracheal wall. Minimum pressures to seal off the lower airways can be lower depending on the patient's trachea size; for example, 20 mm Hg may be adequate to ensure a seal for mechanical ventilation purposes depending on the anatomical variances in individuals. If a low pressure can ensure ventilation control, and if the sealing off of the lower airway is necessary, lower cuff pressures are advisable. Increased cuff pressure against the tracheal wall will reduce the blood flow to the tissue and may cause damage, such as tracheal necrosis or malacia.

The technique for manometry usage requires insertion of the manometer connection into the cuff pilot line. The pressure readout will display on the manometer dial as a digital or LCD (liquid crystal display) readout. The use of manometry to monitor cuff pressures is helpful to identify cuff leakage or rupture (Figure 3-15).

In some institutions, in addition to cuff manometry use, it is the practice to periodically deflate the cuff in order to allow capillary blood flow into the tracheal tissues. This technique is not well tolerated by the patient and is thought to be inadequate to prevent tracheal stenosis.

TRACHEAL CUFF COMPLICATIONS

The primary reason for a cuffed tracheostomy tube is mechanical ventilation. The cuff provides a closed, sealed (or partially sealed)

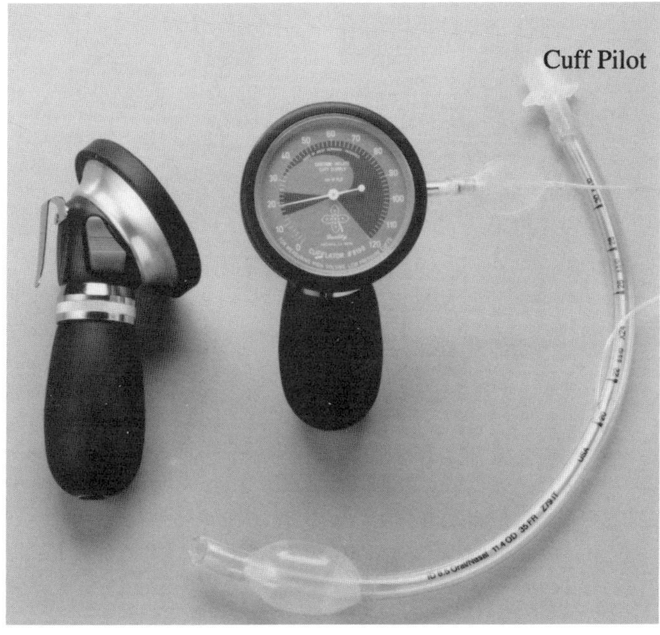

Figure 3-15 Tracheal cuff manometer, Posey Cufflator with endotracheal tube. (Courtesy of Posey, Arcadia, CA.)

airway so the patient gets the maximum volumes he or she needs for adequate respiration and gas exchange.

There are several complications and hazards that may occur with the use of the tracheal cuff (Figures 3-16 and 3-17). These include: partial or total occlusion of the airway, herniation of the tracheal mucosa, tracheal stenosis, granuloma formation, tracheal erosion, tracheal malacia, necrosis, erosion of the innominate artery, and tracheoesophageal fistula. Today, tracheostomy tubes with cuffs are manufactured as low-pressure, high-volume devices, which avoids pressure on the tracheal mucosa by distributing the cuff seal over a larger area of the trachea with lower pressure. Prior to this design, low-volume, high-pressure cuffs were used. High-pressure cuffs contributed to complications by exerting high pressure on the tracheal mucosa. However, complications can occur from improper inflation, such as overinflation of the tracheal cuff, thus losing the effectiveness of the low-pressure cuff. Trauma to the tracheal wall is more easily

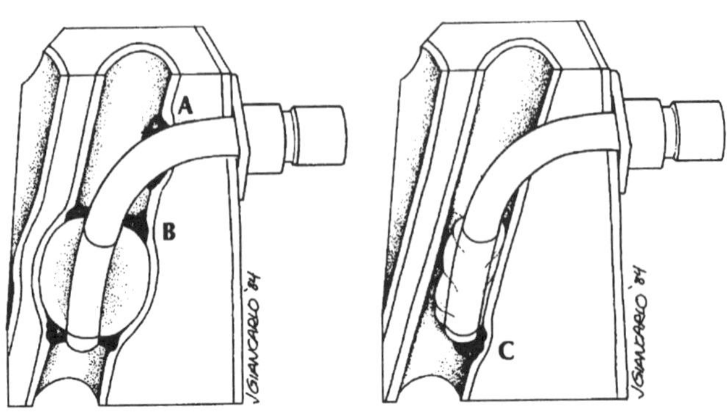

Figure 3-16 Postextubation tracheal stenosis usually occurs at one of three locations. The tracheostomy site (a) is common, and the incidence depends greatly on surgical technique (see text). Endotracheal and tracheostomy tubes usually cause stenosis at the cuff site (b) and less commonly at the location (c) where the end of the tube irritates the tracheal wall. Since the advent of large-volume cuffs, stenosis at site C is limited to indwelling tubes without cuffs or with cuffs deflated. It should be noted that cuff inflation usually ensures the tube end does not come in contact with the tracheal wall. (From Shapiro, B.A., Kacmarek, R.M., and Cane, R.D., Clinical Application of Respiratory Care, *4th Edition, St. Louis: Mosby-Year Book, 1991, Figure 12-2, p. 199.)*

averted with the low-pressure cuffs and the techniques for cuff inflation now being used.

The need for cuff inflation for the ventilator dependent patient must be closely examined in a nonacute, long-term ventilator dependent patient. Bach and Alba[43] in 1990 studied the efficacy of the use of cuffs with the more stable long-term ventilator dependent patients (Table 3-2). They concluded that many patients are maintained with their cuffs unnecessarily inflated and are forced to explore nonverbal means of communication despite the fact that the majority of patients with neuromuscular disease may be successfully ventilated through cuffless tracheostomy tubes. Their study indicated that the vast majority of long-term tracheostomized patients with severe respiratory insufficiency and reasonably competent oropharyngeal muscles can be safely and adequately ventilated up to 24 hours a day with their cuffs deflated or removed. End tidal PCO_2 and SaO_2 can be used to

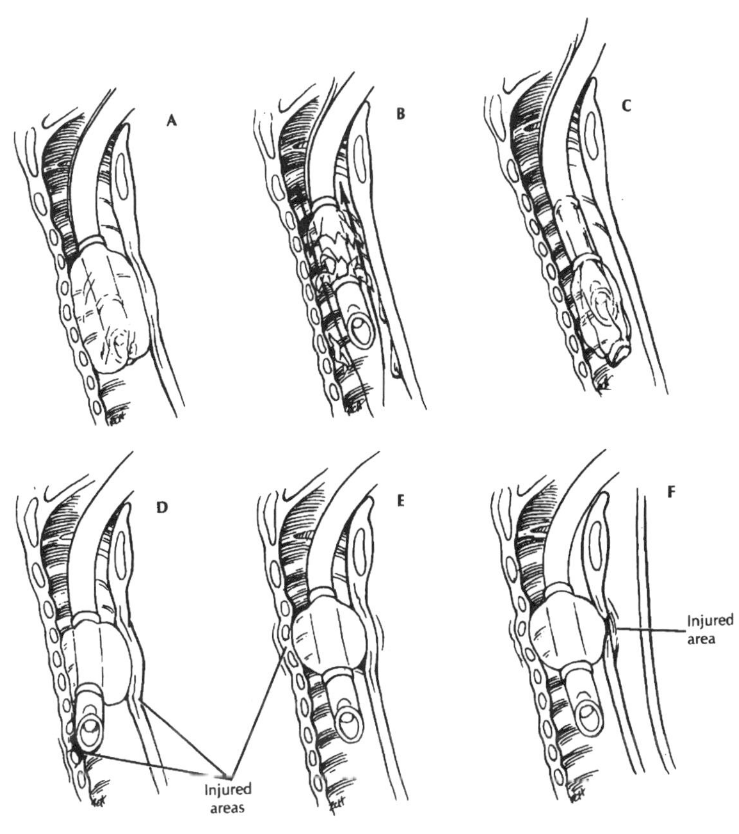

Figure 3-17 Hazards of tube cuffs. ***A****, Cuff overinflation and distention over tube end.* ***B****, Cuff rupture.* ***C****, Cuff slippage.* ***D****, Uneven inflation.* ***E****, Overinflation causing tracheal stenosis and necrosis.* ***F****, Tracheoesophageal fistula. (From Eubanks, D., and Bone, R.C.,* Comprehensive Respiratory Care: A Learning System, *2nd Edition, St. Louis: The C.V. Mosby Company, 1990, Figure 20-30, p. 560.)*

adjust delivered ventilator volumes and FIO_2 both during the daytime and during sleep. Ongoing monitoring of arterial blood gases gives immediate feedback on the status of blood gases.[43]

TRACHEAL CAPS AND PLUGS

The need for tracheal caps and plugs occurs for many reasons, such as weaning, decannulation and speech. Some patients have sleep

Patient	Birth Year	Diagnosis	Onset	Onset TIPPV	Trach No.	VC Supine, ml	VC Predicted, %	Free Time, min
1	1955	Myopathy	1967	1978	4 non	0	0	<1
2	1939	DMD	1941	1978†	6 non	30	1	<1
3	1922	Polio	1954	1983	6 non	40	1.5	<1
4	1967	SCI	1986	1986	8 def	90	2	<1
5	1966	DMD	1968	1987	6 def	260	6	10
6	1936	Polio	1950	1983†	6 non	290	7	<1
7	1973	SCI	1976	1976	4 def	270	9	20
8	1948	Myopathy	1951	1984†	6 non	300	10	5
9	1959	SCI	1979	1979	6 non	690	12	15
10	1934	MND	1976	1987	6 non	650	14	60
11	1963	SCI	1985	1985‡	6 non	980	19	Daytime
12	1978	SCI	1985	1985	4 def	360	16	60
13	1936	Myopathy	1937	1983	6 non	500	18	60
14	1967	DMD	1971	1985	6 non	760	19	60
15	1924	Polio	1925	1984	6 non	624	26	<1
16	1971	SCI	1987	1987	6 non	1920	30	Daytime
17	1949	SCI	1981	1981	6 def	830	30	30
18	1969	SCI	1979	1979	6 non	1710	31	Daytime
19	1942	CMT	1953	1983	4 non	1150	33	60
20	1961	SCI	1976	1976	6 non	1750	33	Daytime
21	1959	SCI	1981	1981	6 non	2800	44	Daytime

*Trach—all are Shiley tracheostomy tubes, cuffless (non) or deflated (def); DMD = Duchenne muscular dystrophy; SCI = spinal cord injury; MND = motor neuron disease; and CMT = Charcot-Marie-Tooth disease.

†Patients dead: No. 2 in 1988, No. 6 in 1987, No. 8 in 1987.

‡Patients weaned: No. 11 in 1988.

Table 3-2 Twenty-One Patients in Order of Increasing Vital Capacity Receiving Overnight TIPPV. (From Bach, J.R., and Alba, A.S., Clinical Investigations in Critical Care, *Chest, 1990, 97:679-683, Table 1 p. 2.)*

apnea and require an open cannula only at night. Others need suctioning access and do not require an open cannula at all times. Assessment of the pulmonary status may allow for a one-way speaking valve to be worn to facilitate vocal communication when a complete plug might compromise the airway.

Some inner cannulas have closed tips and some plugs or caps are inserted over the proximal end of the tracheostomy tube. All patients must be carefully monitored in the beginning phase of occlusion and must be able to remove the cap when required.

TRACHEOSTOMY TUBE TYPES

Metal Tubes

The Tucker, Jackson, Holinger, and Engstrom tubes are examples of metal tracheostomy tubes (Figures 3-19 and 3-20). Metal tubes are made of stainless steel or sterling silver, with an inner cannula, outer cannula, and obturator. Although a cuff may be attached to this tube type, they are usually cuffless. Cuffs on a metal tube are detachable and can create complications if the cuff slides off the end of the tube, causing total occlusion of the lumen. These cuffs sometimes exert higher tracheal pressures. Metal tubes come in more sizes than the nonmetal tubes, and it is important to be aware of the differences in sizes when comparing them to other tubes. The metal tubes are used less frequently because they are rigid, have minimal flange adaptability, are heavier on the stoma site, and are heat/cold

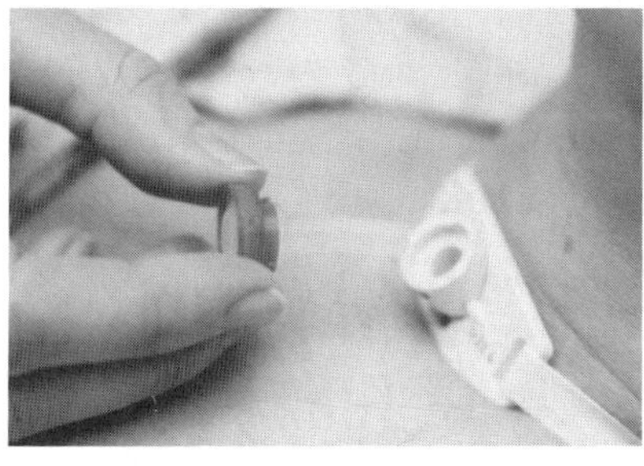

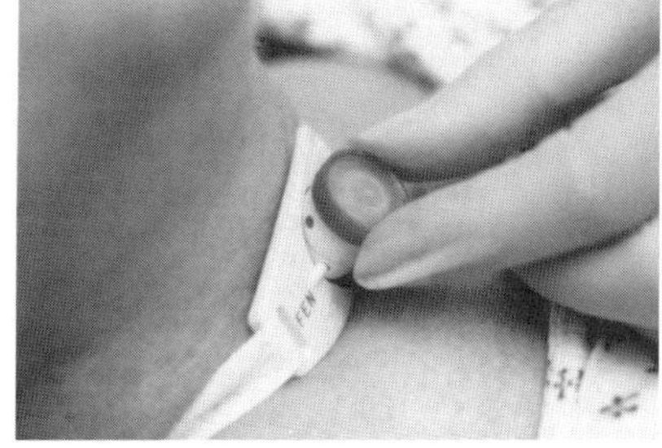

Figure 3-18 Shiley decannulation cap insertion. (Courtesy of Mallinckrodt Medical TPI, Inc. Irvine, CA.)

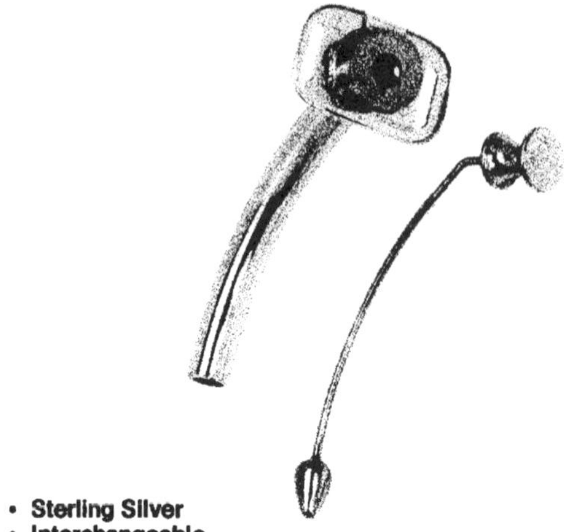

- **Sterling Silver**
- **Interchangeable**

Complete Tube	Size	MM O.D.	MM I.D.	Length	Complete Tube	Size	MM O.D.	MM I.D.	Length
51-2085	000	4.1	2.1	33 mm	**51-2155**	2	6.0	3.3	46 mm
51-2090	000	4.1	2.1	40 mm	**51-2159**	3	7.0	4.4	33 mm
51-2100	00	4.5	2.4	33 mm	**51-2160**	3	7.0	4.4	50 mm
51-2105	00	4.5	2.4	40 mm	**51-2165**	3	7.0	4.4	55 mm
51-2110	00	4.5	2.4	46 mm	**51-2170**	3	7.0	4.4	60 mm
51-2115	0	5.0	2.9	33 mm	**51-2175**	4	8.0	5.3	50 mm
51-2120	0	5.0	2.9	40 mm	**51-2180**	4	8.0	5.3	55 mm
51-2125	0	5.0	2.9	46 mm	**51-2185**	4	8.0	5.3	60 mm
51-2130	1	5.5	3.0	33 mm	**51-2190**	5	9.0	6.1	63 mm
51-2135	1	5.5	3.0	40 mm	**51-2195**	5	9.0	6.1	68 mm
51-2140	1	5.5	3.0	46 mm	**51-2205**	6	10.0	7.1	63 mm
51-2145	2	6.0	3.3	33 mm	**51-2210**	6	10.0	7.1	68 mm
51-2150	2	6.0	3.3	40 mm	**51-2215**	6	10.0	7.1	73 mm

Figure 3-19 Holinger tracheostomy tube. (Courtesy of Pilling, Fort Washington, PA.)

reactive. These tubes are more likely to cause pressure necrosis, increased patient discomfort and skin irritation, and stimulate mucus production in some patients.[44] Skin irritation may be caused by the oxidation that takes place when the tube is exposed to air. These tubes often do not have a 15 mm hub and require a separate adapter; therefore, manual resuscitation can be difficult in an emergency. An intubation adapter, also known as a 15 mm OD endotracheal or anesthesia adapter, can be used to create the 15 mm OD hub. These are inserted into the tracheostomy cannula but will narrow the lumen at the insertion site.

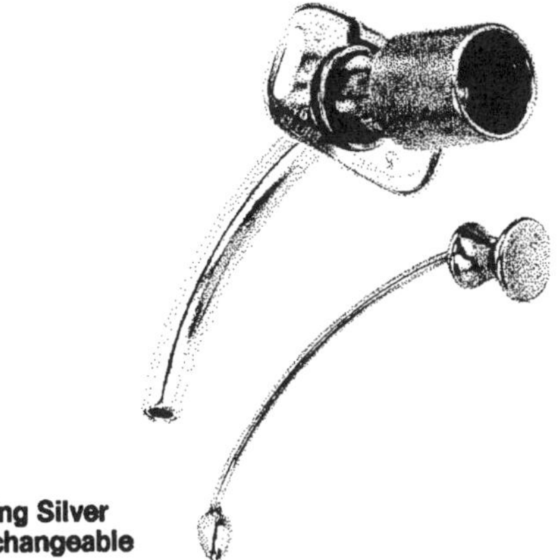

Complete Tube	Size	MM O.D.	MM I.D.	Length	Complete Tube	Size	MM O.D.	MM I.D.	Length
51-2086	000	4.1	2.1	33 mm	**51-2136**	1	5.5	3.0	40 mm
51-2091	000	4.1	2.1	40 mm	**51-2141**	1	5.5	3.0	46 mm
51-2096	000	4.1	2.1	46 mm	**51-2146**	2	6.0	3.3	33 mm
51-2101	00	4.5	2.4	33 mm	**51-2151**	2	6.0	3.3	40 mm
51-2106	00	4.5	2.4	40 mm	**51-2156**	2	6.0	3.3	46 mm
51-2111	00	4.5	2.4	46 mm	**51-2161**	3	7.0	4.4	50 mm
51-2116	0	5.0	2.9	33 mm	**51-2166**	3	7.0	4.4	55 mm
51-2121	0	5.0	2.9	40 mm	**51-2176**	4	8.0	5.3	50 mm
51-2126	0	5.0	2.9	46 mm	**51-2181**	4	8.0	5.3	55 mm
51-2131	1	5.5	3.0	33 mm	**51-2186**	4	8.0	5.3	60 mm

Figure 3-20 Holinger tracheostomy tube with 15 mm adapter. (Courtesy of Pilling, Fort Washington, PA.)

Tracheostomy tube manufacturers in the United States are:

Metal

Pilling
420 Delaware Drive
Ft. Washington, PA. 19034
(215) 643-2600

Dittmar
101 E. Laurel Avenue
Cheltenham, PA. 19012
(800) 523-0850

Gilbert Surgical Instruments
115 Harding Avenue
Bellmauer, NY 08031
(809) 933-2770

Storz
3365 Tree Court Industrial Boulevard
St. Louis, MO. 63122
(800) 325-9500

Disposable

Shiley Tracheostomy Tubes
Mallinckrodt Medical TPI, Inc.
17600 Gillette Avenue
Irvine, CA 92713-9503
(714) 250-0500

Concord/Portex, division of
Smith's Industries
Medical Systems
15 Kit Street
Keene, NH 03431
(603) 352-3812

COMMUNItrach
Spectrum Medical of California
27 Summerwind
Irvine, CA 92714
(714) 551-6610

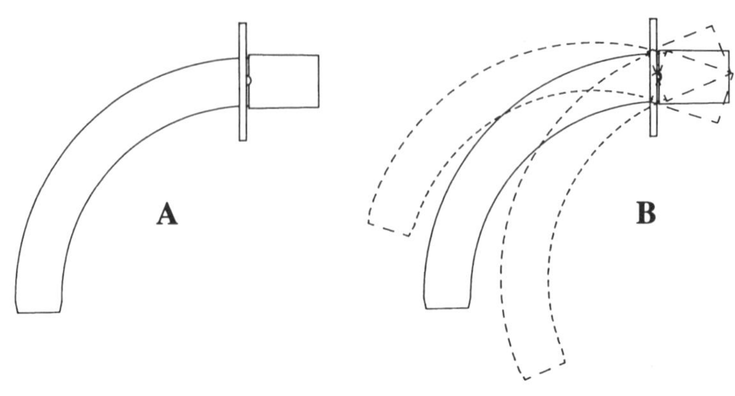

Figure 3-21 ***A****, Metal tracheostomy tubes are rigid.* ***B****, Plastic tracheostomy tubes are flexible to accommodate patient movement.*

Disposable Tracheostomy Tubes

Most other tube types are made with a medical-grade polyvinyl chloride (PVC) that is nontoxic. These are lightweight disposable tubes that are flexible and soften at body temperature (Figure 3-21 B). The most widely used disposable tubes are manufactured by Mallinckrodt (Shiley) and Concord/Portex (Portex). Both companies have tubes with cuffed and cuffless designs and in adult, pediatric, and neonatal sizes, as well as fenestrated tubes. Tube preference is dependent on the institution, the physician, and the medical needs of the patient (Figures 3-22 and 3-23).

Silicone Tracheostomy Tubes

Silicone tubes† are softer than the more rigid polyvinyl chloride tubes. These tubes are less rigid, often adapting better to the patient's anatomy, physical needs, and percutaneous tracheostomies and are manufactured in a variety of types with various cuffs to meet various patient requirements. Some tracheostomy tubes are wire reinforced to give firmness. Tracheostomy tube companies also manufacture custom-made tracheostomy tubes to meet specific patient requirements.

†This manufacturer refused permission to reference or to reprint photographs of these products.

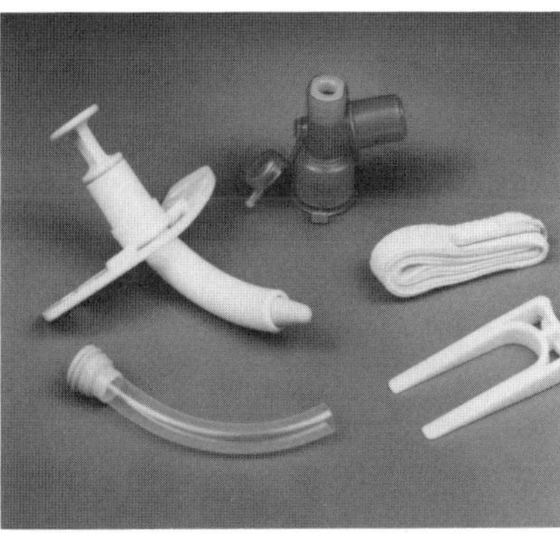

Figure 3-22 Portex disposable cuffless tracheostomy tube. (Courtesy of Concord/ Portex, division of Smith's Industries Medical Systems, Keene, NH.)

Pediatric Tracheostomy Tubes

Pediatric tracheostomy tubes are smaller in size than adult tracheostomy tubes and traditionally are cuffless. Recently, there has been the addition of a pediatric tracheostomy tube line that has cuffed and uncuffed silicone tubes. Cuffless tubes have been used because pediatric airways are small and a cuff has not been necessary for ventilatory purposes. This sometimes necessitates using a larger tube in relation to the diameter of the trachea of a child. In addition, cuffless tubes were not used in order to avoid the risk of tracheal damage from cuff inflation. The paradox of these issues can involve the placement of a large-size pediatric tracheostomy tube to seal the airway for ventilation, which may contribute to undue trauma to delicate pediatric airway mucosa, thus increasing the risk of tracheal stenosis, fistula, and malacia in the pediatric population. The introduction of cuffed tracheostomy tubes is an attempt to use cuff inflation to seal the lower airway for ventilatory control. Extreme care should be taken, and the use of cuff pressure manometry should be used to assist in the prevention of overinflation of the tracheostomy tube cuff and resulting airway trauma.

Pediatric tracheostomy tubes have a sharper angle and a shorter length than adult tubes, which is more compatible to the pediatric anatomy. Flange designs usually allow for short necks and a lower

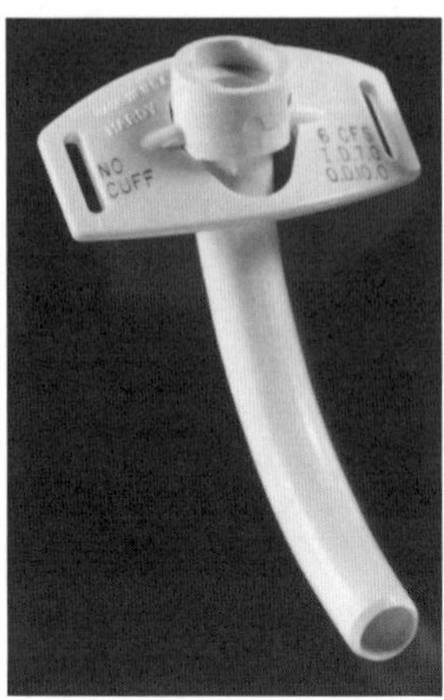

Size	Product Designation	O.D.	I.D.	Length
4	4 CFS	8.5 mm (26 Fr.)	5.0 mm	67 mm
6	6 CFS	10.0 mm (30 Fr.)	7.0 mm	78 mm
8	8 CFS	12.0 mm (36 Fr.)	8.5 mm	84 mm
10	10 CFS	13.0 mm (39 Fr.)	9.0 mm	84 mm
4	4 CFN	8.5 mm (26 Fr.)	5.0 mm	67 mm
6	6 CFN	10.0 mm (30 Fr.)	7.0 mm	78 mm
8	8 CFN	12.0 mm (36 Fr.)	8.5 mm	84 mm
10	10 CFN	13.0 mm (39 Fr.)	9.0 mm	84 mm

Figure 3-23 Shiley cuffless tracheostomy tube. (Courtesy of Mallinckrodt Medical TPI, Inc. Irvine, CA.)

chin point directly above the tracheostomy site. Infants who have soft, fat chins may rest very close to the tracheostomy opening or even occlude it. It is important to ensure that the child's chin does not occlude or obstruct airflow or press the flange downward. That can cause a painful twisting of the tracheostomy tube in the airway and possibly contribute to complications from this movement. It is not always possible to avoid chin proximity, and an extension may be added to the end of the tracheostomy tube to prevent this in the pediatric patient. An extension to the pediatric tube will increase the dead space and the patient should be monitored for signs of CO_2 retention.

Plastic pediatric tubes do not come with inner cannulas for secretion management and will necessitate suctioning with either a bulb syringe or suctioning catheter. Larger metal pediatric tracheostomy tubes come with an inner cannula that can be removed for cleaning. Physicians feel that metal tubes are too rigid to use in delicate pediatric airways, and the use of inner cannulas reduces available airway space for ventilation purposes. Metal tubes may also contribute to innominate artery erosion and tracheoesophageal fistula formation[5] (Figures 3-24 to 3-27).

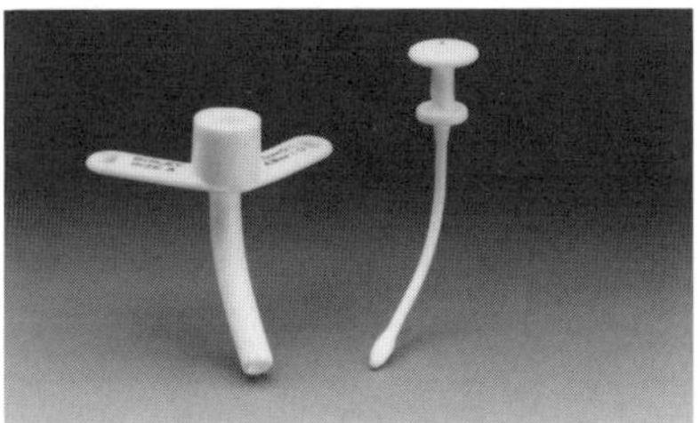

Pediatric Tracheostomy Tubes

Size	Product Designation	O.D.	I.D.	Length
00	00 PT	4.5 mm (14 Fr)	3.1 mm	39 mm
0	0 PT	5.0 mm (15 Fr)	3.4 mm	40 mm
1	1 PT	5.5 mm (17 Fr)	3.7 mm	41 mm
2	2 PT	6.0 mm (18 Fr)	4.1 mm	42 mm
3	3 PT	7.0 mm (21 Fr)	4.8 mm	44 mm
4	4 PT	8.0 mm (24 Fr)	5.5 mm	46 mm

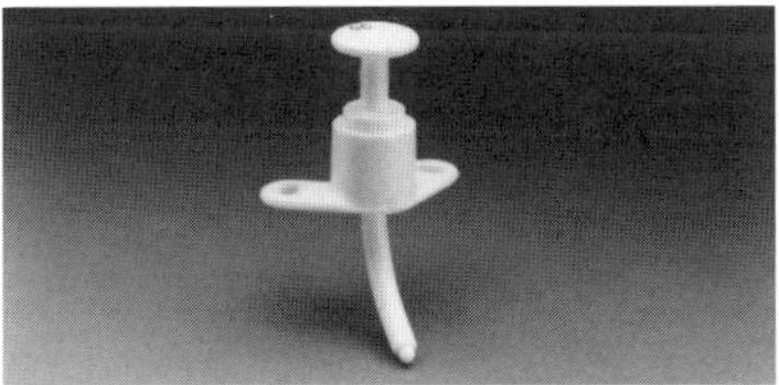

Neonatal Tracheostomy Tubes

Size	Product Designation	O.D.	I.D.	Length
00	00 NT	4.5 mm (14 Fr)	3.1 mm	30 mm
0	0 NT	5.0 mm (15 Fr)	3.4 mm	32 mm
1	1 NT	5.5 mm (17 Fr)	3.7 mm	34 mm

Figure 3-24 Shiley pediatric and neonatal tracheostomy tubes. (Courtesy of Mallinckrodt Medical TPI, Inc. Irvine, CA.)

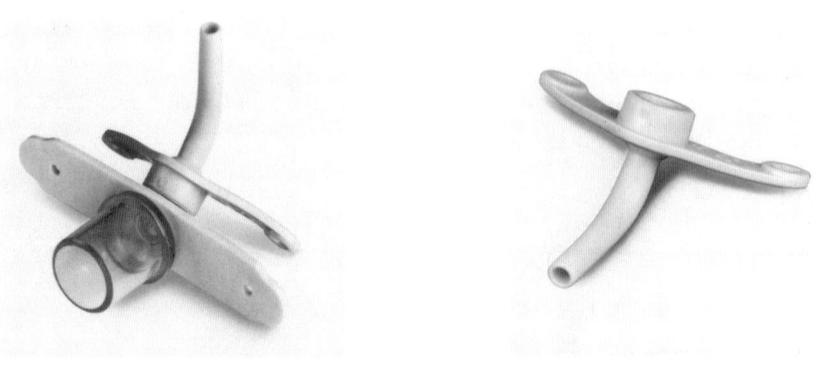

Cat. No	I.D. mm	O.D. mm	(approx.) French	(approx.) Jackson	Length mm	Units Per Case
		O.D. Size Equivalents				
Neonatal Tracheostomy Tubes (with 15mm Connector)						
553025	2.5	4.5	13	00	30	1
553030	3.0	5.2	15	0	32	1
553035	3.5	5.8	16	1	34	1
Neonatal Tracheostomy Tubes (without 15mm Connector)						
554025	2.5	4.5	13	00	30	1
554030	3.0	5.2	15	0	32	1
554035	3.5	5.8	16	1	34	1

Figure 3-25 Neonatal tracheostomy tubes and sizes. (Courtesy of Concord/Portex, division of Smiths Industries Medical Systems, Keene, NH)

Pediatric Tube Placement Considerations

Appropriate airway considerations in pediatric patients are even more crucial than in the adult because length, angle, and outer diameter sizing have a more dramatic impact in more delicate and smaller airways. Pediatric airway management is also more complicated than that of an adult. In addition, pediatric patients are highly reactive to treatment and can degenerate rapidly, making them even more difficult to manage than adults.

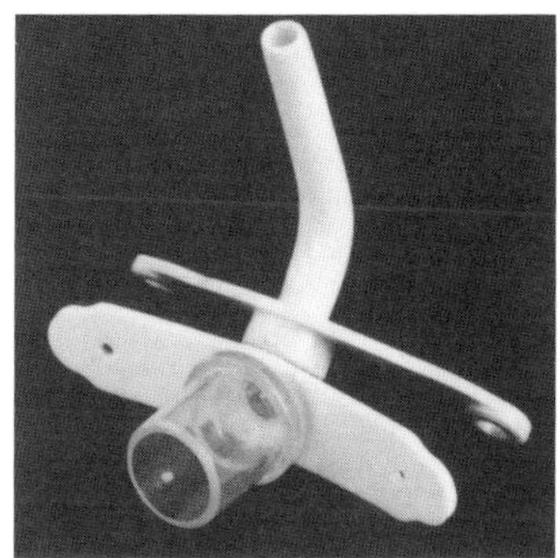

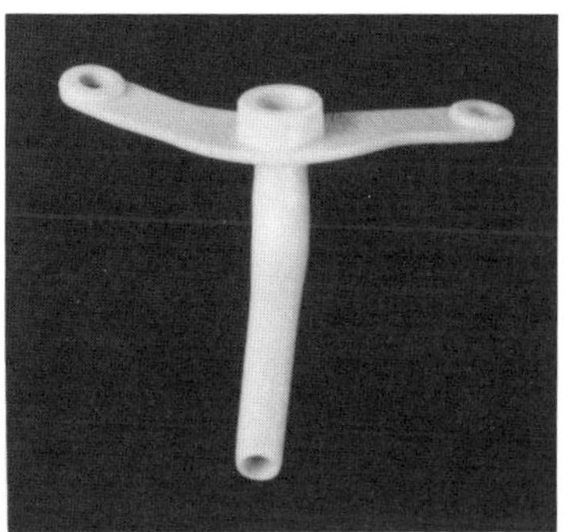

Cat. No	I.D. mm	O.D. mm	(approx.) French	(approx.) Jackson	Length mm	Units Per Case
Pediatric Tracheostomy Tubes (with 15mm Connector)						
555025	2.5	4.5	13	00	30	1
555030	3.0	5.2	15	0	36	1
555035	3.5	5.8	16	1	40	1
555040	4.0	6.5	18	2	44	1
555045	4.5	7.1	19	-	48	1
555050	5.0	7.7	21	3	50	1
555055	5.5	8.3	23	4	52	1
Pediatric Tracheostomy Tubes (without 15mm Connector)						
559025	2.5	4.5	13	00	30	1
559030	3.0	5.2	15	0	36	1
559035	3.5	5.8	16	1	40	1
559040	4.0	6.5	18	2	44	1
559045	4.5	7.1	19	-	48	1
559050	5.0	7.7	21	3	50	1
559055	5.5	8.3	23	4	52	1

Figure 3-26 Pediatric tracheostomy tubes and sizes. (Courtesy of Concord/ Portex, division of Smiths Industries Medical Systems, Keene, NH.)

Fenestrated Tracheostomy Tubes

A fenestrated tracheostomy tube is designed with a precut opening (fenestration) in the back of the outer cannula (Figures 3-28 to 3-30). The fenestration allows air to pass through the hole, as well as around the tube, and pharynx, directing the flow of air through the larynx and pharynx, permitting airflow for speech. The fenestration allots a larger space for respiration, that is, air is passed not only around the tracheostomy tube but through it as well. (The inner cannula is removed.) A cap can be applied to the outer cannula, avoiding finger closure. All staff must be alerted to the fact that the

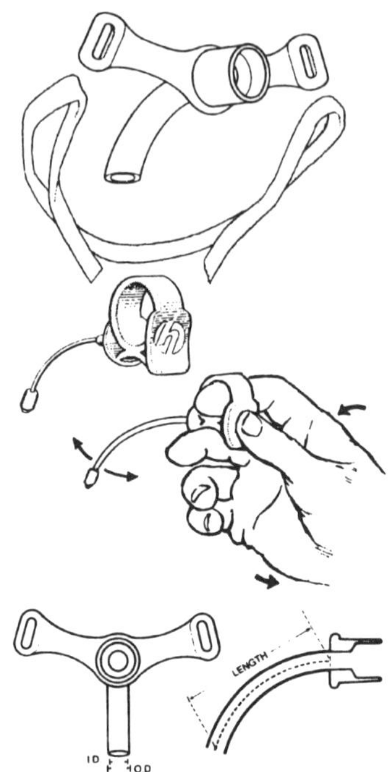

Pediatric Tracheostomy Tube

CODE NO.	I.D. mm	O.D. mm	LENGTH mm	LENGTH JACKSON	JACKSON SIZE APPROX.
20025	2.5	3.6	32		—
20030	3.0	4.3	36	33	00
20035	3.5	5.0	40	36 or 38	0
20040	4.0	5.6	44	40 or 44	1
20045	4.5	6.3	48	44 or 51	2
20050	5.0	7.0	50	52 or 62	3
20055	5.5	7.6	55	52 or 62	4
20060	6.0	8.4	62	56 or 68	5

Neonate Tracheostomy Tube

CODE NO.	I.D. mm	O.D. mm	LENGTH mm	JACKSON SIZE APPROX.
10025	2.5	3.6	30	—
10030	3.0	4.3	32	00
10035	3.5	5.0	34	0
10040	4.0	5.6	36	1

Figure 3-27 Hood pediatric tracheostomy tubes. (Courtesy of Hood Laboratories, Pembroke, MA.)

cuff must be completely deflated or the entire airway could be obstructed. If the cuff is inflated and only the fenestration is open for respiration, the airway may be compromised to the size of the fenestration, which is too small for most adults.

If a fenestrated tube is used when a patient is aspirating, the aspirated material also uses the fenestration to enter the lungs. The primary use for this tube is for weaning and decannulation as well as for speech. It is not well tolerated by all patients, and a speaking valve could be considered at this time. All patients must be carefully monitored as this process is initiated.

There have been several concerns associated with the use of the fenestrated tubes. Fenestration holes are precut and they do not necessarily align well with the tracheal lumen of some patients. The

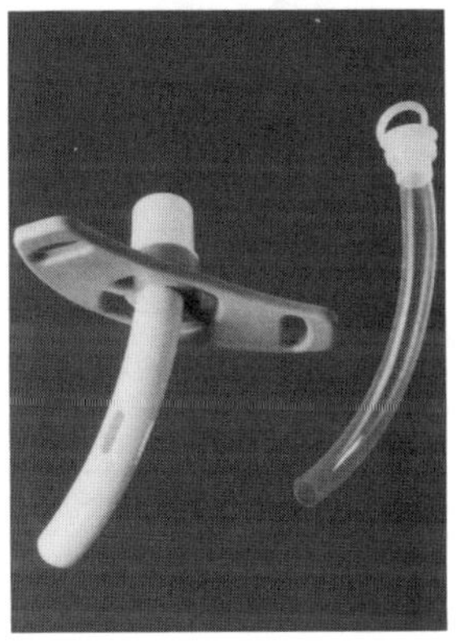

Uncuffed Fenestrated Tracheostomy Tube-D.I.C.			
Reorder No.	I.D. mm	O.D. mm	Length mm
512060	6.0	8.5	67
512070	7.0	9.9	73
512080	8.0	11.3	78
512090	9.0	12.6	84
512100	10.0	14.0	84

Figure 3-28 Concord/Portex fenestrated tracheostomy tube. (Courtesy of Concord/ Portex, division of Smiths Industries Medical Systems, Keene, NH.)

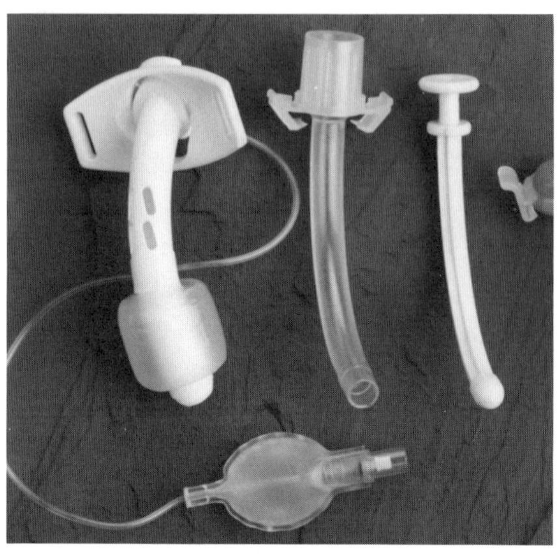

Disposable Cannula Fenestrated Low Pressure Cuffed Tracheostomy Tube

Size	Product Designation	O.D.	I.D.	Length
4	4 DFEN	8.5 mm (26 Fr.)	5.0 mm	67 mm
6	6 DFEN	10.0 mm (30 Fr.)	7.0 mm	78 mm
8	8 DFEN	12.0 mm (36 Fr.)	8.5 mm	84 mm
10	10 DFEN	13.0 mm (39 Fr.)	9.0 mm	84 mm

One sterile Disposable Decannulation Plug (DDCP) is supplied with each DFEN. Additional DDCPs (universal size) can be ordered in cartons of 10.

Figure 3-29 Shiley cuffed fenestrated tracheostomy tube. (Courtesy of Mallinckrodt Medical TPI, Inc. Irvine, CA.)

improper alignment may cause difficulties with irritation of the tracheal mucosa, and the fenestration may become blocked by tissue growth. This tissue growth (granulation tissue) can obstruct the lumen of the outer cannula, and the inner cannula cannot be inserted. There are reports of the fenestrations becoming blocked with secretions and granuloma tissue, therefore defeating the purpose of the fenestration. Siddharth and Mazzarella conclude from their 1985 study of patients with fenestrated tubes, "The insertion of a fenestrated tube was the direct cause of the excessive amount of granuloma that caused

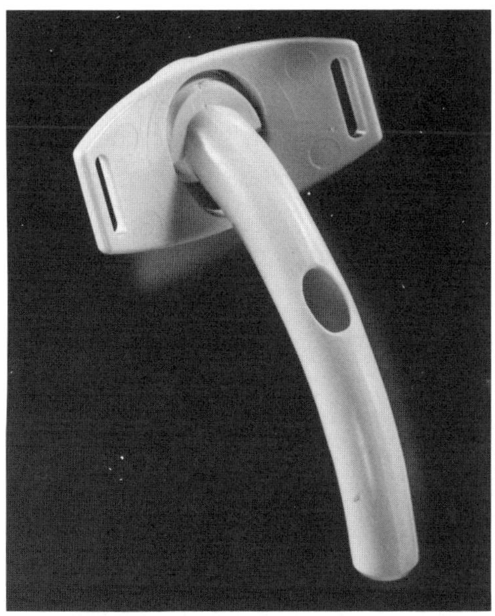

Size	Product Designation	O.D.	I.D.	Length
4	4 CFS	8.5 mm (26 Fr.)	5.0 mm	67 mm
6	6 CFS	10.0 mm (30 Fr.)	7.0 mm	78 mm
8	8 CFS	12.0 mm (36 Fr.)	8.5 mm	84 mm
10	10 CFS	13.0 mm (39 Fr.)	9.0 mm	84 mm
4	4 CFN	8.5 mm (26 Fr.)	5.0 mm	67 mm
6	6 CFN	10.0 mm (30 Fr.)	7.0 mm	78 mm
8	8 CFN	12.0 mm (36 Fr.)	8.5 mm	84 mm
10	10 CFN	13.0 mm (39 Fr.)	9.0 mm	84 mm

Figure 3-30 Shiley cuffless fenestrated tracheostomy tube. (Courtesy of Mallinckrodt Medical TPI, Inc. Irvine, CA.)

tracheal obstruction."[45] Tracheostomy manufacturers will supply made-to-order tubes if the measurement to the mid-trachea is determined.

Talking Tracheostomy Tubes

"Talking" tracheostomy tubes have been in use for many years. The tube is manufactured to allow for ventilation and the ability to speak. Because the cuff occludes the trachea and air does not pass through the vocal cords, the patient remains aphonic. The talking tracheostomy tube provides an outlet located above the cuff, where an artificial air source may be attached to provide a volume of humidified air for vocalization. Patients must be able to deliver some effort and also to mouth words clearly for the mechanism to work successfully. The speech-language pathologist's role of assessing the achievement of speech with this device is vital. He or she can evaluate the patient's ability and motivation required to produce speech and to assist the patient during its use. Talking tracheostomy tubes are discussed more fully in Chapter 7.

Tracheostomy Tubes vs. Laryngectomy Tubes

Laryngectomy tubes are designed for patients whose larynx has been removed. The laryngectomy procedure results in the trachea being rerouted directly out of the stoma site with no access to the upper airway. Due to this anatomical change, laryngectomy tubes are cuffless and shorter in length than tracheostomy tubes (Figure 3-31). Laryngectomy tubes are manufactured in similar types of materials as tracheostomy tubes, including metal, plastic, nylon, and silicone. Laryngectomy tubes cannot be used with tracheostomized individuals because the length needed to traverse tissue from the stoma site to the trachea is insufficient in most individuals.

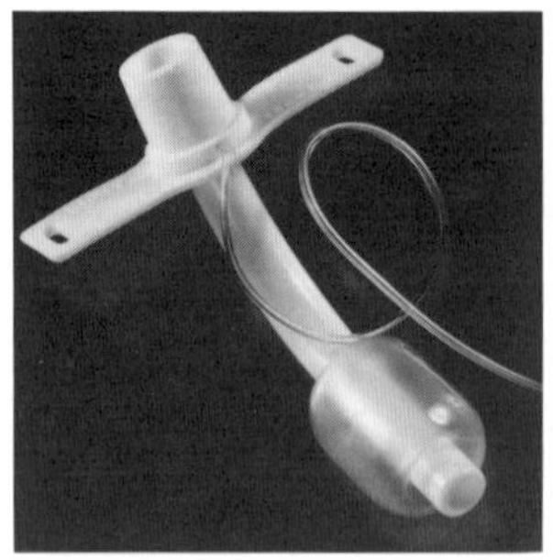

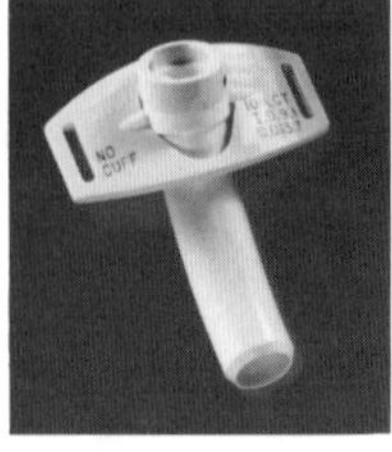

Figure 3-31 Comparison of sizes between tracheostomy tube on the left and laryngectomy tube on the right. (Courtesy of Mallinckrodt Medical TPI, Inc. Irvine, CA.)

TRACHEOSTOMY SUCTIONING

Suctioning is a necessary and very important part of the care of the tracheostomized patient. Suctioning is performed by authorized personnel only (e.g., respiratory therapists and nurses). It is a procedure used to remove secretions from the lower and upper airways.

The oral cavity can be cleared of mucus by inserting a suction catheter or a "Yankauer" suction tip into the patient's mouth, going along the side(s) of the tongue to prevent gagging and into the oral pharynx to remove accumulated mucus and saliva from above the larynx. The area is not sterile, and the same suction catheter should not then be used in the trachea.

If the patient is alert, he or she should be instructed about the procedure. The person suctioning should observe appropriate aseptic technique and wear gloves and other appropriate protective "barriers."

The patient's lungs are often first hyperoxygenated using a manual resuscitation device that delivers oxygen and is connected to the tracheal hub. After washing one's hands, the sterile suction catheter should be opened and gloves applied. This equipment often comes as a kit. The catheter is then attached to the tubing of the suction machine and introduced into the patient's tracheostomy tube, inserting until the patient coughs or an obstruction is felt. One method that is used is to cover the control port of the catheter with the suctioner's thumb to initiate the suctioning process. The thumb is then released and the catheter withdrawn slightly. Suction is applied again for a few seconds and released. This is repeated until the catheter is removed. The patient is then reoxygenated and the suctioning procedure is repeated, if needed. The entire suctioning procedure is not recommended for longer that 15 to 20 seconds, and appropriately sized catheters are recommended. The catheter should then be discarded. The patient's head can be turned to attempt to clear both the right and left mainstem bronchi. Suctioning protocols vary extensively in each facility. Many institutions practice other regular pulmonary exercises for lung clearance to substitute for or accompany suctioning, (e.g., manual cough, assisted cough, or IPPV treatments).

SUCTIONING COMPLICATIONS

Hypoxemia is a serious concern when suctioning because oxygen as well as secretions are evacuated from the airway. In a ventilated patient, the loss of PEEP (positive end expiratory pressure) is an additional complication that causes hypoxemia.

Another side effect of suctioning is cardiac dysrhythmia because stimulation of the carina or bronchi can inhibit cardiac activity and may provoke dysrhythmias. Atelectasis during suctioning occurs when portions of the lung are completely evacuated, causing alveolar collapse.

Pneumonia can be caused when suctioning catheters introduce bacteria into the patient's lower airway. The risk of contamination occurs with each suctioning, increasing the possibility of infection to the patient. Excessive coughing, severe bronchospasm, and laryngospasm during suctioning can be fatiguing, painful, and traumatic for the patient. Increased intrathoracic pressures sufficient to fracture ribs and cause soreness of intercostal and abdominal muscles can occur. Bronchoconstriction and airway resistance may increase due to the direct mechanical stimulation of the respiratory mucosa by the suction catheter.

DECANNULATION

Once the patient has sufficiently recovered from the respiratory insult and has an adequate airway, decannulation (removal of the tracheostomy tube) can be considered (Table 3-3). Before removal of the tracheostomy tube, the primary and possibly secondary reasons for the tracheostomy tube placement should be reviewed. These might include a patient who has a primary problem of airway protection, secondary to vocal cord paralysis in an abducted position or surgical removal of glottal structures. The speech-language pathologist's assessment of the patient's ability to manage secretions and avoid aspiration provides a major contribution to the decision to decannulate. This may involve teaching new swallowing techniques, and the patient must exhibit the required skill before the tube is removed.

1. Diagnoses necessitating tracheostomy placement significantly improved
2. Airway sufficiently patent
3. Ability to respirate adequately
4. Appropriate vocal cord function or lack of aspiration
5. Ability to handle secretions

Table 3-3 General Decannulation Guidelines.

There are various techniques utilized to achieve decannulation (Table 3-4). Downsizing of the tracheostomy tube is often used as a weaning method. That is, the patient gradually has smaller and smaller-sized tracheostomy tubes placed. With each smaller tracheostomy tube placement, the patient's respiratory status is re-evaluated until the tube is finally removed. Decannulation is indicated when auscultation of the chest emits clear breath sounds and mucus is manageable and free of infection. The patient should also be able to carry out activities of daily living without shortness of breath. Sometimes a laryngoscopy or bronchoscopy will be performed before the removal of the tracheostomy tube to inspect for the integrity of the anatomy as well as the movement of the vocal cords. Examination of the lower respiratory tract might be required if the patient is having trouble during the decannulation process. Many times the examination of arterial blood gases as well as spirometry are utilized.

Other decannulation methods might include the use of cuffless tubes, capping, a fenestrated tube, and a one-way speaking valve.

1. Cap or plugged inner cannula
2. Fenestrated tube with cap
3. Downsizing of tracheostomy tube
4. One-way valve usage
5. Cuffless tube use

Table 3-4 Decannulation techniques.

Upper airway usage and functions may be assisted with the use of one-way speaking valves that will assist in airway patency assessment as exhaled volumes can now be measured. The process of decannulation may be of long or short duration, according to the patient's needs. Both metal and plastic tracheostomy tubes may be used for decannulation purposes simply because they are cuffless and more air can pass around the tube during inhalation and exhalation. Fenestrated tubes allow air through and around the tube as previously discussed. Plugging an uncuffed tube forces the air around the tube only and, if well tolerated, is a sure signal that the patient's condition allows removal of the tube.

Stenosis at the stoma or at the site of the cuff as well as tracheomalacia are complications that can be noted at the time of decannulation. When a tracheostomy tube is removed, stenotic tissue flaps or the softened tracheal wall may remain, obstructing the airway that the tracheostomy tube had been stenting open. Recannulation is necessary to avoid airway compromise. Stenosis can occur at a much later date, months or even years later.

Particularly with children, careful preparations must be made before decannulation can take place. Sometimes there is a psychological dependence on the tube, and education and counseling must precede removal of the tube. Because of the small airway, decannulation almost always takes place in a hospital setting. Careful monitoring of the airway must be done, distress noted immediately. Reinsertion of the tracheostomy tube or even intubation of the child may be necessary. The child is usually observed for 24 to 48 hours following removal of the tube.

TRACHEOSTOMY CARE

The care of the tracheostomy tube and adjacent skin, stoma care, humidification, pulmonary cleaning technique (pulmonary toilet), and other related procedures vary widely. Some basic principles apply.

The most important aspect is to maintain a clear patent airway for adequate respiratory function. Clearing secretions by suctioning or by other proven techniques is a high priority and is performed only by authorized personnel. A routine schedule for clearing the tracheostomy tube is usually provided as a baseline of care, and the frequency is then increased according to the patient's demands. If an inner cannula is in place, it should also be cleaned or replaced at regular intervals.

Humidification is also a major requirement. Moisture and often oxygen are provided via the ventilator tubing or by an appliance that hooks or attaches to the tracheostomy tube. Extra saline solution is often instilled during suctioning or when required. Ambulatory patients may instill saline at regular intervals to moisten the area when they are not wearing a tracheostomy mask over the lumen of the tube. Dryness, crusting, coughing, and sometimes bleeding are symptoms of the area being too dry.

The tube must be secured snugly to the neck. If the tube is loose, the risk of inadvertent decannulation is high. The tube might also slip into the pretracheal tissues. Loose tubes also can be the cause of granulation tissue formation and stomal stenosis from the constant movement in and out and side to side. Many devices are used to keep the tube secured in its opening.

Clean, dry skin and stoma are important to prevent inflammation and infection of the tissues around the tracheostomy tube. At times, the application of antibiotic ointment to these areas is necessary.

Often dressings of various types are inserted between the tracheostomy tube flange and the skin. This provides a cushion of comfort and acts as a wick to absorb the drainage from around the tracheostomy tube.

Orderly, routine, and careful management of patients with tracheostomies will decrease the risk and possible complications that can occur.

REFERENCES

1. Frost, E.A.M., "Tracing the tracheostomy." *Ann Otol*, 1976; 85:618-624.

2. Mclelland, R.M.S., *Progress in Anesthesiology*, Proceedings of the 4th World Congress of Anesthesiologists, Amsterdam: Excerpta Medica, 1970; pp.195-196.

3. Wright, J., *A History of Laryngology and Rhinology*, 2nd Edition, Philadelphia: Lea & Febiger, 1914; pp. 23, 29.

4. Gordan, B.L., *The Romance of Medicine*, Philadelphia: F.A. Davis, 1947; p. 461.

5. Meyers, E.N., and Stoal, S.E., *Tracheotomy*, New York: Churchill Livingstone, 1985; pp. 1-12.

6. Lyons, A.S., and Petruceli, R.J., *Medicine: An Illustrated History*, New York: Harry N. Abrams Inc., 1978.

7. Goodall, E.W., "The story of tracheotomy." *Br J Child Dis*, 1934; 31:167-253.

8. Galen, *Introductio Seu Medicus*, Kohn, C.G., (trans), Leipzig, 1827; 14:743.

9. Aretaeus, *The Therapeutics of Acute Diseases*, Adam, F., (trans), London: The Sydenham Society, 1856; Chap. 7, p. 406.

10. McKenzie, M., *Diseases of the Pharynx, Larynx, and Trachea,* New York: W. Wood and Co., 1880; p. 397.

11. Vesalius, A., *De Humani Corporis Fabricia Libri Septem*, Basel: Oporinus, 1543; p. 658.

12. Fabricius, H., *Opera Chirurgica*, Vol VI, Frankfurt, 1660; Para 1, Cap. 44, p. 155.

13. Bonetus, T., *Sepulchetum Sive Anatomica Practica*, T.I. Lib. 2 De Respiratione Laesa, Obs. I, Geneva: 1700; p. 483.

14. Heister, L., *General System of Surgery*, 8th Edition, London: 1768; 8:52.

15. Louis, M., *Memoire sur la Bronchotomie,* Presented before the Royal Academy of Surgery, Paris: April 1759.

16. Sharp, J., *A Treatise of the Operations of Surgery*, 4th Edition, London: 1761; p. 187.

17. Van Swieten, G., *Commentar in Herniann Boerharii Aphorism*, Aph 813, 1741: 42.

18. Martin, G., "Philosophical Trans," cited by McKenzie, M., *Diseases of the Pharynx, Larynx, and Trachea*, New York: W. Wood and Co., 1880; 6:398.

19. Herholdt, J.D., and Rafn, C.E., *Life Saving Measures for Drowning Persons*, Copenhagen: H. Tikiob, 1796; p. 52.

20. Biehat, C., *The Surgical Works, or State of the Doctrine and Practice of P.J. Desault*, Vol 1, Philadelphia: Thos Dolson, 1814; pp. 299-234.

21. Favier, M., *Memoires de l'Academic Royale de Chirurgie*, T.V., Paris: 1819; p. 356.

22. Home, F., *An Enquiry into the Natural Causes and Cure of Croup*, Edinburgh: Kincaid and Bell, 1765.

23. Bretonneau, P., *Des Inflammations Speciales du Tissu Muquex et en Particulier de la Diphterite, ou Inflammation Pelliculaire, Connue - Sous le Nom de Croup, d'Angine Maligne, d'Angine Gangreneuse, etc.*, Paris: Crevot,1826.

24. Trousseau, A., *Lectures on Clinical Medicine*, Vol. 2, Cormack, J.R., (trans), London: The New Sydenham Society, 1869; p. 598.

25. Billroth, Luecke H., *Deutsche Chirurgie; Die Tracheotomie, Laryngotomie und Extirpation des Kehlkopfes*, Stuttgart: 1880.

26. Conway, E., "On tracheotomy in croup." *Edinburgh Med J*, January and May, 1860.

27. Erichsen J.E., *The Science and Art of Surgery*, Philadelphia: Henry C. Lea,1869; p. 919.

28. Norton, A.H., *A Text Book of Operative Surgery and Surgical Anatomy*, London: Long, Bailliere, Tindall and Cox, 1886.

29. Jackson, C., and Jackson, C.L., *The Larynx and Its Diseases*, Philadelphia: W.B. Saunders Co., 1937.

30. Jackson, C., "High tracheotomy and other errors -- The chief causes of chronic laryngeal stenosis." *Surg Gynecol Obstet*, 1923; 32:392.

31. Wilson, J.L., "Acute anterior poliomelitis treatment of bulbar and high spinal types." *N England J Med*, 1932; 206:887.

32. Galloway, T.C., "Tracheotomy bulbar poliomyelitis." *JAMA*, 1943; 23:1096.

33. Hazard, P., et al., "Comparative clinical trial of standard operative tracheostomy with percutaneous tracheostomy." *Critical Care Medicine*, 1991; 8.

34. Seldinger, S.I., "Catheter replacement of the needle in percutaneous arteriography: A new technique." *Critical Care, Acta Radiol*, 1953; 39:368.

35. Schachner, A., Ovil, J., Sidi, J., et al., "Rapid percutaneous tracheostomy." IL: The American College of Chest Physicians, 1992; 102:4.

36. Bergbom-Engberg, I., and Haljamae, H., "Assessment of patients' experience of discomforts during respirator therapy." *Critical Care, Acta Radiol*, 1989; 1069-1072.

37. Nash, M., "Swallowing problems in the tracheostomized patient." *Otolaryngolic Clinics of North America,* Vol. 21 (4), 1988.

38. Leverment, J.N., Pearson, F.G., and Rae, S., "A manometric study of the upper esophagus in the dog following cuffed tracheostomy tube." *Br J Anaesth*, 1976; 48:83-89.

39. Sasaki, C.T., Suzuki, M., Horiuchi, M., et al., "The effect of tracheostomy on the laryngeal closure reflex." *Laryngoscope*, 1977; 87:1428-1433.

40. Scott, M., et al., "Modified barium swallow." *Videofluoroscopy*, 1992.

41. Ferris, B.G., Mead, J., and Opie, L.H., "Partitioning of respiratory flow resistance in man." *J Appl Physiol*, 1964; 19:653.

42. Sorli, J., Grassino, A., Lorange, G., et al., "Control of breathing in patients with chronic obstructive lung disease." *Clin Sci Molecular Med*, 1978; 54:295.

43. Bach, J.R., and Alba, A.S., "Tracheotomy ventilation." *Chest*, 1990; 97:679-683.

44. Caldwell, S., and Sullivan, K., "Artificial airways." In Burton, G., and Hodgkin, J., (Eds.), *Respiratory Care - A Guide to Clinical Practice*, 2nd Edition, Philadelphia: J.B. Lippincott Co., 1984.

45. Siddharth, P., and Mazzarella, L., "Granuloma associated with fenestrated tracheostomy tubes." *Am J Surg*, 1985; 150:279-280.

46. Light, R.W., Aten, J.L., et al., "Decannulation procedures for patients with chronic tracheostomies."*Chest*, 1989; 96:257s.

BIBLIOGRAPHY

Downes, J.J., and Schreiner, M.S., "Tracheostomy Tubes and Attachments in Infants and Children." *International Anesthesiology Clinics*, 23:4, 1985.

Feldman, S.A., and Crawley, B.E., *Tracheostomy and Artificial Ventilation in the Treatment of Respiratory Failure*, 2nd Edition, Baltimore: Williams & Wilkins, 1872; p. 20.

Fowler, S.M., Simon, B.M., and Handler, S.D., "Communication development in children." In *Tracheotomy*, New York: Churchill Livingstone, 1985: 271-284.

Goldstein, M.A., *The Laryngoscope*, St. Louis: Tindall & Cox, Vol XIX, Jan.-Dec., 1909.

Goodall, E.W., "The story of tracheostomy." *Br J Child Dis*, 1934; 31:12-176.

Heffner, J.E., "Managing difficult intubations in critically ill patients." *Respiratory Management,* 1989; 19(3): 53-55.

Hutchinson, R.C., and Mitchell, R.D., "Life-threatening complications from percutaneous dilation tracheostomy." *Critical Care Medicine*, January, 1991, Vol. 19, No. 1, p. 118-120.

Jackson, C., and Jackson, C.L., *The Larynx and Its Diseases*, Philadelphia: W.B. Saunders Co., 1937.

Kersten, L.D., *Comprehensive Respiratory Nursing*, Philadelphia: W.B. Saunders Co., 1989.

Koltai, P.J., and Nixon, R.E., "The story of the laryngoscope." *Ear Nose and Throat Journal*, 1989; 68:494-500.

Kozak, L.J., Norton, C., et al., "Hospital use patterns for children in the United States." *Pediatrics*, 1987; 80:481-490.

Lim, R.A., Salem, M.R., and Davis, G., "Airway obstruction with a fenestrated tracheostomy tube." *Anesthesiology*, 1979; 50:72-73.

Lyons, A.S., and Petrucelli, J.R., *Medicine: An Illustrated History,* New York: Harry N. Abrams, Inc., 1978.

McKenzie, M., *Disease of the Pharynx, Larynx, and Trachea*, New York: William Wood and Co., 1880.

Mayo, W.J., Ochsner, A.J., et al., *Surgery, Gynecology and Obstetrics*, Michigan: The Surgical Publishing Company of Chicago, January-June 1921:32.

Murphy, D.A., and Popkin, J., "Tracheal collapse in tracheostomized infants: Resistance by reference to flow rates in a variety of tracheostomy tubes." *Journal of Pediatric Surgery*, 1971; 6:314-322.

Sinfield, A., DiVito, J., and Brandstetter, R.D., "Airway obstruction from over inflation and herniation of tracheostomy tube balloon." *Heart and Lung*, 1989; 18:260-262.

Tepas, J.J., Heroy, J.H., Shermeta, D.W., and Haller, D.W., "Tracheostomy in neonates and small infants: Problems and pitfalls." *Surgery*, 1981; 89:635-639.

Trousseau, A., "Lecture XX: Diphtheria: Tracheotomy, lectures on clinical medicine." Cormack , J.R., (trans), London: The New Sydenham Society, 1869; 2:594-617.

Trousseau, A., "Lectures XX: Diphtheria: Treatment of diphtheria and croup, lectures on clinical medicine." Cormack, J.R., (trans), London: New Sydenham Society, 1869; 2:569-593.

CHAPTER IV

RESPIRATORY CARE

Mary F. Mason, *M.S., C.C.C.-SLP*

Jo Ann Irene Frey, *B.S.N., R.N., C., C.R.R.N.*
Pulmonary Nurse Clinician
Pulmonary Rehabilitation Coordinator
Pulmonary Rehabilitation, Pulmonary Services
Good Samaritan Hospital
Cincinnati, Ohio

Beverly Fornoff, *B.S., R.R.T.*
R. Adams Cowley Shock Trauma Center
Maryland Institute for Emergency Medical Services Systems
University of Maryland Medical System
Baltimore, Maryland

Edited by:

Anthony Oppenheimer, *M.D., F.A.C.P., F.C.C.P.*
Chief, Pulmonary Medicine
Los Angeles Kaiser Permanente Medical Center
Physician Coordinator of Kaiser Permanente Regional
Ventilator Home Care Program
Associate Professor of Medicine
University of California School of Medicine, Los Angeles
Los Angeles, California

Pope L. Moseley, *M.D., M.S.*
Associate Professor
Department of Internal Medicine
Division of Pulmonary, Critical Care, and Occupational
Medicine and the Department of Exercise Science
University of Iowa
Iowa City, Iowa

INTRODUCTION

This chapter is written to be introductory in nature and to familiarize the speech-language pathologist with the terminology, equipment, and treatment utilized in respiratory and pulmonary medicine.

It is to the benefit of the respiratory-compromised patient and the health care team members to have a basic knowledge as to the function and purpose of each of the disciplines involved in the care of this complex patient.

The information provided in this chapter will assist the speech-language pathologist in building a working relationship with the respiratory team members, which can enhance and expedite the opportunity for early intervention with the intensive care unit and respiratory compromised patients to meet their communication needs. All members of the health care team will benefit from educating other team members as to the function and purpose of their individual contribution. This sharing of knowledge will facilitate the most appropriate diagnosis and treatment for the medically complex patient with a tracheostomy or who is ventilator dependent.

HISTORY OF MECHANICAL VENTILATION

The history of mechanical ventilation can be traced to the 16th century when Wesele Vesalius first gave a detailed account in "de Humani Corporis Fabrica, 1555" of the resuscitation of a sow via tracheotomy. With the placement of a reed, which he blew through, Vesalius was able to observe the resulting respiration.

In the late 1700s, societies for resuscitating drowning victims were organized in Europe. Creative methods of resuscitation included blood letting, fumigation (blowing smoke into the rectum), chest-belly compression, and stimulants.[1] By 1776, the use of fireplace bellows was advocated until complications such as pneumothorax caused this treatment to be discontinued.

The 1800s brought arterial and venous oxygen, carbon dioxide analyses, and spirometry, as well as the identification of the process of oxygen and carbon dioxide transport.[2,3] Intense research in acid-base chemistry took place in the 1920s and 1930s with Werner Forsmann developing the first technique for cardiovascular study by performing the first cardiac catheterization on himself in 1928.[1,4]

The 19th century and early 20th century yielded numerous negative pressure devices. Tanks that could create a negative pressure were developed with a vacuum resulting from the manipulation of an outside device such as a bellows or a motor. Negative pressure within the chamber caused the diaphragm to drop, allowing inspiration to follow. These were the forerunners of negative pressure devices, such as the iron lung.

A negative pressure chamber that enclosed both the patient and the surgeon was used by Sauerbruch for thoracic surgery in 1904.[5] The first portable body respirator to encase the patient's body with his head outside of the chamber was developed by Drinker and Shaw around 1929[6] and became the first iron lung.

The late 19th century also provided research into the use of mechanical ventilation via tracheostomy tube and endotracheal tube. These ventilators were piston driven and delivered positive pressure to facilitate respiration. The term *positive* refers to a pressure gradient higher than normal atmospheric pressure. *Positive* also refers to the act of pushing the air into the lungs. Air is positively pressured or "pushed" into the lungs for inspiration and air is passively exhaled. This technique provided the basis for the development of the positive pressure ventilators.

With World War II, the need to maintain personnel on submarines for extended periods of time and the need to support aviators for high-altitude flying created the stimulus for further research that led to the more sophisticated positive pressure ventilation we use today.[7]

During the 1950s, the need to provide treatment to the staggering number of individuals who had fallen victim to the polio epidemic contributed to advances in artificial ventilation via the widespread use of the iron lung (negative pressure ventilation) and positive pressure ventilators. Positive pressure ventilators became more sophisticated and were able to provide more precise ventilation to patients with severe respiratory failure when negative pressure ventilation did not provide adequate support and an invasive procedure (i.e., a tracheostomy or endotracheal intubation) was required.

By 1960, positive pressure ventilation was widely used in hospitals, thus improving survival rates for patients with respiratory failure. The improving clinical skills of medical professionals increased the successful management of acute and chronic respiratory patients. The practice of respiratory therapy as a separate technical medical specialty began during the 1950s and 1960s.

In 1967, adult respiratory distress syndrome (ARDS) was identified and a treatment was developed that provided ventilation with positive end expiratory pressure (PEEP).[8]

During the 1970s, advances in computer microprocessors used in ventilation equipment contributed to more precise ventilatory control and increased available patient data feedback. This was due to sophisticated breath waveform, volume, and pressure monitoring systems. In addition, an increased number of ventilator modalities and breath types that could be delivered by the ventilator were developed. Also, more alarm options were developed, which contributed to patient safety and the effectiveness of the critical care unit team and increased the survival rates of patients as well as the number of chronic ventilator dependent patients.

The 1980s and 1990s have brought about further evolution in ventilator equipment as computer technologies have continued to enhance the sensitivity and function of these machines. Additional ventilator modalities have become available, such as synchronized intermittent mandatory ventilation (SIMV) and the use of continuous positive airway pressure (CPAP). These modes will be described later in this chapter. Noninvasive continuous patient monitoring techniques such as pulse oximetry and transcutaneous carbon dioxide monitoring also continue to improve and contribute to the increased survival rate with respiratory failure patients.

Rapidly advancing medical technologies and highly trained clinical personnel, combined with an ever-growing and aging population increases the use of sophisticated lifesaving techniques such as mechanical ventilation and contributes to the growing number of acute and chronic ventilator dependent patients.

Some acute care hospitals have developed step-down units or subacute units to care for the chronic ventilator dependent patient. This is due to the highly expensive care and equipment that the intensive care unit or critical care unit patient requires. Higher nurse-to-patient ratios, specialized personnel such as respiratory therapists and specialty nurses, and, of course, the expensive equipment and monitoring techniques provided in the intensive care unit and the cardiac care unit make this type of patient very costly to the hospital. To help contain the high cost of maintaining ventilator dependent patients, subacute units have been developed where patients who need less nursing time and less sophisticated equipment can also receive the concentrated efforts of a team devoted to weaning therapies or long-term rehabilitation training.

The expanding population of patients requiring extremely expensive care has also resulted in a growing number of skilled nursing facilities (SNFs) and subacute specialty hospitals designed and equipped to handle the stable ventilator dependent patient. These facilities require more skilled personnel than a typical nursing home to provide the complicated care and respiratory equipment monitoring that mechanically ventilated patients require. Although the cost of care from these subacute care facilities is substantially less than the cost of acute care hospitals, this type of specialized care does add greatly to cost of care delivered by skilled nursing facilities. Government reimbursement rates (Medicare and Medicaid) may be the primary funding source for these facilities. Federal and state budget policies dictate the future use of these facilities for this patient population.

GOALS OF MECHANICAL VENTILATION

The goal of mechanical ventilation is to temporarily support a patient in respiratory failure. This can occur as a result of respiratory distress, respiratory arrest, drug overdose, alcohol overdose, anesthesia, surgery, or acute trauma. In some cases mechanical ventilation is used to provide long-term support when a patient cannot be weaned from the ventilator.

Mechanical ventilation can reduce the workload or output of other body functions, such as the work of the heart (cardiac function) or kidneys (renal output), or to temporarily rest the respiratory muscles which can become fatigued due to chronic or acute neuromuscular or respiratory conditions.

Mechanical ventilation provides the pulmonary system with the support needed to maintain an adequate level of alveolar ventilation and oxygenation, to restore normal acid base balance and increase oxygen transfer and oxygenation to the body organs and tissues. Normal blood gas values are as follows:

1. Arterial oxygen pressure (PaO_2)
   Normal Range: 80-100 mm Hg

2. Carbon dioxide pressure of arterial blood ($PaCO_2$)
   Normal Range: 35-45 mm Hg

3. pH (acid/base) balance of the body's metabolism
   Normal Range: 7.35-7.45

RENAL SUPPORT

The pH level of the blood is regulated by the renal system. A disorder of the renal system has a direct impact on the acid-base (pH) regulation of the body, and this increases the burden on the respiratory system. Mechanical ventilation may be required in order to support the body in an effort to normalize the pH balance of the blood by the regulation of hydrogen ion and bicarbonate levels.

After these goals have been satisfied, an immediate and ongoing assessment of the viability of weaning the patient from the ventilator (to reduce or eliminate need for ventilator support) must take place to avoid further medical complications caused by mechanical ventilation.

CARDIOPULMONARY RELATIONSHIP

It is a goal of mechanical ventilation to support cardiac function and workload. Cardiac failure often results in a build up of lung fluid that impairs ventilation and oxygenation. As blood flow decreases, perfusion of lungs and gas exchange are directly affected by the performance of the heart. Congestive heart failure results from fluid-filled lungs (pulmonary edema). Respiratory arrest can result as the body ceases to be able to meet its respiration requirements necessitating ventilatory support.

COMPLICATIONS OF MECHANICAL VENTILATION

Infection

Complications from mechanical ventilation can include infection related to endotracheal or tracheal intubation; nosocomial infection from the hospital environment; infection from the patient's own natural upper airway bacteria contaminating lower airways; and infection from improperly maintained ventilator equipment. Infections can be life-threatening, such as sepsis or pneumonia, or chronic, as with pseudomonas, proving difficult to manage and thus further compromising a patient's respiratory system and recovery.

Pneumothorax

Pneumothorax is due to air entering the pleural space between the lung and the chest wall. This results in lung collapse. This condition can lead to difficulty reinflating the lung, resulting in atelectasis (discussed below). This can be caused by ventilator mismanagement. There are many predispositions to pneumothorax such as necrotizing lung pathology, secretion retention, duration of ventilation, peak cycling pressures, mean alveolar pressure, minute ventilation requirement, and positive end-expiratory pressure. Pneumothorax is usually managed by inserting a chest tube to remove the air from the pleural space, helping the lung to reinflate until the cause resolves.

Atelectasis

Atelectasis can be an acute chronic condition where portions of lung alveoli continue to collapse. This is a frequent occurrence in both the pediatric and adult ventilator dependent patient. If lung collapse persists, alveoli become more difficult to reinflate. Sometimes positive end expiratory pressure (PEEP) is used to treat or prevent atelectasis and help keep the alveoli expanded and open.

Bronchopulmonary Dysplasia

Bronchopulmonary dysplasia is a condition that can result from lung injury in infants and neonates, due to mechanical ventilation of under-developed or severely damaged lungs. Alveoli are overinflated, distended, and injured. Fibrosis and loss of normal alveoli impair ventilation.

Oxygen Toxicity

High levels of supplemental oxygen (usually over 60%) can cause lung injury. This is related to the oxygen concentration and the length of time supplemental oxygen is administered (oxygen exposure), as well as to the patient's condition. Oxygen is a substance that can cause severe complications or even death when not appropriately utilized. A different problem can occur when oxygen administration is not monitored carefully and it depresses respiratory drive. This can result in CO_2 elevation and acute respiratory failure.

Acid-Base Balance

The acid-base balance or pH of the blood is normally 7.35 to 7.45. This reflects the body's ability to control the hemodynamic systems as related to chemical metabolic balances, specifically blood gases. This acid/base relationship directly affects the autonomic regulatory ability of the body and can be altered by mechanical ventilation

Acidosis is the excessive acidity of body fluids and is caused by an increase in hydrogen ion concentration as a result of CO_2 retention, which affects the body's acid-base balance, or pH of the blood. This can result from hypoventilation. Respiratory acidosis is caused by respiratory failure, neuromuscular disease, chronic obstructive pulmonary disease or central nervous system depression. Metabolic acidosis is caused by lactic acidosis, ketoacidosis or renal failure.

Alkalosis is the acute reduction of plasma bicarbonate with proportionate reduction in plasma CO_2 levels. Respiratory alkalosis is caused by hypocapnia (decreased CO^2 level in the blood), or by hyperventilation, central nervous system disorders, and anxiety. Alkalosis is caused by hypokalemia (chlorine deficiency in the blood), hypochloremia (extreme calcium deficiency in the blood), vomiting, steroids, or diuretics. This can result when oxygen levels are too low or from hyperventilation due to incorrect ventilator parameters causing hypercapnia. Basically, an imbalance in ventilation can cause an imbalance in acid-base levels, that is, alkalosis can be caused by hyperventilation and acidosis can be caused by hypoventilation.

Respiratory Muscle Fatigue

Inappropriate ventilation rates and modes can result in the fatigue of supportive musculature. This inhibits the patient's spontaneous breath rate, which increases ventilator dependency and inhibits weaning efforts.

Respiratory muscle fatigue can be due to one or more of the following:

Lung or neuromuscular disease
Poor ventilator management that increases work of breathing
Muscle disuse, deconditioning, or atrophy

Barotrauma

The pressure applied during mechanical ventilation can cause lung injury, decreased blood flow, or pneumothorax. The higher the pressures used, and the more underlying disease that is present in the lungs, the more risk of barotrauma. Hyperinflation with air-trapping may cause pressure injury increasing the size of bullae and enlarge alveolar areas, distending into fewer, less efficient, and larger areas for ventilation. Persisting hyperinflation can cause lung rupture and pneumothorax.

Gastric Distention or Vomiting

Air entering the stomach can produce vomiting and increase the risk of aspiration of stomach contents. This is also referred to as *gastric insufflation*. Aspiration into the lungs can cause severe damage from acidic gastric fluids, an aerobic infection, or from an obstructing foreign body.

Decreased Cardiac Output

Mechanical ventilation can be useful in decreasing cardiac output requirements by relieving the respiratory muscle work of breathing. This can decrease a critical burden on an unstable cardiovascular system during severe illness. However, intermittent positive pressure ventilation, (IPPV) also called positive pressure ventilation (PPV) can cause increased intrapulmonary pressure that decreases blood flow from the lung into the heart. PPV can cause pulmonary venous blood vessels to partially collapse, with increased right cardiac pressures and decreased venous return to the left ventricle. This can result in decreased cardiac output and hypotension.

Psychological Dependency

The psychological stress level or psychological dependency of the ventilator dependent patient can result in high levels of fear and anxiety. These factors can greatly decrease the patient's success with rehabilitation and weaning from the ventilator.

Chemical or Narcotic Dependency

Chemical or narcotic dependency from chronic medication used to reduce the discomfort of mechanical ventilation may result in a drug-dependency problem. Sedative or narcotic drugs can decrease respiratory drive and interfere with weaning.

Hyperinflation

Hyperinflation, or lung overinflation, can result in lung alveolar damage or rupture (pneumothorax), as well as decreased venous return of blood to the left ventricle of the heart.

Hypoinflation

Hypoinflation, or lung underinflation, can result in lung collapse or atelectasis as alveoli collapse and become more difficult to reinflate.

Inefficient matching of ventilation and blood flow results in abnormal gas exchange and hypoxemia.

Tracheal or Bronchial Mucosa Damage

Tracheal or bronchial mucosa damage that can occur from the use of mechanical ventilation includes edema, necrosis, surface loss of cilia, blister formation, erosion, epithelial mucosa loss, and tracheoesophageal (TE) fistula (TE fistula results primarily from endotracheal tube or tracheostomy tube cuff overinflation). This airway damage can be caused by trauma from intubation, lack of humidified air, rapid air flow, inappropriate suctioning technique, and infection.

Intracranial Hemorrhage

Intracranial hemorrhage is a serious and common complication in the neonatal population but is infrequently seen in adults. It can be an effect of ventilator positive pressure, leading to decreased venous return, causing blood to accumulate in the cranium, and thus increasing intracranial pressure, causing hemorrhage.

Increased Airway Resistance

Airway resistance can increase from excessive use of saline (fluid) that accumulates in airways, increasing resistance to airflow and making ventilation more difficult to achieve. Airway resistance also results from excess secretions (need for suctioning), bronchospasm (need for bronchodilators), and adult respiratory distress syndrome (stiff lungs). Other causes of airway resistance include:

- Airway inflammation or infection
- Intraluminal secretions
- Smooth muscle bronchoconstriction or bronchospasm (asthma)
- Increased lung water due to adult respiratory distress syndrome or congestive heart failure

Increased Secretions

Secretions can increase due to infection or other inflammatory processes, or due to liquefaction and mobilization from the smaller airways or an increase in production and may be pushed distally further into the lungs, making them difficult to remove. If secretions are not removed, they increase airway resistance and decrease the effectiveness of mechanical ventilation, and may become infected.

Increased Work of Breathing

Work of breathing (WOB) increases when a patient fights the ventilator by attempting to breathe against ventilator-delivered breaths or is unable to coordinate spontaneous breathing efforts or when the ventilator is not adjusted optimally. During the last decade progress in ventilator management has focused on many aspects that need to be considered in order to avoid increased work of breathing.

Nosocomial Infections

Cross contamination from other medical equipment or poor hygiene techniques (such as failure to wash hands before starting patient care or contact with the patient's own upper airway bacterial flora) can precipitate a nosocomial infection, further compromising the medical status of the ventilator dependent patient. There are many sources of infection during the medical care process itself. These include contact with the tracheostomy stoma, intravascular lines, heated nebulizers, and so forth.

VENTILATION EQUIPMENT

Noninvasive

Noninvasive methods of ventilation should be used when they are effective since they are safer and usually do not interrupt speech, swallowing or coughing (Figure 4-1). Experience with these techniques is increasing. These methods include:

Mouth or nasal positive pressure ventilation (PPV)
Continuous positive airway pressure (CPAP)

Chest shell (cuirass) or iron lung*
Exsufflation belt (Pneumobelt)
Pulmo wrap*
Rocking bed
Glossopharyngeal breathing
BiPap®

Negative Pressure Ventilation

Negative pressure ventilation is a noninvasive type of ventilation that does not require endotracheal tube placement or tracheostomy tube placement in order to establish an airway (Figures 4-1 and 4-2). This type of ventilation historically preceded the invention of positive pressure ventilators. Negative pressure refers to the creation of a less than atmospheric pressure within a chamber. This creates a vacuum or negative pressure outside the chest and abdomen, causing airflow into the lungs and expands the chest. Expiration occurs passively due to elastic recoil of the lung and thorax. Negative pressure ventilators apply negative pressure around the thorax for the inspiratory phase of respiration. Although negative pressure ventilators are noninvasive, ventilation cannot be as precisely controlled or readily measured as with positive pressure ventilators. Recently, there has been an increased interest in negative pressure devices in an attempt to avoid invasive procedures. This is primarily in the neuromuscular and spinal cord injury population, but there has also been some success in chronic pulmonary obstructive disease.

Devices that currently incorporate the use of negative pressure ventilation are the iron lung, chest shell (cuirass), and the pulmo wrap (poncho). All of these devices incorporate the use of a chamber that produces a negative pressure around the thorax, causing the chest to expand and inspiration to take place.

Complications from negative pressure ventilation include difficulty with patient access interfering with patient care, immobilization of patient affecting daily living activities, soreness in areas where the seal of negative pressure must be maintained and organ distention from pressure placed on the abdomen. Negative pressure can cause

*Negative intermittent pressure ventilation

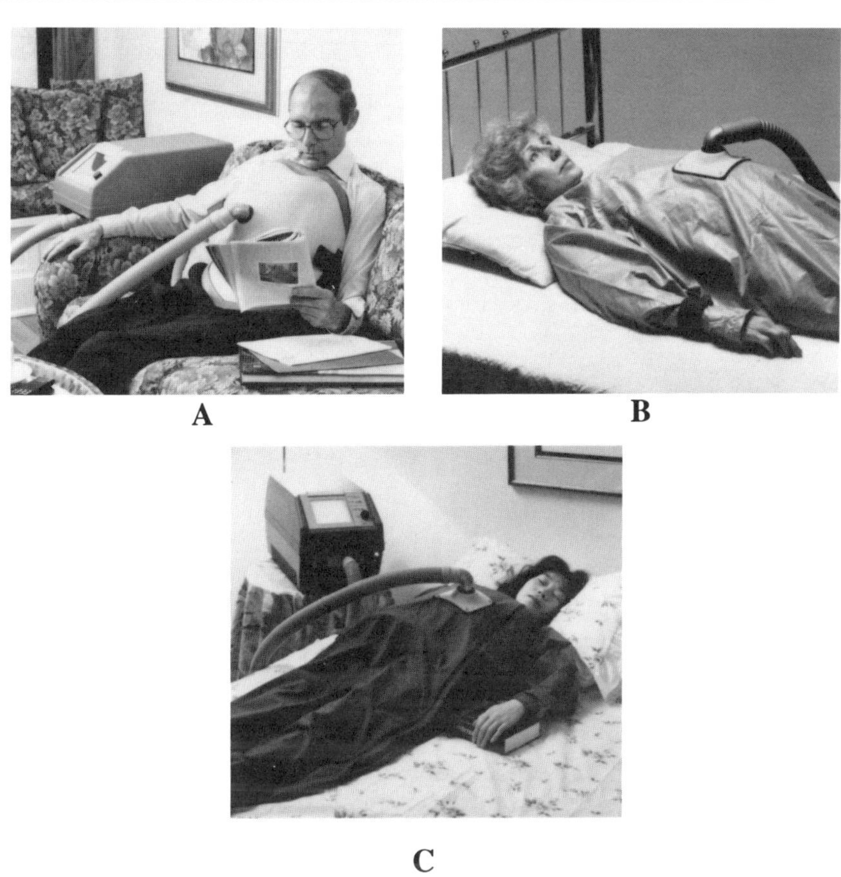

A B C

*Figure 4-1 **A,** Chest shell and cuirass shell. **B,** Pulmo wrap. **C,** NU-MO suit. (Courtesy of Lifecare®, Lafayette, CO.)*

airway collapse (airway obstruction blocking airflow during sleep), resulting in obstructive sleep apnea. This is a complication that has been recognized more and more in patients receiving chronic negative pressure ventilation and thus may require a switch to a positive pressure ventilation mode such as BiPAP®.

Positive Pressure Ventilation

Positive pressure ventilation is achieved by applying above-atmospheric pressure (or pushing air) into the airway to inflate the

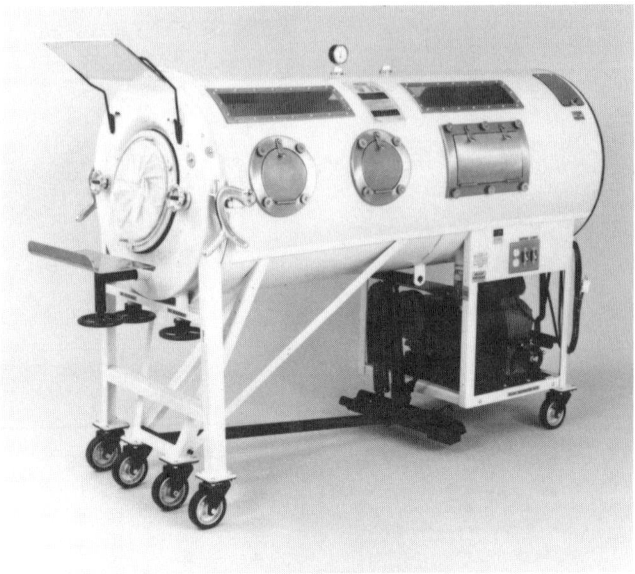

Figure 4-2 Iron lung. (Courtesy of Lifecare®, Lafayette, CO.)

lung. Commonly an artificial airway such as an endotracheal tube or tracheostomy tube is used to connect the patient to the ventilator. Recently, there has been increased interest and experience with a variety of methods for noninvasive intermittent positive pressure ventilation. The most common methods involve use of a mouth-piece, nasal or face mask, or nasal pillows.

Bi-Pap®

Bi-Pap® refers to a method of noninvasive ventilation used with either continuous positive pressure or intermittent pressure delivered by nasal mask or mouth piece (Figure 4-3). This method has been used as a treatment for sleep apnea or progressive respiratory failure in order to avoid tracheostomy and can be used with tracheostomy for intermittent positive pressure ventilation.

Recently, there has been some use of Bi-Pap® (or other methods of noninvasive ventilation) in emergency care to help stabilize patients with acute respiratory failure in order to avoid the application of invasive procedures such as endotracheal intubation.

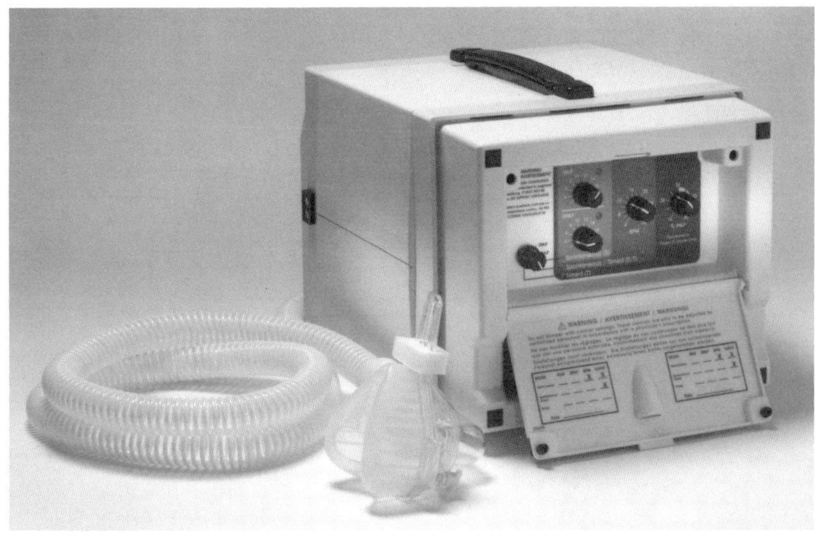

Figure 4-3 The BiPap S®. (Courtesy of Respironics, Inc., Murrysville, PA.)

Critical Care Ventilators

Critical care hospital ventilators have more patient alarm systems and data displayed for monitoring purposes. Readouts specific to the patient's prescribed parameters such as airway pressures, tidal volumes, inspiratory and expiratory ratio, breaths per minute, high-pressure limits, disconnect/low-pressure settings, and type of ventilator modes are available. Critical care ventilators are usually larger and more sophisticated than small portable ventilators. Many critical care ventilators have built-in microprocessors that can be utilized to provide constant data printouts for detailed patient assessment and monitoring (Figures 4-4 to 4-6).

Portable Ventilators

Portable ventilators are much smaller and somewhat less complex than critical care ventilators (Figures 4-7 and 4-8). These ventilators are available to deliver positive or negative pressure and are generally smaller machines so that they can be readily accessible for transport, rehabilitation purposes (i.e., can be mounted on a wheelchair), and home care. Small units are available to drive nega-

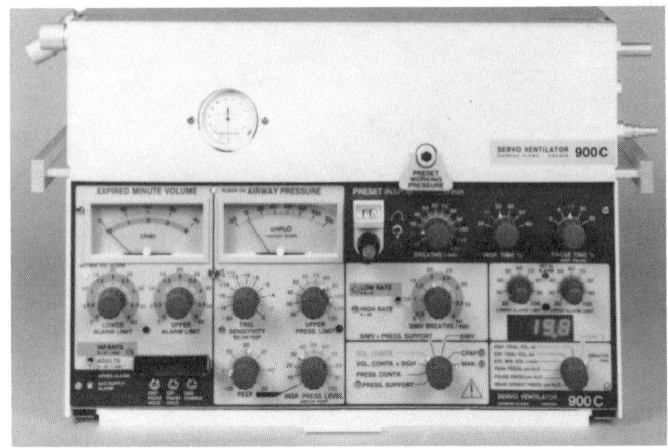

Figure 4-4 The Servo 900C. (Courtesy of Siemens Medical Systems, Inc., Danvers, MA.)

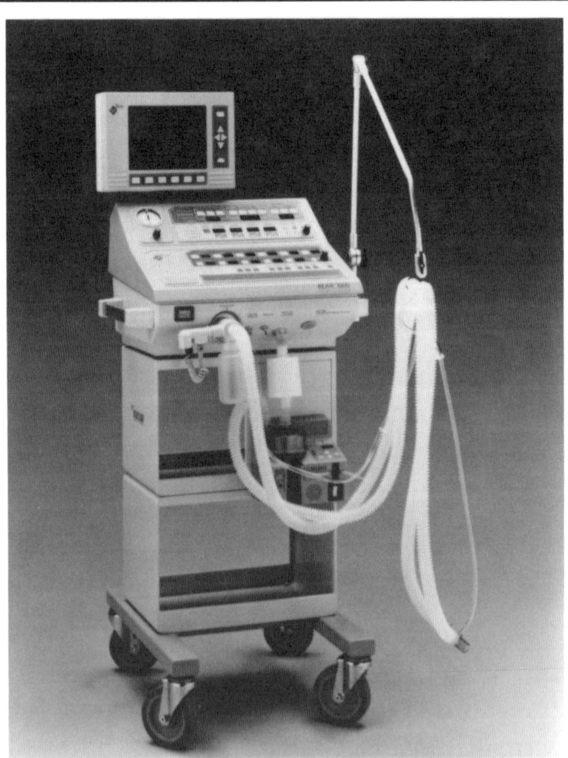

Figure 4-5 The Bear 1000. (Courtesy of Bear Medical Systems, Inc., Riverside, CA.)

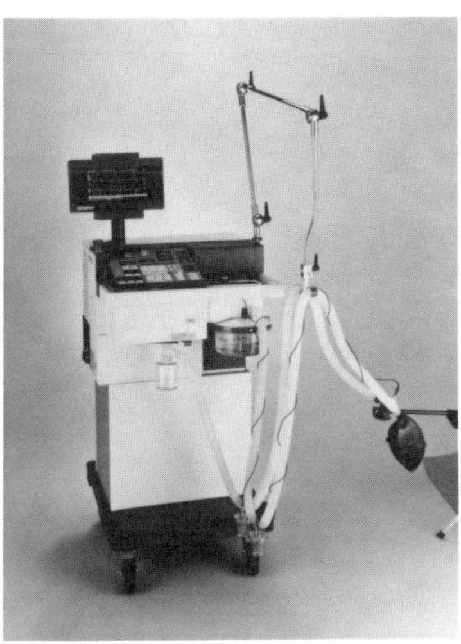

Figure 4-6 Puritan Bennett 7200. (Courtesy of Puritan Bennett Corporation, Lenexa, KS.)

tive pressure ventilation, and others are positive pressure drivers. Portable ventilators provide the same basic functions and alarm systems as critical care ventilators but usually have less patient data available and may have fewer ventilator modes. Portable ventilators cost less than critical care ventilators. They are used for transport, weaning, and long-term ventilator dependent patients. Portable ventilators have most ventilation modes and alarms available but they do not provide the extensive data that critical care ventilators provide. They are easier to operate, have internal batteries, and can be used with external portable batteries or standard electrical outlets (Figures 4-7 and 4-8).

Pediatric Ventilators

Pediatric ventilators are critical care ventilators that are designed to work with smaller airways, smaller tidal volumes, higher breathing rates and may be pressure regulated. They deliver much smaller volumes at faster breath rates to accommodate pediatric requirements. They are usually smaller than adult critical care ventilators but have essentially the same ventilatory modes available (Figure 4-9). Some larger critical care ventilators are available that can be used with

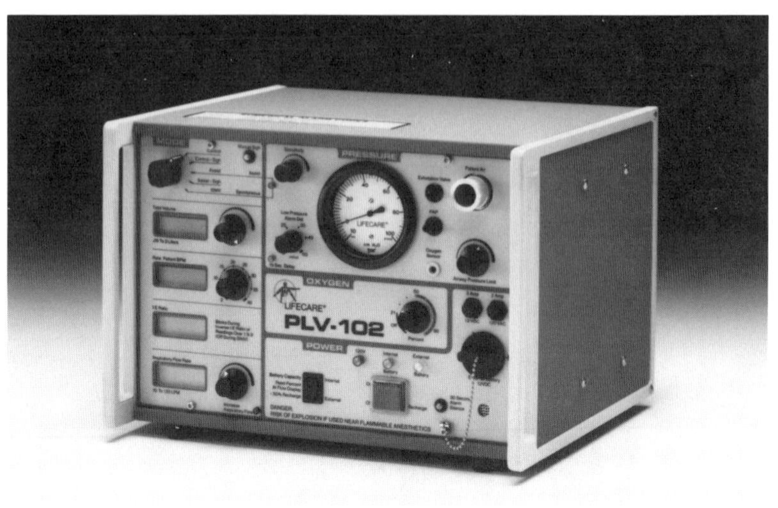

Figure 4-7 Lifecare ventilator PLV 102. (Courtesy of Lifecare®, Lafayette, CO.)

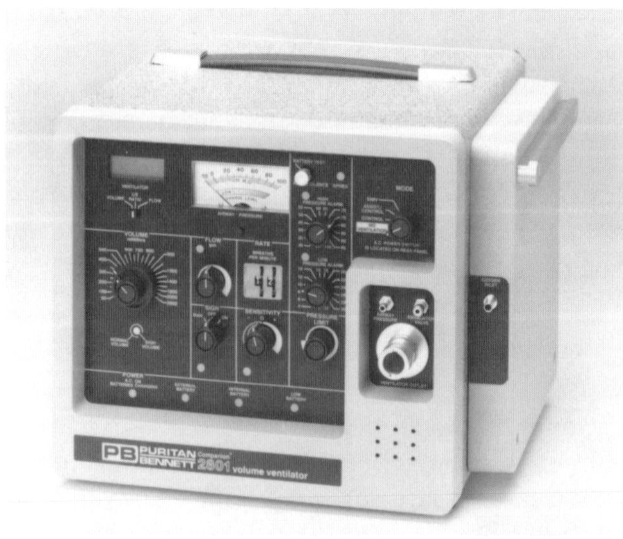

Figure 4-8 Companion 2801. (Courtesy of Puritan Bennett Corporation, Carlsbad, CA.)

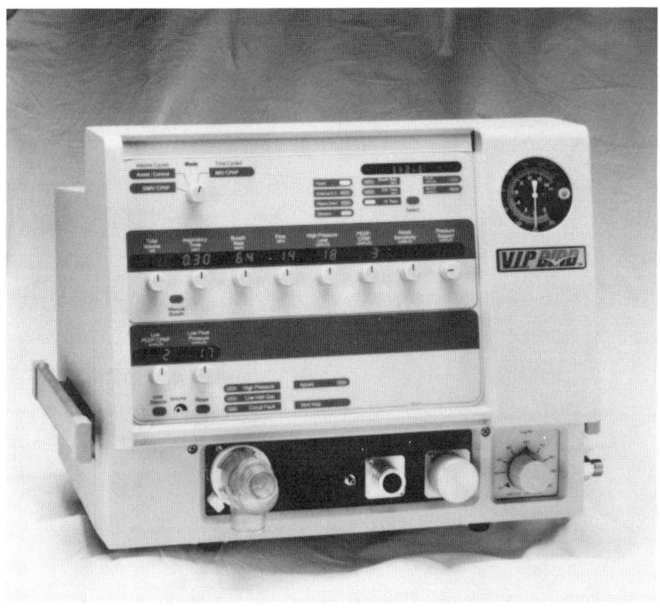

Figure 4-9 V.I.P. Bird® ventilator. (Courtesy of Bird Products Corporation, Palm Springs, CA.)

pediatric patients. Depending on the child's age and needs, the ventilators used vary and many are volume set. Pediatric home care ventilators are usually volume ventilators, but some can be set up with pressure limit mode.

High-Frequency Ventilation or Jet Ventilation

High-frequency ventilation (HFV) or jet ventilation operates differently than negative and positive pressure ventilation. This method uses ventilation rates of over 60 breaths per minute. CO_2 exchange can take place with tidal volumes less than patient dead space (tidal volume area of lungs at resting state). In some hospitals, jet/high-frequency ventilation is used primarily for CO_2 removal and does not work well for patients with oxygenation difficulty. Airflow is laminar and bi-directional (Figure 4-10). Inspiration occurs through the center airway with simultaneous exhalation. Gas diffusion occurs with enhanced gas dispersion, increased turbulent flow movement of gas and bulk convection current. This method may promote rest for the cardiopulmonary system as it uses small tidal volumes of air requiring minimal chest excursion. Circulant currents provide for the mixing of gas and molecular diffusion at terminal air spaces (alveolar level). High-frequency ventilation is used primarily in the neonatal population and is under investigation in the adult population. Rates are typically limited to 150 breaths per minute. The theory of jet ventilation is to move air in and out of the lung while using as little patient tidal volume as possible. A jet incorporates the use of a flow interrupter at about 600 cycles per minute. The jet oscillator uses a piston or cone at about 900 cycles per minute. The theory is to reduce or minimize the volume of inflation and deflation while still adequately oxygenating patients who have intolerably high airway pressures (i.e., neonatal ventilator dependent patients).

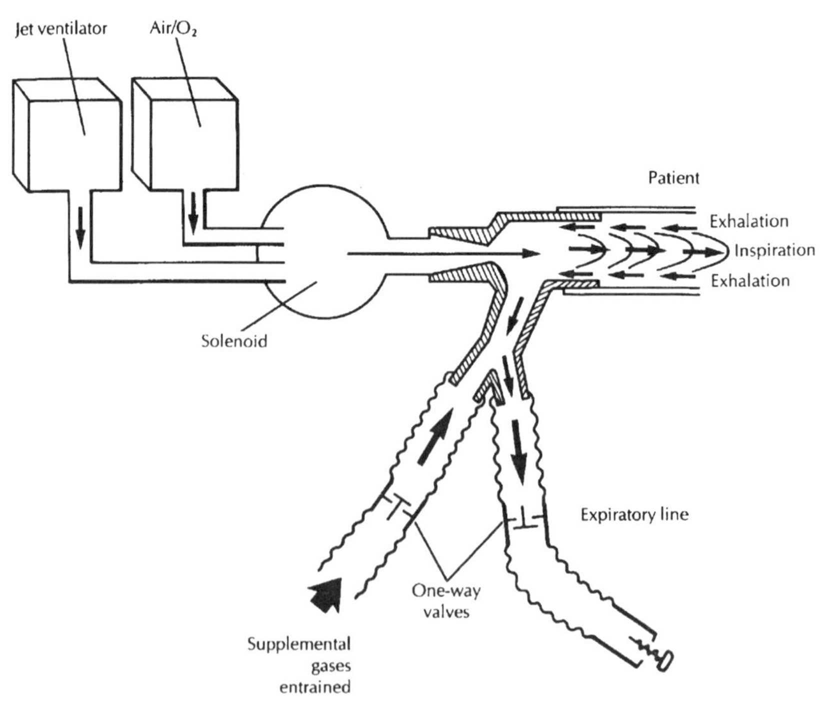

Figure 4-10 Schematic representation of high-frequency jet ventilator. (From Eubanks, D., and Bone, R.C., Comprehensive Respiratory Care: A Learning System, *2nd Edition, St. Louis: The C.V. Mosby Company, 1990, Figure 23-85, p. 753.)*

Use of jet ventilation theoretically decreases the incidence of barotrauma and improves ventilation and oxygenation in certain disease states (i.e., hyaline membrane disease, a condition that occurs with neonatal ventilator dependent patients, involves alveolar cell injury). In theory, it reduces risk of intracranial pressure and increases ventilation in lungs having low compliance or bronchopulmonary fistula.

The use of high-frequency jet ventilation is controversial. While initial trials gave hope that jet ventilation would be useful in decreasing airway pressures, there are a number of studies that suggest jet ventilation is no better at preventing barotrauma than more conventional modes of positive pressure ventilation. There are also studies that show no difference in the time of healing of bronchopleural fistula using conventional versus jet ventilation.

There are some drawbacks to jet ventilation. Due to the high rate of jet ventilation, small volumes and concurrent airflow pattern are not effective in maintaining airway patency. In addition, as a result of these concurrent bidirectional airflow and high-frequency rates, one cannot use the ventilator speaking valve (Passy-Muir) or other types of traditional weaning therapies. High-frequency ventilation provides poor humidification and medicated aerosol delivery, retards mucociliary transport, and does not allow for maintenance of positive end expiratory pressure requirements in those requiring additional pressures for ventilation.

Extracorporeal Membrane Oxygenation

Extracorporeal membrane oxygenation (ECMO) is a highly invasive procedure using long-term heart and lung bypass and is still an experimental therapy that is of unproven benefit in patients with respiratory failure. This method was first used in neonates for the management of intractable respiratory failure not manageable by conventional therapies. ECMO is delivered venovenous (VV) or venoarterial (VA). Venous perfusion is performed via the internal jugular vein with a single, double-lumen catheter or via the internal jugular, femoral, or umbilical veins with two catheters. Blood is obtained from a patient and diffused (CO_2 removal and oxygenation).

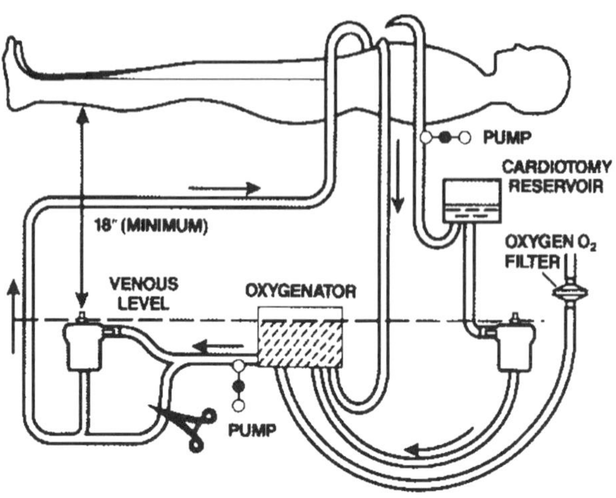

Figure 4-11 ECMO diagram. (Courtesy of Pall Biomedical Corporation, East Hills, NY.)

This procedure involves venovenous bypass cannulation of the right atrium through the right internal jugular vein or iliac vein. Alternatively, it can be done with venoarterial bypass cannulation of the right internal jugular vein for venous drainage and cannulation of the right common carotid artery or femoral artery for arterial return.

Equipment used in this technique includes a regulated pump, membrane lung, heat exchanger, tubing, and connectors (Figure 4-11).

PRINCIPLES OF MECHANICAL VENTILATION

Work of breathing is the energy expended by the respiratory muscles to expand the lungs and overcome airway resistance. Ventilation can be achieved with the assistance of positive pressure. Air is forced into the lungs with an above-atmospheric pressure. With negative pressure, there is a chamber with a less-than-atmospheric pressure. Negative pressure, or vacuum, is created, causing the diaphragm to drop and respiration to result. Negative pressure actually has a direct effect on the chest wall (expanding it, causing a pressure drop in the lungs). Exhalation is a passive process.

TERMINOLOGY OF VENTILATORY MODES AND STRATEGIES

The following are descriptions of commonly used modes of ventilation. The mode refers to the type of breath support provided by the ventilator. Mode is the combination of the type of breath pattern, pressures maintained, and size of breath or volume to be maintained with a ventilator dependent patient.

Assist Control

Assist control provides a ventilator-assisted breath each time the patient tries to initiate a breath. Assist control requires a preset back-up rate. If a patient's breath rate drops below the preset level, the ventilator will provide controlled breath support. With this mode, breaths may be initiated by the patient's own inspiratory effort. A pressure sensor responds to the patient's inspiratory effort, and this results in a breath triggered from the ventilator (Figure 4-12). In addition to the assisted breaths, the ventilator delivers a controlled preset number of breaths/inflations per minute. This mode is commonly used with stable patients or as a step toward weaning from ventilator dependence. It is designed to reduce work of breathing for a patient but facilitates weaning and ensures delivery of full tidal volume. The assist control mode is, in effect, a controlled mandatory ventilation mode (see the following paragraph) in a non-spontane-

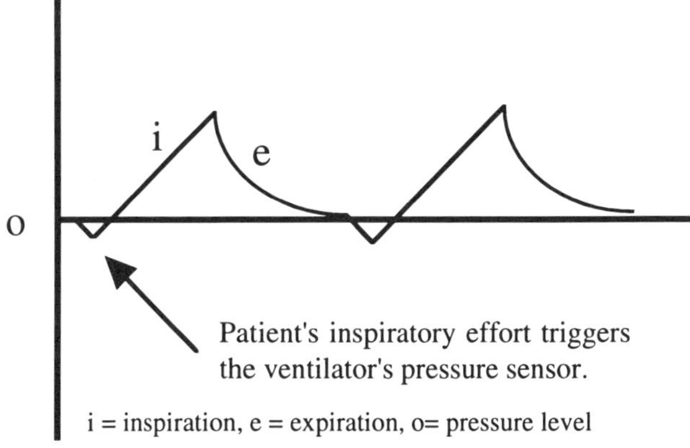

Figure 4-12 Breathing pattern for assist/control.

ously breathing patient due to mandatory back up breath rate. Since most patients will initiate some ventilation, the assist control mode is also commonly used in critically ill patients who require controlled ventilation. In fact, assist control may provide efficient ventilation because it provides a full ventilator breath every time the patient initiates respiration. This mode is also commonly used for long-term ventilatory maintenance.

Controlled Mandatory Ventilation (CMV)

This mode is a specific strategy/type of positive pressure ventilation. This mode of ventilation can be used for critically ill patients who lack spontaneous breath efforts and require totally controlled ventilation. CMV (Figure 4-13) is not often used because patients who make even slight spontaneous efforts will not trigger the ventilator as they will in the assist control mode. CMV is most often used with acute cases of respiratory failure, surgery, or trauma. Very often this mode may be used in conjunction with sedation and/or paralytic agents to eliminate the patient's work of breathing or resistance to the ventilator and to ensure a specific minute volume (rate per minute multiplied by volume).

Intermittent Flow Expiratory Ventilation (IFEV)

This mode requires endobronchial catheter delivery of fresh gas during the expiratory phase. This eliminates equipment and anatomic

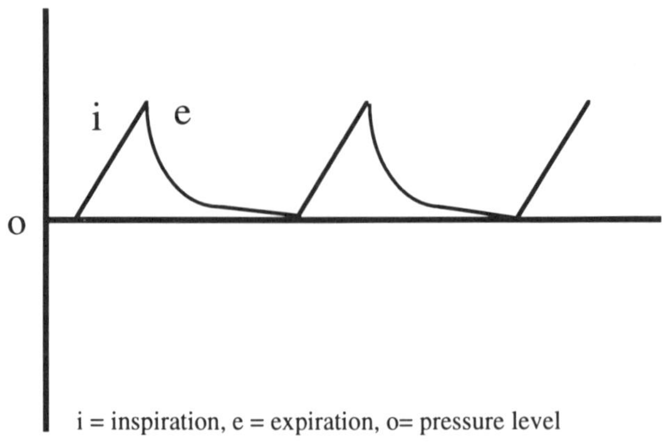

Figure 4-13 Breathing pattern for controlled mandatory ventilation.

deadspace, permitting a reduction in tidal volume and reduced peak airway pressures. It also minimizes pulmonary excursion (movement of the chest) while flushing out CO_2 from end expiratory gas. *End expiratory* refers to the amount of air left in the lungs at the end of the expiratory phase.

Intermittent Mandatory Ventilation (IMV)

This mode allows spontaneous breathing through a ventilator circuit (tubing set-up) and in addition provides a set number of ventilator breaths (Figure 4-14).

This mode can be used as a step toward weaning a patient from the ventilator as it allows for spontaneous patient effort between mandatory breaths. However, the set ventilator-delivered breath may interfere or conflict with spontaneous efforts made by a patient in some situations.

Synchronized Intermittent Mandatory Ventilation (SIMV)

Technical advances have improved intermittent mandatory ventilation (IMV) by the development of synchronized intermittent mandatory ventilation (SIMV). This mode allows for spontaneous breathing while delivering a set mandatory breath rate (Figure 4-15). In addition, this mode will sense a patient's spontaneous breath and

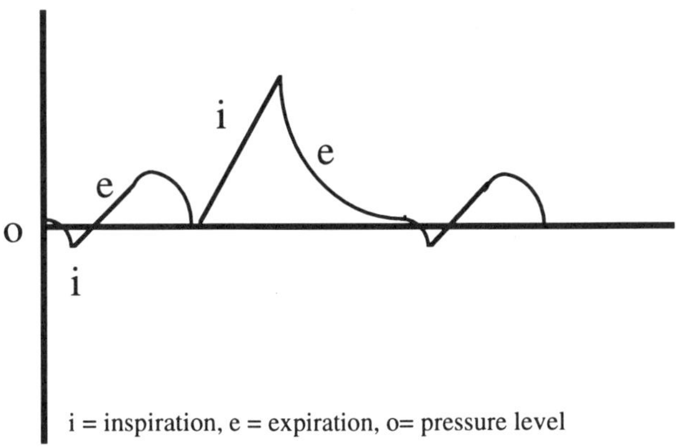

Figure 4-14 Breathing pattern for intermittent mandatory ventilation.

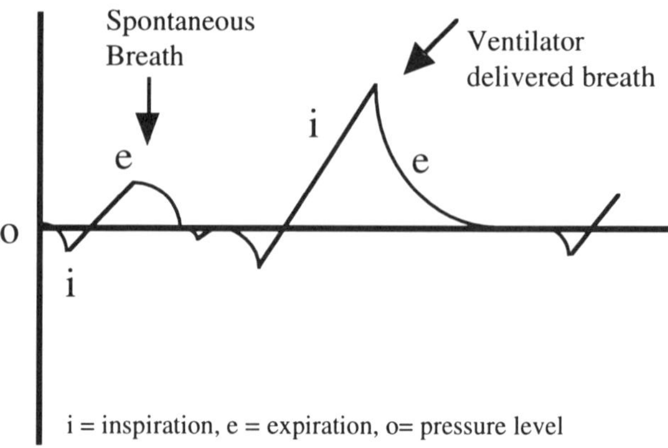

Figure 4-15 Breathing pattern for synchronized intermittent mandatory ventilation.

deliver the mandatory breath in coordination with the spontaneous effort so as not to interfere with the patient's work of breathing. It has proven to be a widely used mode and works well with weaning intervention.

Mandatory Minute Volume (MMV)

Mandatory minute volume refers to a mandatory breath per minute rate that is utilized with traditional mandatory tidal volume delivery to achieve a minimum amount of ventilation. Other modes such as SIMV are more commonly used.

Positive End Expiratory Pressure (PEEP)

The normal anatomy of the lungs allows for a slight residual pressure gradient after the end of inspiration. This naturally provides for easier reinflation due to less alveolar surface tension interface in the lungs thus reducing the work of breathing during the inspiratory phase. Positive end expiratory pressure (PEEP) can be used with other mechanical ventilation modes. This added pressure is coordinated with a ventilator breath to maintain constant end expiratory pressure (Figures 4-16 and 4-17). Patients with diseased lungs or acute respi-

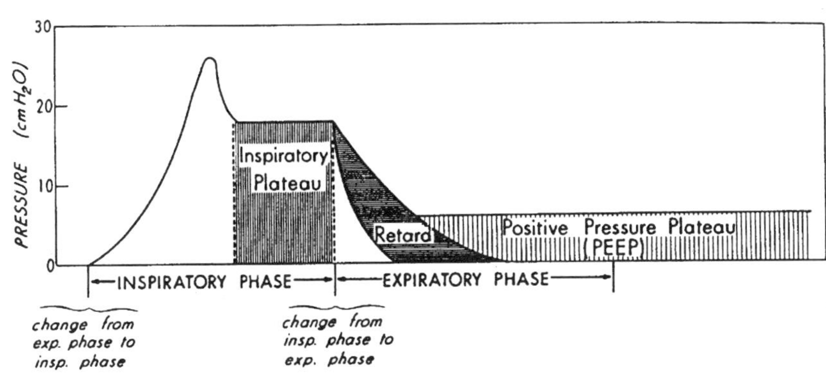

Figure 4-16 Phases of the mechanical ventilator cycle, with and without PEEP and retard. (From Burton, G.G., Hodgkin, J.E., and Ward, J.S., Respiratory Care: A Guide to Clinical Practice. *3rd Edition, Philadelphia: J.B. Lippincott Company, 1991, Figure 21-1, p. 508.)*

ratory failure may benefit from PEEP to assist in ventilation, to prevent lung alveolar collapse or atelectasis, or to improve oxygenation.

Complications from PEEP can include alveolar enlargement and or rupture (Figure 4-18).

Pressure Support Ventilation (PSV)

Breaths initiated by the patient are supported by a preset positive pressure (above PEEP levels if in use). This was designed to overcome airway resistance and assist the patient in spontaneous breathing. It can be used without ventilator cycling modes to help with spontaneous breathing efforts for weaning purposes. As a patient initiates a spontaneous breath, this breath is then supported by applying a certain pressure level to assist in the work of breathing and to overcome equipment deadspace (deadspace is the amount of air not involved in gas exchange, for example, air in the ventilator tubing). It is important to point out that under any pressure ventilation mode, ventilator volumes will vary. Because ventilator volumes vary, gas exchange can be altered tremendously, depending on lung compliance.

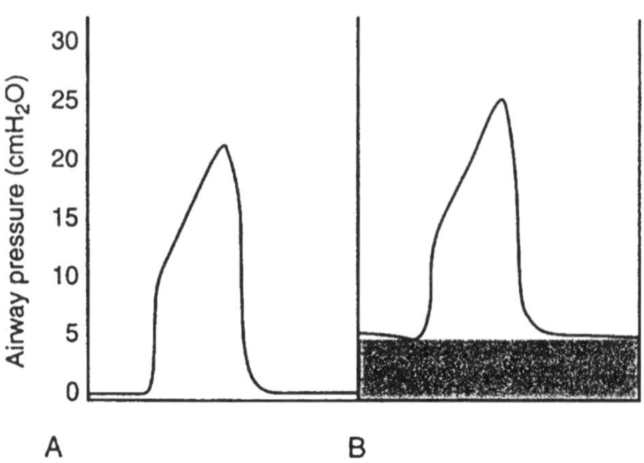

Figure 4-17 The effect of PEEP on airway pressure, as demonstrated in one of the first clinical reports of its use in severe oxygenation failure. Tracheal pressure measurements were made during volume-limited ventilation with an Ohio 560 ventilator. A, Airway pressure increases progressively during inspiration and then falls quickly to zero (ambient). B, With addition of 5 cm H_2O PEEP the same tidal volume (VT) is delivered but with a starting and ending pressure kept positive to the extent of the added PEEP; both peak and end-expiratory pressures are higher than they were before PEEP was added. (From Pierson, D.J., and Kacmarek, R.M., Foundations of Respiratory Care, *New York: Churchill Livingstone, 1992, Figure 65-1, p. 724.)*

Pressure Control

Pressure control pressure limits the amount of gas delivered to a patient from a ventilator breath. This may prevent hyperinflation of the lungs and any damage to lung alveolar tissue as a result. It can be used to compensate for leaks related to a partially deflated tracheostomy cuff or cuffless tracheostomy. Traditional tidal volumes are not used. It is similar to pressure ventilation used for neonates. This mode ventilates a patient's lungs by delivering a preset positive pressure and time for inspiratory phase. Tidal volumes vary upon airway resistance and lung compliance to positive pressure. While pressure control ventilation does overcome some of the high airway pressure of volume control ventilation, these press-cycled modes are more difficult to manage correctly because of the gas exchange problem as tidal volumes may not be achieved based on ventilator inspiratory drive.

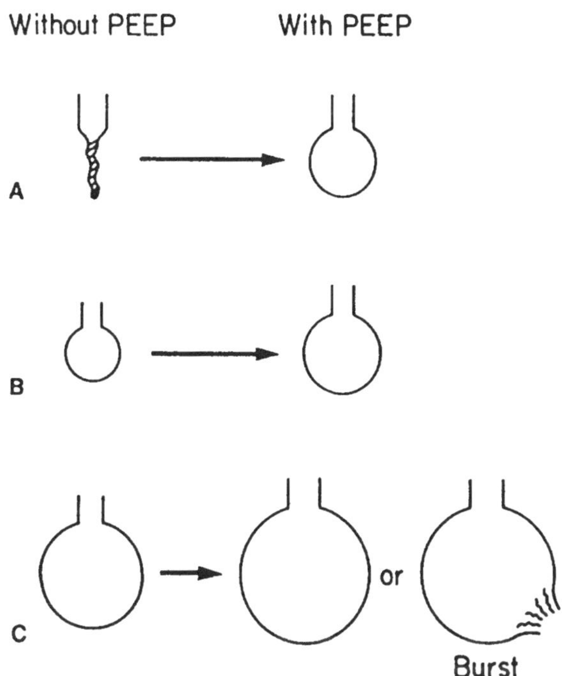

Figure 4-18 Postulated alveolar effects of PEEP. A, If the lung contains alveoli that are collapsed or fluid-filled, PEEP may reinflate them or displace the fluid into the interstitium. B, Alveoli that are at low volume and thus at increased likelihood of collapse may be resorted to normal volume with application of PEEP. C, However, alveoli that are normal in size or already enlarged would be expected to be further overinflated by the addition of PEEP, possibly leading to rupture (barotrauma). (From Pierson, D.J., and Kacmarek, R.M., Foundations of Respiratory Care, *New York: Churchill Livingstone, 1992, Figure 65-3, p. 725.)*

Continuous Positive Airway Pressure (CPAP)

Continuous positive airway pressure can be used as a weaning technique or can be delivered noninvasively with the use of a nasal mask, as with nocturnal nasal ventilation used in sleep apnea therapy. A continuous pressurized airflow is used to provide additional support for a patient who is post ventilator dependent. This mode is often used as a weaning therapy and requires the patient's ability to sustain spontaneous breath rate and tidal volume. CPAP is similar to PEEP except that CPAP is referred to as PEEP when it is used in conjunction with a mechanical ventilation mode such as in SIMV, pressure control, or assist control. CPAP is used to prevent airway collapse or to improve oxygenation by preventing atelectasis increasing the functional residual capacity during spontaneous ventilation only.

Continuous Flow Ventilation (CFV)

Continuous flow ventilation is designed as a weaning option and can be used in conjunction with intermittent mandatory ventilation. This is similar to CPAP but does not utilize prescribed pressure levels. Instead, a prescribed flow rate is used to supplement ventilator breaths.

VENTILATOR ALARM SYSTEMS

High-Pressure Alarm

High-pressure alarms may indicate obstruction from increased airway resistance (often from secretions or bronchospasm) or a decrease in lung compliance (such as from heart failure or adult respiratory distress syndrome). Other causes include lung collapse, the ventilator circuit tubing kinking, or water build-up in the circuit creating an obstruction and increasing pressures. A high-pressure limit refers to the upper range of appropriate airway pressure parameters that must be maintained to safely ventilate a patient.

Low-Pressure/Disconnect Alarm

Low-pressure or disconnect alarms indicate patient removal from the ventilator. When pressure within the ventilator circuit drops below a set limit and is not reinitiated after a certain time, the low-pressure alarm sounds. Normally, a patient connected to the ventilator will create a back pressure between the ventilator and the patient's lungs. The ventilator must sense the pressure in the circuit rising and falling past the low-pressure setting. After each breath, pressure in the circuit and lungs will drop to zero, or PEEP level, then rise again as the next breath is given. If the patient disconnects or there is a disconnection in the ventilator circuit, the pressures may not rise at all, therefore causing the low-pressure alarm to activate.

Parameter Alarms

These types of alarms are based on prescribed patient parameters that must be maintained within set limits or these alarms will activate (for example: airway pressures or volume).

Apnea Alarm

Apnea alarms indicate an apneic state of a patient, that is, a patient has no spontaneous breathing effort. This alarm senses respiratory effort from a patient to ensure that the patient is breathing spontaneously. This is used in vulnerable, spontaneously breathing patients as a safety precaution or sometimes if an "assist" ventilator mode is used.

MONITORING AND VENTILATOR SETTINGS

Tidal Volume

Tidal volume is the amount of air (volume) in a regular breath. Commonly, critical care unit ventilators are set to deliver 10 to 15 ml per kg of ideal body weight, (usually 500 to 1000 ml). The tidal volume may be increased if there is an upper airway leak from cuff deflation or from the use of a cuffless tracheostomy tube. The expired tidal volume can be measured through the upper airway to determine what tidal volume the ventilator delivered and what will be needed to compensate for an airway leak.

Respiratory Rate

The normal adult respiratory rate is 10 to 15 breaths per minute. Higher settings may sometimes be needed. Pediatric respiratory rates are significantly higher depending on patient age and size.

Inspiratory Flow Rate

Inspiratory gas flow is controlled typically from 40 to 60 liters per minute. Higher flow rates may be used in more severely diseased patients if these are needed to maintain adequate ventilation. (Higher flow rates mean increased expiratory time. High flow rates cause more turbulent flow, which increases airway pressure and reduces expiratory time.)

Inspiratory Time: Expiratory Time Ratio (I:E Ratio)

Inspiratory time is normally 0.5 to 1.5 seconds. Expiratory times may be 2 to 5 times the inspiratory time. Typical I:E ratios are 1:2 to 1:5. For example, it will take five times longer to exhale than the time required for one inspiratory breath.

Sigh Volume or Sigh Breath

A sigh volume is often 1.5 to 2 times a patient's tidal volume. A sigh breath or sigh volume mimics a yawn in normal breathing. A sigh breath is used for hyperinflation before or after suctioning and has been used in efforts to prevent atelectasis (alveolar consolidation/collapse). It is usually used at physician discretion.

Sensitivity Setting

Sensitivity setting refers to the amount of negative pressure a patient must generate in order to trigger ventilator breaths. If a setting is too sensitive, - 0.25 to - 0.50, it may trigger ventilator automatic cycling, causing the ventilator to deliver unneeded breaths. If a sensitivity setting is too low, requiring an increase in patient effort, it may increase the work of breathing causing hypoventilation (lack of ventilation), fatigue, and discomfort.

AIRWAY PRESSURES

Peak Airway Pressures

Peak airway pressures are parameters (limits to the range of pressures) that are determined. This is the highest measured airway pressure during the inspiratory cycle of the ventilator. The pressure limit alarm may be set 10 cm above the patient's measured peak airway pressure. Any pressures above this setting will result in the activation of the ventilator alarm system.

Mean Airway Pressures

This term refers to the average pressure in the patient's lungs. This allows for the establishment of normal parameters to be maintained by a ventilator dependent patient and for tracking trends of change. This can be affected by volume, rate, and inspiratory time, as well as by lung compliance.

MONITORING

The following are basic monitoring techniques and devices used with mechanical ventilation.

Arterial Blood Gases

Arterial blood gas levels are determined from an arterial blood sample obtained from an arterial puncture (using needle and syringe) or an indwelling arterial cannula. This is an invasive technique and will only document the status of blood gases at the time the sample is taken. It does not indicate patient condition patterns or fluctuations as readily as does a continuous monitoring system. This method is considered to be the most conclusive for a single point in time.

Arterial Probe

Arterial probes are invasive and costly. An electronic probe is inserted into an artery for continuous monitoring of blood gas levels.

Pulse Oximetry

Pulse oximetry was introduced in the 1980s and measures arterial oxygen saturation (SaO_2), pulse rate and pulse amplitude (Figure 4-19). It is a noninvasive measurement and is generally reliable and widely used. Manufacturers estimate measurement error within +/- 2% for levels between 70 and 100%. It may not be as reliable with hypoxic patients at values lower than 70%, as it has a +/ -3% measurement error.

An oximeter oxisensor emits a red and infrared light. This light transilluminates tissues. Pulsating expansion and contraction of arterial blood tempers the amount of light absorbed, and the sensor records the change. The sensor is usually clipped to a finger, toe, or ear lobe, where highly capillarized tissues exist and the ratio of light absorbed can be measured. The majority of light is absorbed by connective tissue, skin, bone, and venous blood. The amount of light absorbed by these substances is constant with time and does not vary during the cardiac cycle. With each heart beat, there is a small increase in arterial blood, which results in an increase in light absorption.

The reliability of oximetry measurements can be affected by movement, low blood pressure, ambient light, interference with absorbers from fingernail polish, skin pigmentation, anemia, dyes, and dyshemoglobinemias (carbon monoxide, methemoglobin, fetal hemoglobin). A major disadvantage of this device is that CO_2 and pH

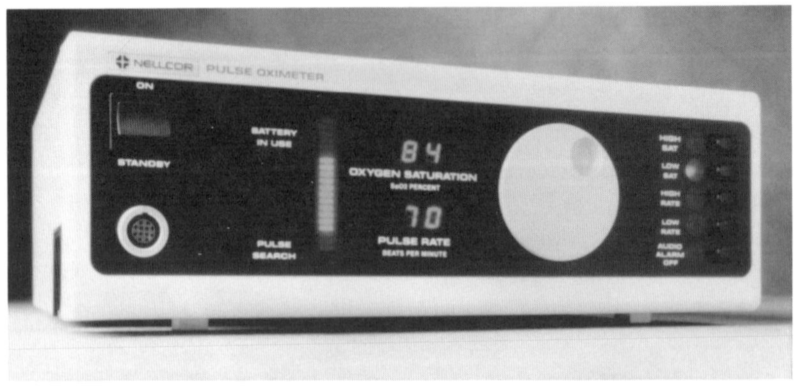

Figure 4-19 Nellcor N-100® Pulse Oximeter. (Courtesy of Nellcor, Inc., Hayward, CA.)

are not measured. Since carbon dioxide is a sensitive measure of gas exchange, pulse oximetry is no substitute for arterial blood gas determination in the critically ill patient.

Co-oximetry

Co-oximetry uses reflective pulse oximetry and tissue transillumination based on spectrophotometric analysis of optical absorption properties of the blood combined with the principle of photoplethysmography. Spectrophotometry is the use of a spectroscope constructed to measure the angular deviation of a ray of light produced by diffraction grading that indicates wavelength. Photoplethysmography measures light perception. This method uses sensors placed on the neck, thigh and scalp.

Transcutaneous Oxygen/Carbon Dioxide Monitoring

Transcutaneous oxygen and carbon dioxide monitoring uses noninvasive heated electrodes applied to the skin to monitor blood gas levels.

Capnography

Capnography is the in-line (within ventilator circuitry/tubing) monitoring of CO_2 levels during tidal breaths. This method uses an infrared analyzer or a mass spectrometer for processing. A normal expired carbon dioxide waveform is called a *capnogram.* End-tidal PCO_2 measurements allow noninvasive continuous monitoring that may correlate with arterial $PaCO_2$ trends.

Wright Spirometry

Wright spirometers are commonly employed rotary or turbine devices used to measure airflow. These bedside portable devices can be attached to the ventilator circuit or used with a mouthpiece for oral measurements. They are typically used to measure a patient's expired tidal volume or vital capacity, either with independent breathing or while on a ventilator.

Impedance Pneumography (IP)

Impedance pneumography measures changes in electrical impedance between two points. Electrocardiographic electrodes are placed at the anterior to mid-axillary line at the level of the patient's chest. This technique is most widely used to monitor respiration. A low-amplitude, high-frequency alternating current is sent through the chest and returns a voltage for calculation of impedance. Impedance thus increases as the lungs fill with air and decreases as the lungs empty. It can be used to estimate tidal volume. Please note that posture will affect an impedance pneumography reading.

VENTILATOR WEANING TECHNIQUES

Typically, as a patient's condition stabilizes, changes will be made to the mode and strategy of mechanical ventilation. These changes are made in an effort to allow a patient to increasingly achieve spontaneous and independent breathing. An example of this would be changing from a fully dependent mode such as controlled mandatory ventilation (CMV) to synchronized intermittent mandatory ventilation (SIMV), or assist control with intervals of CPAP that requires spontaneous breathing participation from the patient. The more competent a patient's breathing ability and rate (breaths per minute), the fewer back-up breaths or mandatory breaths will need to be delivered from the ventilator in SIMV and IMV ventilator modes.

Continuous Positive Airway Pressure (CPAP)

Continuous positive airway pressure (CPAP) can be used when a patient is attempting to maintain time off the ventilator as a weaning option. CPAP involves the use of continuous flow and airway pressure that augment and support the spontaneous breathing efforts of the patient.

Blow-by Systems or T-Piece Trial

Blow-by systems or T-piece trials involve a low flow of air set up to blow by the tracheostomy tube. Airflow enters into one side of the set-up and flows out of the other side. This airflow is usually not from a ventilator but from an outside air source such as an all-purpose nebulizer. The patient is breathing by his own efforts but the airflow, often with supplemental oxygen, avoids rebreathing of expired air from the tubing.

Pressure Support

Ventilator breaths are augmented by a certain amount of pressure to aid in any patient effort to breathe spontaneously. This technique can be used with ventilator modes such as IMV and SIMV. As the patient initiates a breath, pressure is added to that breath (either on or off the ventilator). This should reduce the work of breathing and aid in weaning efforts.

When a patient is spontaneously breathing through the ventilator circuit (tubing), the ventilator can sense breathing efforts (negative pressure) and support these breath efforts with pressurized airflow.

Passy-Muir Ventilator Speaking Valve

These are one-way valves for in-line use with ventilator dependent patients, primarily to establish speech. However, studies have indicated there are additional secondary benefits. Use of these valves will facilitate the reestablishment of exhalation through the vocal cords and pharynx in tracheostomy patients and ventilator dependent patients. Transition to this type of breathing should assist in building a patient's confidence in using the upper airway for exhalation and for secretion management through oral expectoration. Ability to produce a productive cough can provide clearing of lower airway secretions and can help prevent potential atelectatic results of secretion accumulation. In addition, patient confidence and well-being are enhanced when verbal communication can be reestablished. Patency of the airway may also be more readily assessed with use of exhalation. Furthermore, due to the reestablishment of exhalation and the physiology of a closed system, breathing normally against the upper airway structures creates an Auto-PEEP or physiological PEEP (see description of PEEP earlier in this chapter). This expiratory retard, or physiological PEEP, can improve the ability of a patient to oxygenate more normally, thus allowing for a reduction or elimination of lower levels of required PEEP from ventilator settings; this in turn can support and expedite weaning efforts.

1. May enable or improve (smooth) verbal communication; avoids possible contamination of tracheostomy stoma with finger occlusion to allow speech

2. Helps to clear secretions that might otherwise accumulate around the tracheostomy tube or cuff

3. May enable a cough to help clear lower airway secretions

4. May produce a physiological PEEP effect that can prevent expiratory airway collapse; this may improve oxygenation and assist with weaning

OXYGEN THERAPY

Oxygen is stored in cylinders or liquid tanks. Anhydrous or dry air from these storage sources may be humidified prior to patient use. Small bubble diffuser humidifiers have been widely used in the past for this purpose. These humidifiers are usually not heated and are of a more simplified design to be used with small-bore tubing, but there is little scientific evidence that they are effective. They may result in extra expense and another source of oxygen leak. When increased moisture is needed, large-bore tubing should be used with a more effective system (Figure 4-20).

Oxygen is a substance must be prescribed by a physician. The goal of oxygen therapy is to increase alveolar oxygen tension so as to provide a satisfactory arterial oxygen saturation without depressing ventilatory drive and without causing acute CO_2 retention. This may decrease the work of breathing required to maintain adequate blood gas levels for the cardiopulmonary system.

Oxygen is administered in the fractional inspired oxygen concentration (FIO_2) as the clinical standard (or as a percent or flow rate).

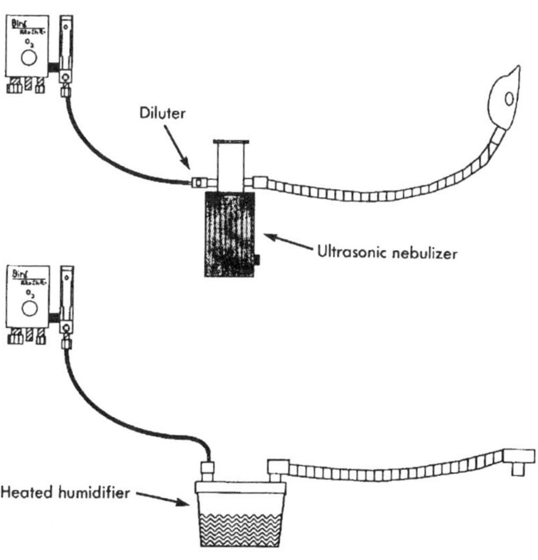

Figure 4-20 A simple dilution device can be used for low-resistance systems such as an ultrasonic nebulizer or a wick-type humidifier. With higher-resistance systems, a controller must be used to provide stable oxygen concentration. Flow must meet or exceed the patient's peak inspiratory flow requirements. (From McPherson, S.D., Respiratory Therapy Equipment, *4th Edition, St. Louis: The C.V. Mosby Company, 1990, Figure 4-49, p. 105.)*

Atmospheric ambient air is approximately 20.9% oxygen. Thus, for therapy, oxygen may need to be increased in relation to total inspired gas flow (e.g., to 22 to 50%). Oxygen therapy involves the mixing of gases of primary room air and oxygen. Oxygen may be needed for emergency treatment of trauma or during ambulance transport. It is administered through high-flow systems and low-flow systems, which are either non-rebreathing or rebreathing systems. Ventilator delivery is an example of a high-flow nonrebreathing system. The reservoir or nasal cannula is low flow, which utilizes the anatomical reservoir of the nose, nasopharynx, and oropharynx.

Another oxygen-delivery option is transtracheal oxygen administered through a small permanent tracheal cannula. This is used for people who have a high oxygen requirement due to hypoxemia, to improve 24-hour compliance, or to improve appearance cosmetically as it is hidden under clothing.

HUMIDITY

The unique and efficient architecture of our natural physiology provides a warming and humidification system by utilizing the specialized upper airway structures of the nasopharynx, oropharynx and trachea, where ambient air is exposed to large moist surface areas of mucous membrane. Ambient air is 100% humidified and warmed to body temperature at the alveolar level. The majority of air humidification occurs in the nasopharynx, where it is estimated that inspired gas reaches a humidity of 90 to 95% at the level of the carina (bifurcation of the trachea). The level at which gases become fully saturated at body temperature is referred to as the *isothermic saturation boundary* (ISB).

As a result of tracheostomy or mechanical ventilation via a tracheostomy or endotracheal tube, the normal upper airway structures used to heat and humidify ambient air are bypassed, requiring humidification to be supplied by the tracheobronchial mucous blanket. Exposure to dry and cold gases can cause losses of heat and water in the bronchial mucosa, leading to airway damage. In neonates, this can cause a drop in body temperature and cause hypothermia (i.e., cold stress syndrome).

Insufficient humidification of inspired gases can cause damage to the tracheobronchial tree, including impairment and eventual destruction of ciliary function; mucosal ulceration; reactive hyperemia (congestion of an unusual amount of blood); retained thickened secretions; decreased compliance (lung function); atelectasis; intrapulmonary shunting (obstruction to alveolar access); cellular damage to the epithelium (airway surface); bacterial infiltration of mucosa; necrosis (tissue death) of ciliated pulmonary epithelium; incrustation; and even pneumonia.

Excessive heat and humidity can also damage airways, resulting in mucosal burns or edema (swelling). This can cause airway obstruction or bronchospasm. Excessive humidification can cause an overabundance of secretions, creating airway obstruction and difficulty maintaining bronchial hygiene.

Aerosol Therapy

Aerosols are defined as the suspension of very fine particles of liquid in a gas. Usually these particles consist of isotonic saline, with a particle size of less than 3 mm in diameter. This size of particle will effect the deposition into the pulmonary tree. *Aerosol stability* refers to the ability of particles to maintain suspension and how long that period will be. This relates to the size and type of particles, concentration, and ambient humidity. *Instability* refers to the tendency that particles have to be removed from a suspended state (Figure 4-21). In order for particles to penetrate into the pulmonary tree, they must achieve adequate or optimum suspension. Particles have a natural tendency to coalesce or join together. As an aerosol travels down the tubular structures of the pulmonary tree, particles bump into each other and combine to form larger and larger spheres until they drop out

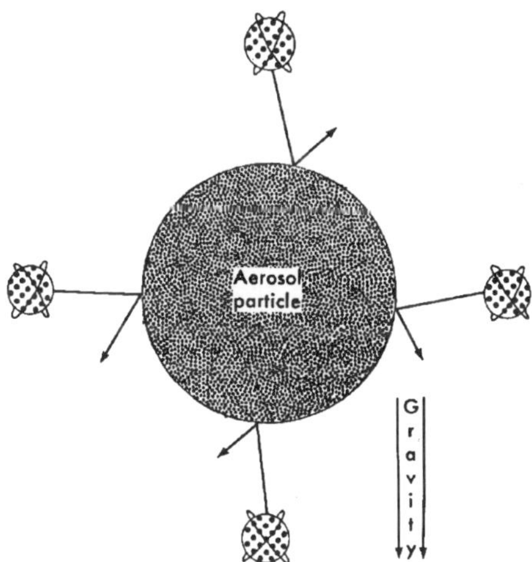

Figure 4-21 Molecular bombardment from all sides tends to provide equalizing force, surrounding the aerosol particle and holding it in suspension. The opposing force to this equalization is gravity. The larger the particle and its mass, the greater gravity's effect and the less stable is the particle. (From McPherson, S.D., Respiratory Therapy Equipment, *4th Edition, St. Louis: The C.V. Mosby Company, 1990, Figure 4-21, p. 91.)*

of suspension. How fine an aerosol can remain in turbulent flow affects its ability to deliver treatment deep into the pulmonary tree (Figure 4-22).

Deposition of aerosols is dependent on other issues as well, including the water content in gases, airway resistance, and ventilatory pattern or mode. Breath depth and rate can also affect particle deposition. One goal is to deliver moisture to the medium-sized and possibly smaller airways. Particle size and stability must allow the water to reach these airways and then to deposit there by impact or by gravitational settling.

Aerosol therapy can be delivered noninvasively to non-ventilator dependent patients (Figure 4-23) or delivered through the ventilator circuit. The goals of aerosol therapy are to induce the mobilization of the mucous blanket for clearance of the tracheobronchial tree, to deliver medication or humidity and to improve bronchial hygiene.

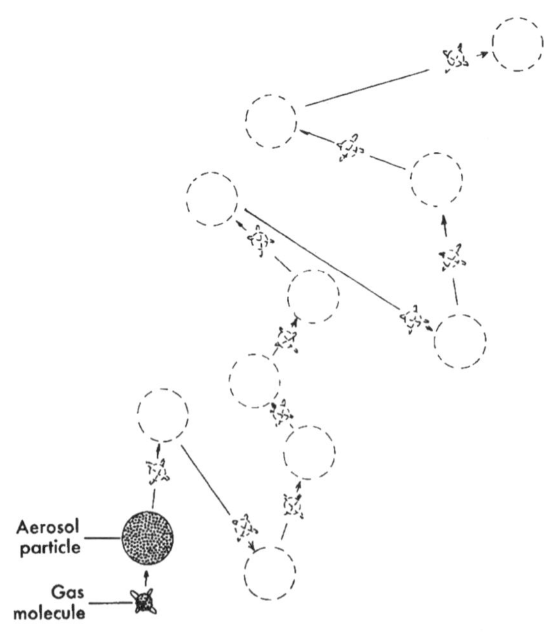

Figure 4-22 The smaller an aerosol particle is, the more influence bombardment by gas molecules has on its path of travel and the greater the brownian movement. (From McPherson, S.D., Respiratory Therapy Equipment, *4th Edition, St. Louis: The C.V. Mosby Company, 1990, Figure 4-22, p. 92.)*

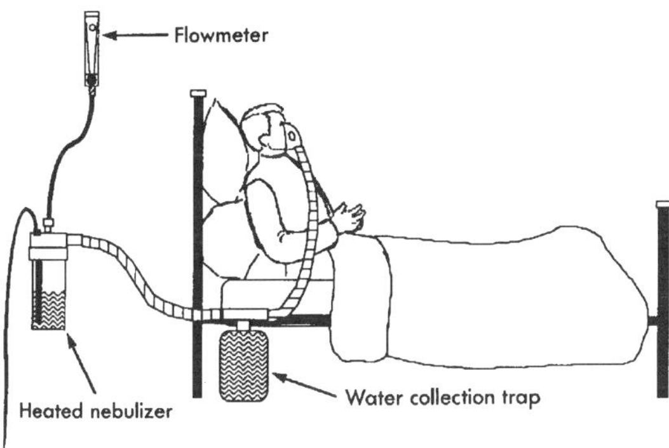

Figure 4-23 Method for delivering heated aerosol. (From McPherson, S.D., Respiratory Therapy Equipment, *4th Edition, St. Louis: The C.V. Mosby Company, 1990, Figure 4-48, p. 105.)*

Nebulizers

An atomizer is a uniform particle device used to produce small particles. Devices used to make and deliver particles from atomizers are called *nebulizers.* They can be manual, pneumatic, or electrical devices. Pneumatic devices use a pressurized gas source jet or hydromatic. Electrical devices are ultrasonic and use vibrations to produce small particles. Both types of devices create particles by the use of a high-stream gas flow against a flow of fluid. This gas flow blows the fluid over a baffle, causing particle breakdown (Figures 4-24 and 4-25).

Hydronamic Nebulizer

Hydronamic nebulizers use a film of water that is blown over a hollow sphere, where a small opening in the sphere shoots gas at a high level of velocity, breaking the stream of water into fine particles. A series of baffles can be used to ensure particle uniformity. This system allows for high-volume aerosol therapy (Figure 4-26).

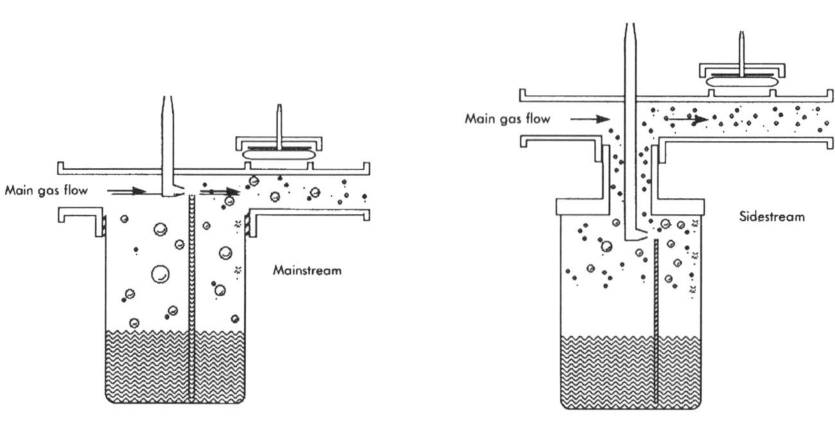

Fig 4-24 Main gas flow passes through the mainstream nebulizer and carries aerosol particles with it. Aerosol drifts into the main gas flow with a sidestream nebulizer, producing smaller particles. (From McPherson, S.D., Respiratory Therapy Equipment, *4th Edition, St. Louis: The C.V. Mosby Company, 1990, Figure 4-29, p. 95.)*

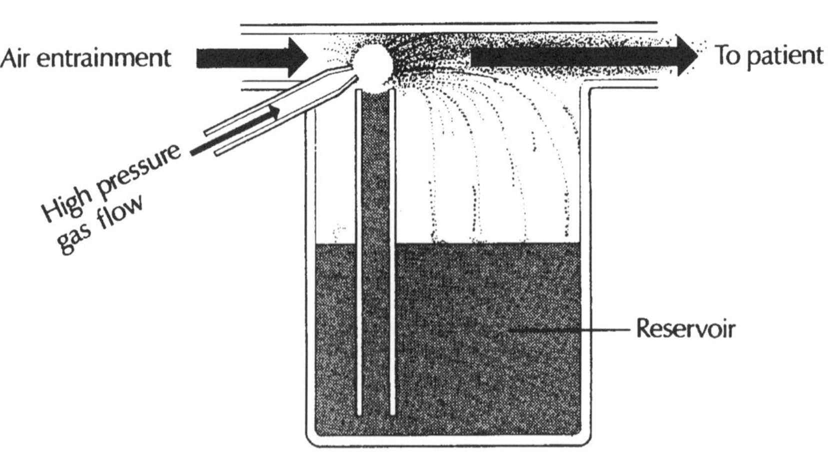

Figure 4-25 Model of reservoir mainstream jet nebulizer. (From Shapiro, B.A., Kacmarek, R.M., & Cane, R.D., Clinical Application of Respiratory Care, 4th Edition, St. Louis, Mosby-Year Book, 1991, Figure 4-6, p. 67.)

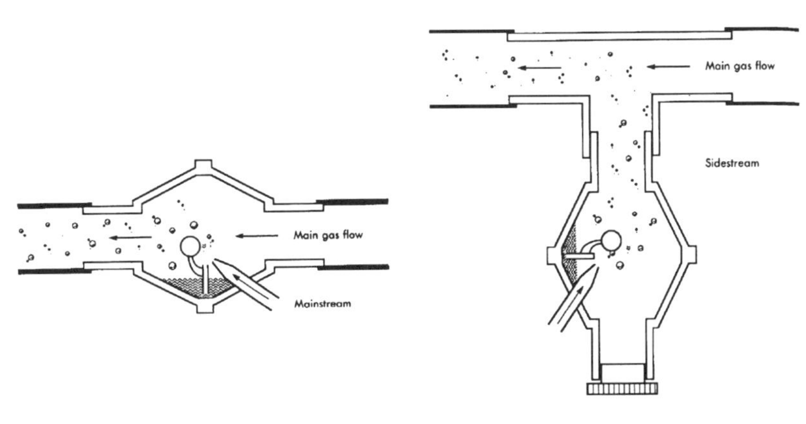

Figure 4-26 Bird micronebulizer can be used as a sidestream nebulizer. (From McPherson, S.D., Respiratory Therapy Equipment, *4th Edition, St. Louis: The C.V. Mosby Company, 1990, Figure 4-34, p. 98.)*

Ultrasonic Nebulizer (USN)

Ultrasonic nebulizers use electrical current and high oscillating discs. Energy waves in an ultrahigh-frequency electrical current pass through a piezoelectric transducer and transmit from the disc through the water copulant (Figure 4-27). These waves form an ultrahigh-frequency vibration through a thin plastic membrane that allows particles to break from the water copulant as a blower distributes the particles to the patient. This is a very efficient device, delivering very dense mists and ensuring particle size within 0.5 to 3 mm 90% of the time, in contrast with other systems which only approach 55%. An ultrasonic nebulizer can sometimes deliver more water than is safe or desired.

Jet Nebulizers

Jet nebulizers utilize high-speed gas delivery over a tube immersed in a reservoir and with a series of baffles creating smaller and smaller particles. This system can be easily combined with oxygen therapy and maintains temperature within a water heater. An all-

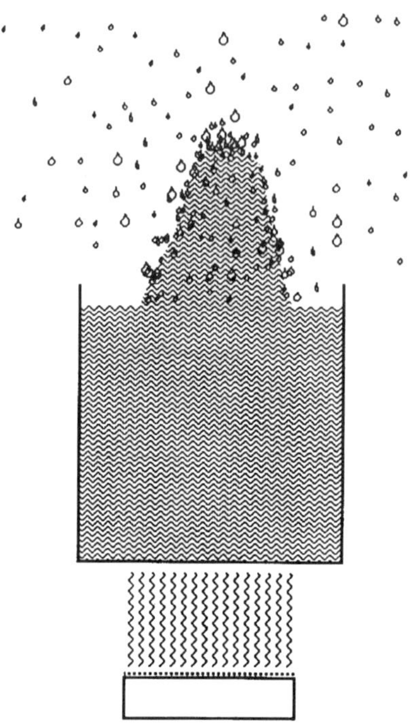

Figure 4-27 Electric energy supplied to a piezoelectric transducer produces sound waves. When sound waves hit the water's surface, aerosol is produced. (McPherson, S.D., Respiratory Therapy Equipment, *4th Edition, St. Louis: The C.V. Mosby Company, 1990, Figure 4-43, p. 103.)*

purpose nebulizer combines a jet nebulizer action, a heater, and an oxygen diluter.

Humidification Systems for Ventilators

Humidification systems are usually heated sterile water reservoirs or a heat-exchange filter device incorporated into a ventilator circuitry system.

Passover Humidifiers

Passover humidifiers are the simplest and least efficient form of humidifier. Airflow passes over a heated reservoir of water (Figure 4-28).

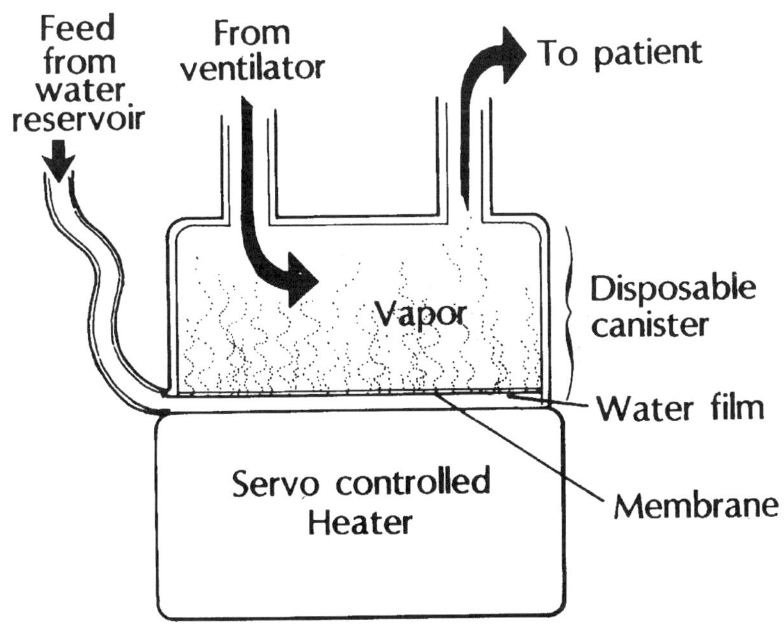

Figure 4-28 Schematic of a servo-controlled passover heater. (From Shapiro, B. A., Kacmarek, R.M., and Cane, R.D., Clinical Application of Respiratory Care, *4th Edition, St. Louis: Mosby-Year Book, 1991, Figure 4-1, p. 59.)*

These devices offer little resistance to gas flow and are the most commonly used type of humidification.

Bubble Humidifiers

With bubble humidifiers, airflow passes through a reservoir of water via a diffuser (Figure 4-29). The diffuser breaks up air into small bubbles, allowing for gas-water interface. This water reservoir can be heated to body temperature. Heated reservoir equipment provides an increased risk for producing nosocomial infection. The higher the heat used, the more complete the humidification of gas will be. Bubble humidifiers are inefficient and usually do not allow for complete humidification of gas. They can inhibit gas flow as air is forced through the diffuser and water. Gas passes through too quickly to pick

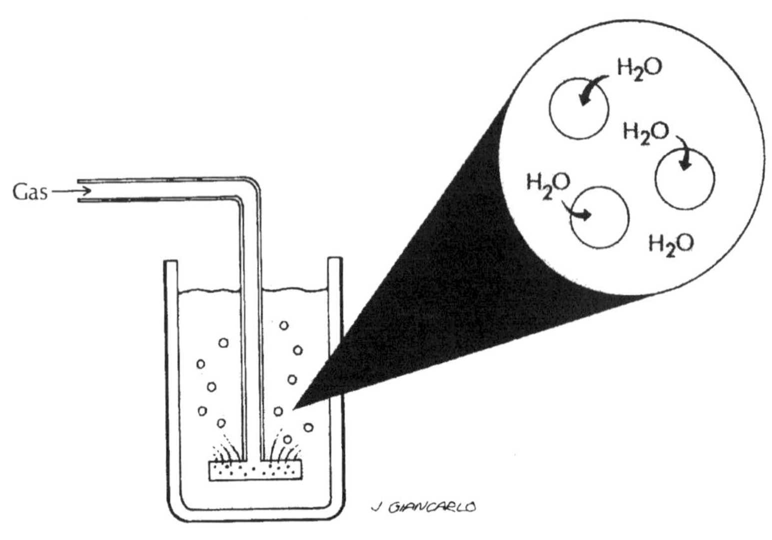

Figure 4-29 Principle of a bubble diffusion humidifier. (From, Shapiro, B.A., Kacmarek, R.M., and Cane, R.D., Clinical Application of Respiratory Care, *4th Edition, St. Louis: Mosby-Year Book, 1991, Figure 4-2, p. 60.)*

up much moisture. The higher the flow rate, the poorer is the humidification.

Wick Humidifiers

With wick humidifiers, a wick of water-absorbent material is used to increase gas-water contact. The wick lies in the reservoir of water against a heat source. Some resistance occurs. This method allows for easy temperature control and will respond more rapidly to changes in airflow than a bubble humidifier. This method often consists of two components: a wick and a water canister with a heat source control module under the water canister.

Vapor Humidifiers

The principle behind vapor humidifiers is that water vapor passes through a special material that allows only the flow of water vapor to pass through. Water vapor is then exposed to incoming air. Water is delivered in small amounts to the platen, which is superheated to create a vapor.

Warmth

Mechanical ventilation uses dry, ambient air that lacks adequate warmth to maintain core body temperature. It bypasses normal physiological structures that warm and humidify inspired air (the oronasopharnyx). To compensate for this, heated wire circuits are frequently used with humidification devices to maintain a more universal air temperature. Heated humidifiers monitor airway temperature via a probe connected to the inspiratory circuit. Other options include heat moisture exchange filters and heated reservoir humidifiers (Figure 4-30).

Heat Moisture Exchange Filters

The heat-moisture exchanger (HME) is also referred to as an "artificial nose." The basic theory of operation is that air flows through a filter material that collects expired humidity and heat from the patient. This filter then uses the collected moisture and heat to heat

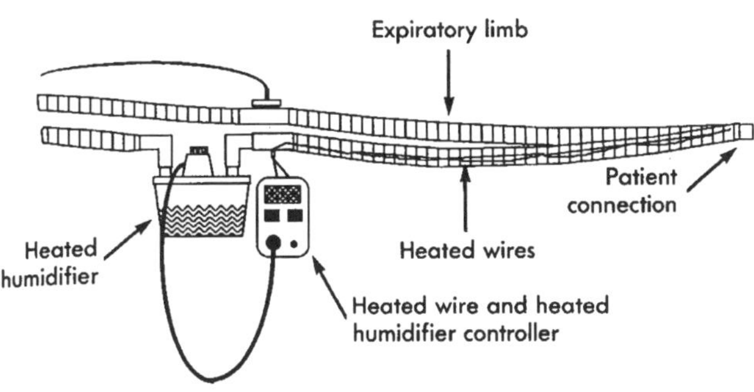

Figure 4-30 Heated wire circuit. The controller acts as master for both humidifier and heated wire to minimize rainout, delivering gas to patient at the body temperature. (From McPherson, S.D., Respiratory Therapy Equipment, *4th Edition, St. Louis: The C.V. Mosby Company, 1990, Figure 4-17, p. 89.)*

and humidify the next inspired breath (Figures 4-31 and 4-32). The material within the HME filter is usually a fiber that may or may not be hygroscopically treated with lithium chloride or calcium chloride and is referred to as a *hydroscopic condenser humidifier* (HCH). If either type of filter possesses bacteria-filtering capability, it may be referred to as a hydroscopic *condenser humidifier filter* (HCHF) or *heat-moisture exchange filter* (HME).

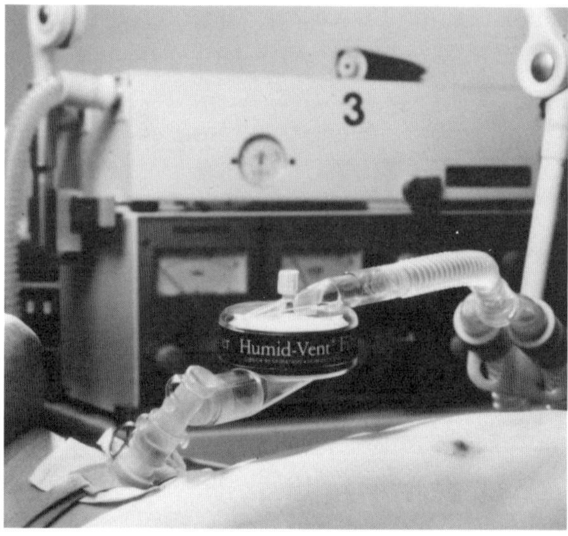

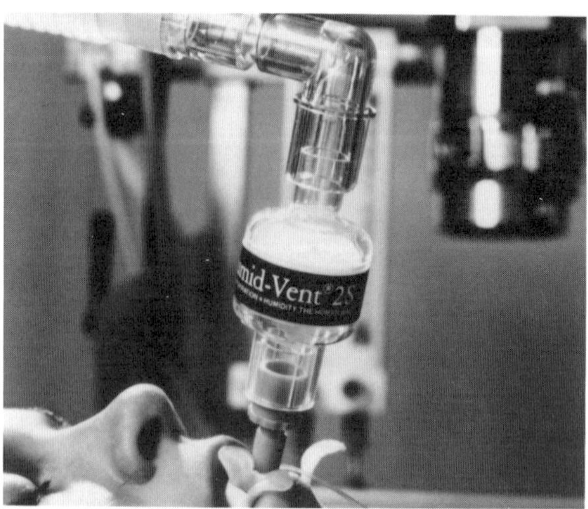

Figure 4-31 Humid-Vent 2S Flex. (Courtesy of Gibeck-Dryden, Indianapolis, IN.)

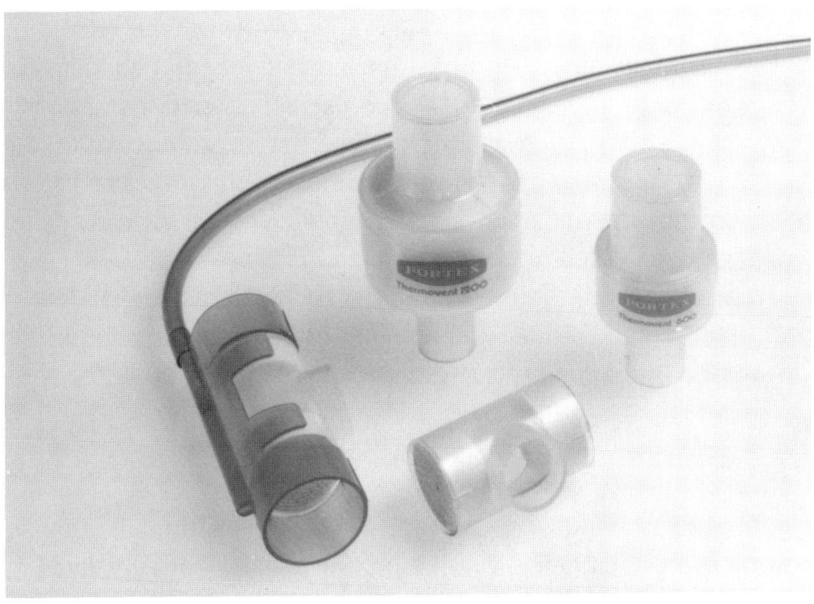

Figure 4-32 ThermoVent heat and moisture exchangers for ventilated or spontaneously breathing patients help minimize loss of heat and moisture. (Courtesy of Concord/Portex, Keene, NH.)

Heat-moisture exchange devices are passive, inexpensive, convenient, eliminate rainout, and may reduce bacterial colonization in ventilator circuitry. Due to the necessity of requiring entire exhaled volumes for breath rehumidification, these devices may not be appropriate for patients with upper airway leaks or cuff deflation or if a Passy-Muir ventilator speaking valve is in use, because all exhaled volumes are rerouted normally through the upper airway and will not travel through the HME. In addition, an HME may not provide sufficient heat for some patients' requirements or for patients requiring therapeutic amounts of humidity. They also add additional deadspace (that of the filter) to the ventilator set-up.

Advantages and Disadvantages of Humidification Systems

Generally, humidification systems are safe, reliable, and efficient; however, complications can include cost, rainout (condensation in tubing), resistance to airflow, bacterial infection, and leaks, or their use may be contraindicated in conjunction with the use of other devices. Rainout of moisture results as gas cools and condensation occurs in the tubing. Sometimes the use of water traps is helpful. However, this may still require frequent emptying of circuits or traps. This can increase the growth of bacteria in tubing. Other limiting factors include maintenance of water supply, cost of wicks, canisters, sterile water and electrical costs.

Adequate fluid intake is essential for ventilator dependent patients, and frequent monitoring for signs of inappropriate humidification such as thickening secretions or airway injury should be made.

VENTILATOR CIRCUITS

The term *ventilator circuit* refers to the connection of tubing and equipment for mechanical ventilation use. Much as an electrician will incorporate the use of a wiring configuration to accomplish the task of supplying electricity, so too must a ventilator have appropriate connections and tubing to accomplish the task of delivering air. Most ventilator circuits require the use of two lines. One line is referred to as the *inspiratory line* and the other is referred to as the *expiratory line*. These two lines can be used to measure inspiratory values and expiratory values, respectively, as well as for gas flow. In addition, the use of two lines prohibits the rebreathing of CO_2 saturated gases that are exhaled by the patient.

The inspiratory and expiratory lines are connected at a "Y"-shaped connection close to the patient, where both lines join to form one short piece of line leading to the patient. This circuit also uses an exhalation valve, which may be internal (inside the ventilator) or external (part of the circuit). Figure 4-33 is a diagram of a basic ventilator circuit set-up.

As patients stabilize, are weaned from the ventilator, or transfer to a home care setting, a single-line circuit may be used to simplify connection to the ventilator and to eliminate the cumbersome bulk of tubing. This usually utilizes an exhalation valve that will dump exhaled air out of the ventilator tubing to prevent the patient from rebreathing exhaled CO_2. Please note that a patient using a Passy-Muir

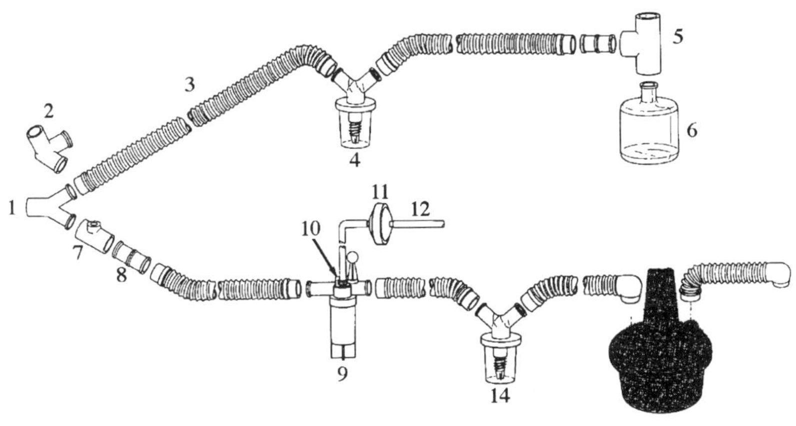

Figure 4-33 Ventilator patient tubing circuits. 1. Wye, straight. 2. Wye, angled. 3. Flex tubing. 4. Water trap, in circuit. 5. Tee adapter. 6. Vial collector. 7. Coupling, temperature probe. 8. Connector, tube junction. 9. Nebulizer. 10. Tube hanger for simplified patient tubing circuit with nebulizer. 11. Bacteria filter coupling, nebulizer. 12. Tube nebulizer. (Courtesy of Puritan Bennett, Lenexa, KS.)

ventilator speaking valve will not be rebreathing CO_2 but will be exhaling normally through the upper airway. In this case, the use of an exhalation valve serves no purpose.

MOBILIZATION OF SECRETIONS

Bronchial Hygiene Therapy

If a patient is unable to mobilize and manage secretions, this requires intervention strategies from clinicians to facilitate removal of secretions that obstruct ventilation and promote infection. Normal body actions to remove secretions include cough after a deep breath, physical exertion, and the lung's mucociliary transport mechanism. The reduction or impairment of mucociliary transport comes as a result of epithelial cilia damage or functional obstruction. This can be due to external causes such as smoking, pollution, or anhydrous gas inhalation or due to internal conditions such as infection, obstruction, dehydration, hypoxia, and electrolyte imbalance. With retained secretions a patient is at risk of airway obstruction including alveolar obstruction, infection risk, inflammation, and atelectasis. All of these can lead to a decrease in effective ventilation and an increase in work of breathing.

The terms *pulmonary bronchial* or *bronchial hygiene* refer to the reduction and management of secretions. This can be accomplished with a variety of methods, alone or in coordination with several methods. In addition, medications can contribute greatly to secretion management. These will be discussed later in this chapter. The next section will review bronchial hygiene techniques, including coughing, intermittent positive pressure breathing, incentive spirometry, forced expiratory technique, postural drainage, chest physical therapy, positioning, and improving chest mobility. Before we review each technique, one should be acquainted with the goals of bronchial hygiene therapy:

To maintain and restore mucous blanket
To hydrate dried retained secretions
To promote expectoration of retained secretions
To humidify inspired gases
To deliver medications deep into the pulmonary tree

Intermittent Positive Pressure Breathing (IPPB) Therapy

IPPB is a therapeutic modality from the 1950s and 1960s that is generally not supported by scientific studies and thus is not usually recommended.

The goals of intermittent positive pressure breathing therapy are to promote and improve the cough mechanism, to improve the distribution of ventilation, and to deliver medication. This is done by a manipulation of inspiratory/expiratory ratios, an increase in airway pressure, and an increase in tidal volume. IPPB is delivered by a pressure-cycled ventilator with a prescribed pressure limit using a mouthpiece and nose clips.

Hazards can include excessive ventilation, resulting in hyperinflation and a feeling of faintness in the patient. Excessive oxygenation can occur due to oxygen being used as a pneumatic air source, especially in diseased lungs that need hypoxic drive to breathe spontaneously. Compressed air machines can resolve this problem. Impedance of venous return can result from improperly applied therapy causing bradycardia, tachycardia, dyspnea and an anxious patient. Corrections in inspiratory and expiratory time and in patient position and patient reassurance may be needed. Also, an increase in intracranial pressure may result as venous return/drainage from the head is congested due to the increase in airway pressures. Another complication can be barotrauma. Although pressures from IPPB are not high enough to cause barotrauma in diseased lungs, a combination of the cough mechanism and IPPB can result in the rupture of blebs, causing barotrauma in patients with lung disease. Hemoptysis (blood in sputum) may be present for no other reason than an increase in ventilation area and the expectoration of retained secretions. However, a physician should be informed of this matter before treatments continue to rule out presence of a tumor or left heart failure. Bronchodilator usage may be needed with IPPB treatments in patients with highly reactive airways and in those who may be prone to bronchospasm from increased airway resistance. Other possible complications include nosocomial infection from improperly maintained equipment and gastric distention occurring when an improperly informed or uncooperative patient swallows air. Also, psychological dependence can occur as patients report feeling relieved after treatments are given, although there may be no need physiologically for the treatment at that time.

Chest Physical Therapy (CPT)

Chest physical therapy is most useful for neuromuscular weakness and postoperative care. It should be coordinated with the administration of postoperative pain medication. It is usually not needed if there is an effective cough.

Chest physical therapy, is used to assist bronchial hygiene by preventing the buildup of and the mobilization of bronchial secretions, improving the cough mechanism, and improving the distribution of ventilation within the lungs. In addition, it is used to improve cardiopulmonary reserves along with exercise and physical conditioning.

Chest physical therapy techniques include postural drainage in which bronchial hygiene is assisted by positioning the body to expedite drainage of secretions, which seeks to improve oxygenation as well as increase ventilated areas.

Caution must be used to avoid intracranial pressures when in the head-down position, and other surgeries may inhibit the application of posturing. Chest percussion is used with postural drainage to loosen secretions. Percussion is achieved by clapping cupped hands rhythmically over a lung area. The energy wave from the clap travels through the lung wall to loosen secretions. This should be done without pain or discomfort to the patient on the bony prominences. Chest vibration is similar, involving the technique of placing the hands on the chest wall and causing a rapid vibratory motion in the arms while compressing the chest wall gently in the direction of the ribs, primarily during the expiration cycle. Again, caution should be taken to select appropriate patients; for example, chest vibration may be contraindicated in brittle (critical) patients, fragile post-surgery patients, or patients with sensitive tissue, such as liver, kidneys, female breast tissue or vital organs.

Voluntary Cough

Cough instruction should be provided to educate a patient in breathing correctly and using the cough technique that can be of greatest assistance in clearing bronchial secretions. A patient can be instructed to take several deep inspiratory breaths before cough to support the generation of back pressure. Placing the hands on the abdomen may also assist coughing efforts. Positioning also can play an important role in effective coughing. A patient should be in an upright, prone, slightly forward position with some arm support. Arm support may be difficult for patients with neurological impairment. Also, as secretions exit out the tracheostomy site, the use of one arm may be required to hold a tissue to catch the secretions.

Normally, coughing occurs out of the oral cavity where secretions are swallowed or expectorated. Coughing is more difficult and less productive in tracheostomized patients. This is due to several factors. Because expectoration back pressures are readily bled out of the tracheostomy site, they do not build up against the upper airway structures as normal coughing would. As a result, these expectoration forces are unavailable or reduced to support coughing efforts. Using a one-way speaking valve (Passy-Muir) in appropriate candidates can be helpful in returning normal cough functions. Care should be taken to secure the speaking valve adequately so as to avoid valve blow-off. When using a one way valve, a patient should be instructed to cough normally out the upper airway and oral cavity instead of through the tracheostomy tube site. Use of a one way speaking valve may not always be possible in patients with an ongoing infection or increased secretions. Removal of speaking valve may be necessary periodically and suspension of valve usage may be required until secretion management improves. Depending on design, one-way valves may have occlusion problems and cough release features that require secretion removal through tracheostomy tube site and are not assistive in functional coughing. Literature provided by the manufacturers of these devices should be reviewed to determine if they recommend using their device for cough enhancement and bronchial hygiene improvement.

Patients will often have additional pain from surgery and be reluctant to cough. Using a pillow to hold onto abdominal muscles and/or used to sprint them or having the therapist hold a slight pressure on the incision site can help support muscles during coughing. Usually, a patient is told to take several breaths. Then, on a deep breath, he or she is to hold that breath for a count of three. Next, while forcefully contracting the abdominal muscles, the patient expels air with an open glottis. Two coughs in succession can be used to expectorate and mobilize secretions.

Cough stimulation can be utilized with a deep breath delivered from the ventilator in conjunction with vibrations and compression. This should provide a high velocity of air from the bronchial tree to mobilize secretions into the trachea for suctioning. Cough stimulation may be needed in patients who are intubated, have glottic disease, or have muscular incompetence.

Manual Cough

This technique is also known as *quad cough* or *diaphragmatic cough*. This type of assistive coughing is used with patients with insufficient expiratory muscle strength or impaired diaphragmatic ability such as high-level spinal cord injury or advanced neuromuscular disease.

The therapist places his or her dominant hand on the patient's abdomen between the xiphoid process at the bottom of the sternum and the umbilicus. Care should be taken to place the hand two inches below the xiphoid process as it is the tip of sternum and can be broken easily. The remaining hand is placed on top of the first hand's fingers as in cardiopulmonary resuscitation. The patient is then instructed to inhale as deeply as possible and then to exhale and attempt to cough. As the patient attempts to exhale and cough, the therapist pushes quickly, firmly, and forcibly in coordination with cough attempts (Figure 4-34). Patient position can vary depending on cough ability. Also, some patients can be taught to manually self-stimulate cough while sitting, standing, or in a supine position by placing arms across the abdomen and bearing forcibly up and in, leaning forward during coughing.

Incentive Spirometry

Sustained maximal inspiration therapy or incentive spirometry is used to encourage maximal lung inflation, prevent atelectasis, prevent accumulation of secretions, assist the cough mechanism, and detect early the onset of acute pulmonary disease. This technique may be taught preoperatively to ensure patient compliance and understanding of technique.

This therapy can be used as often as every hour to help ensure maximal lung inflation and to fight atelectasis and secretion buildup. Lung expansion should improve the forced vital capacity needed for an effective cough. Inability to perform incentive spirometry may indicate onset of disease complications such as atelectasis or pneumonia even before clinical signs are obvious (e.g., fever, heart rate

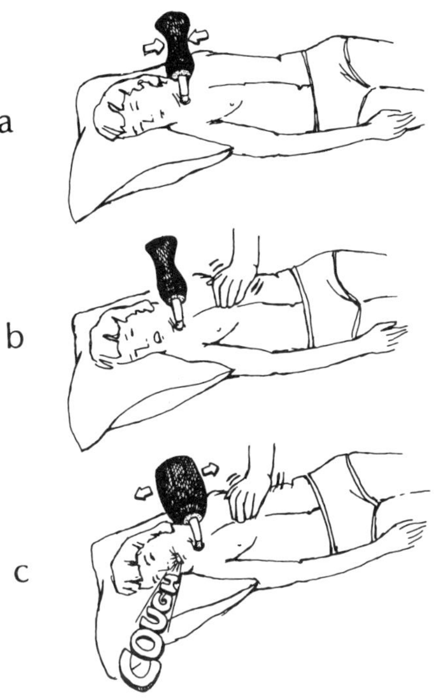

Figure 4-34 Schematic representation of cough stimulation by a manual ventilator and chest physical therapy techniques. ***A,*** *A deep breath is provided and inspiration maintained while* ***B,*** *chest compression and vibration are started.* ***C,*** *A sudden release of the positive pressure allows expiration and may allow high-velocity airflow approaching that of a true cough. (From Shapiro, B.A., Kacmarek, R. M., and Cane, R.D.,* Clinical Application of Respiratory Care, *4th Edition, St. Louis: Mosby-Year Book, 1991, Figure 6-9, p. 102.)*

change, respiratory rate change). Incentive spirometry is usually most successful with a cooperative and motivated patient. In addition, a thorough explanation of the procedure, equipment, technique, and goals to the patient will help ensure effective treatment. Treatment typically will be every hour for 30 to 60 seconds, with each maneuver repeated four or five times, for no more than 5 minutes each hour. Patient performance and progress should be monitored a minimum of twice a day.

Forced Expiratory Technique

Forced expiratory technique causes less airway compression and lower pulmonary pressure than coughing. In patients who experience pain with coughing, bronchospasm, or uncontrolled paroxysmal coughing, this method can be helpful to mobilize secretions. Incorporating this technique with chest physical therapy (percussion) and/or postural draining may make both types of therapies more productive in secretion expectoration. The patient should be instructed to take a deep inspiratory breath and after beginning exhalation, produce two to three forceful exhalation bursts with the mouth and throat open. Instruction should be given to use forceful abdominal contractions during forced exhalation attempts. It can be beneficial to instruct the patient to say "Ha-Ha-Ha" or "Hu-Hu" while attempting forced expiratory technique. These attempts are best followed by a period of rested diaphragmatic breathing to prevent the occurrence of bronchospasm.

Postural Drainage

As mentioned earlier, patient positioning can affect the accumulation of secretions in the lungs, prohibiting optimum distribution of ventilation and the mobilization of secretions. For postural drainage a patient is positioned so that lung areas treated are superior to (above) the bronchi draining the lung lobes or segments. This promotes gravitational drainage to clear secretions. Figures 4-35 and 4-36 are diagrams indicating how secretion drainage and mobilization can occur via gravity from consolidated areas of the lungs by changing patient positions. Treatment should be prior to or at least one hour after meals to prevent reflux or vomiting. It should be determined with auscultation and chest x-ray which lung segments require drainage. Hydration and medication treatments should be implemented to assist in drainage of secretions. Patients should try to maintain positions for 3 to 15 minutes, and longer in certain circumstances. It is common practice to begin with the most congested segment and to leave the patient in that same position if appropriate at the end of the session to promote drainage. Therapists should begin with apical segments and move thereafter on to the lower lobes. Only involved lung segments

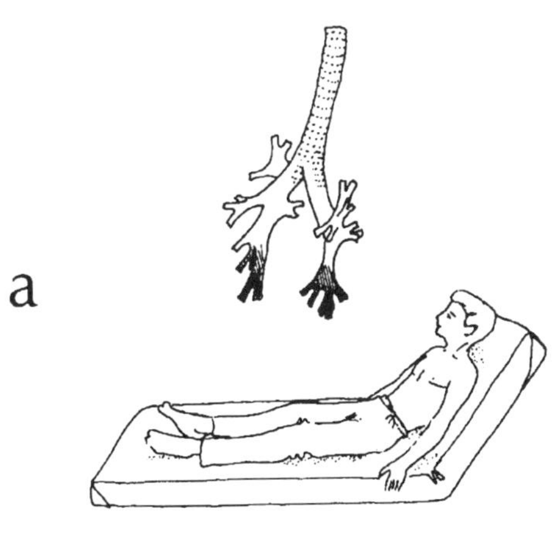

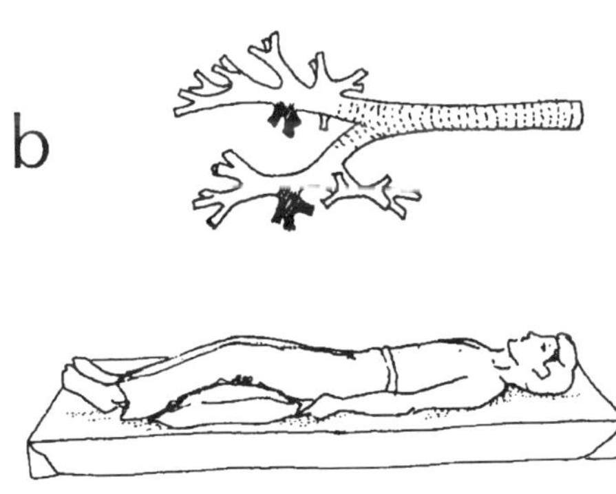

Figure 4-35 Common body positions for ill or convalescent patients. ***A,*** *Common "hospital bed" position. Note that the shaded segmental and subsegmental bronchi of the posterior basilar segments of the lower lobes have no gravity drainage. These are the areas of the lung most commonly involved with atelectasis and pneumonia in the acutely ill patient.* ***B,*** *Supine position; there is absence of gravity drainage of the apical segments of the lower lobes. (From Shapiro, B.A., Kacmarek, R.M., and Cane, R.D.,* Clinical Application of Respiratory Care, *4th Edition, St. Louis: Mosby-Year Book, 1991, Figure 6-2, p. 97.)*

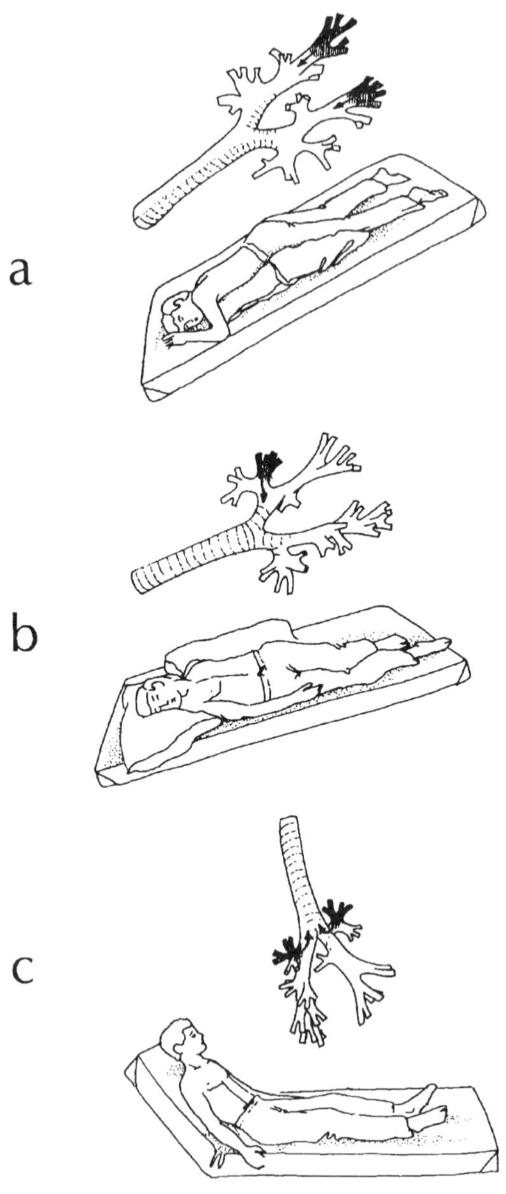

Figure 4-36 Common postural drainage positions for ***A,*** *posterior basilar segments;* ***B,*** *middle lobe and lingula; and* ***C,*** *apical segments of upper lobes. (From Shapiro, B.A., Kacmarek, R.M., and Cane, R.D.,* Clinical Application of Respiratory Care, *4th Edition, St. Louis: Mosby-Year Book, Figure 6-3, p. 98.)*

should be drained. The patient should be instructed to relax and breathe slowly.

Clinical indications for postural drainage usually involve the impairment of secretion clearance, increased secretion production and retainment, and an impairment in coughing ability. Diseases and conditions that might benefit from postural drainage include, but are not limited to, cystic fibrosis, acute atelectasis, lung abscess, bronchiectasis, and ventilator dependency. Also, postural drainage may be used for appropriate post-surgical patients and patients experiencing prolonged bed rest. Precautions must be taken for recent surgeries and healing tissue areas (e.g., skin grafts or spinal fusion) and for the head-down position which affects venous return to the head and can cause increasing intracranial pressures. Contraindications also include lack of patient tolerance; unstable cardiac status; head, thoracic, or spinal surgery; tracheoesophageal fistula; esophageal reflux; recent meals; tension pneumothorax; bronchopleural fistula; frank hemoptysis; pulmonary edema, pulmonary embolus; orthopedic procedures; elevated blood pressure; chest fractures; seizures; and open wounds.

Metered Dose Inhaler

Metered dose inhalers release a specific amount of propellant gas with a precise amount of medication. A high velocity of the gas and medication is mixed and discharged through a small opening (Figure 4-37). This inhaler should be used at the beginning point of a slow, deep inhalation. Most studies show that only 10% of the medication reaches the lung because the majority of medication falls in the oropharynx or remains in the device. Many hospitals are now

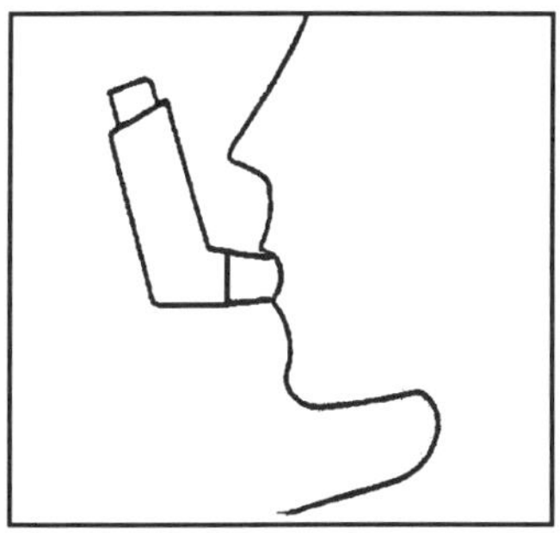

Figure 4-37 Metered dose inhaler.

using a spacer device that improves technique and enhances deposition. For most people the metered dose inhaler is the most effective technique for medication inhalation (bronchodilators, steroids, and/or cromolyn).

Assessing Effectiveness of Bronchial Hygiene Therapy

The effectiveness of any of the above therapies (Table 4-1) can be assessed by auscultation, sputum production, work of breathing and blood gas measurements. Through the use of auscultation, breath sounds are evaluated to interpret effective aeration of the lung. For example, in the case of bronchial asthma, auscultation would demonstrate improvement of the condition if normal breath sounds were heard along with good aeration of all areas of the chest. Use of accessory muscles, rate of breathing and ventilatory pattern will reveal work of breathing and changes in blood gases. Blood gas measurements should improve if retained secretions are mobilized allowing for improved gas exchange at alveolar sites. However, in some instances, benefits from therapy may not be reflected by blood gas changes. Pulmonary function studies may improve, indicating that therapy has been effective, however changes may not always occur in every patient. In addition, the improvement of bronchial hygiene may be seen radiographically as portions of the lung become clear of infiltrates and densities.

MEDICATIONS

Selected Pulmonary Medications

Pulmonary medications typically work to reduce secretion levels, relieve airway obstruction (bronchodilators), regulate nervous system (breath rate), and relieve allergic reactions.

Decongestants

Decongestants are among the most widely used medications. They decrease upper airway edema and stimulate alpha receptors that can increase blood pressure. Some decongestants may act as anti-

Findings	Therapy*
Thick/tenacious secretions with or without wheezing	
Retained with adequate VC	USN/CPT + BD
Retained with inadequate VC	USN (± CPT) + BD
Able to mobilize	USN ± BD
Wheezing with thin secretions	NEB BD ± CPT
Wheezing without secretions	NEB BD
Absorptive atelectasis	USN/CPT (± BD)
Benefit of doubt	
Postoperative fever	USN + IS
Post-thoracotomy	USN/CPT + IS
Chronic lung disease with questionable acute symptoms or findings	USN + BD
No identifiable bronchial hygiene problem	
Postoperative	IS
Bedridden	IS
No increased risk of pulmonary disease	No therapy
Frequency of therapy	
Tachypnea, shortness of breath, or distressful symptoms	Every 4 hr (twice for every 8-hr shift)
Patient not in distress	QID (twice on day and evening shifts)

*Abbreviations: USN, ultrasonic nebulized 0.5N saline solution; CPT, chest percussion, vibration, postural drainage, and cough assist; BD, bronchodilator; NEB BD, nebulized bronchodilator; IS, incentive spirometry.

Table 4-1 Bronchial Hygiene Regimen. (From Shapiro, B.A., Kacmarek, R.M., and Cane, R.D., Clinical Application of Respiratory Care, *4th Edition, St. Louis: Mosby-Year Book, 1991, p. 105.)*

inflammatory drugs and may have secondary side effects such as central nervous system depression leading to lower respiratory rate, sleepiness, and reduced cognitive status.

Mucolytic Drugs

Mucolytic drugs are thought to assist in the movement and removal of mucous secretions. Expectorants are one group of these drugs which encourage the release of secretions by initially increasing secretion levels leading to a reduction in mucus levels and viscosity as result of secretion expectoration. Mucolytic drugs decrease mucous viscosity, although some, such as acetylcysteine, may induce bronchospasm.

Wetting solutions such as saline, water and hypertonic solutions may increase the viscosity of secretions, helping to loosen them for expectoration or suctioning. These agents may also increase the volume of secretions, and use must be carefully monitored to produce an effective pulmonary hygiene regimen to reduce bronchial secretion levels. In addition, use of salt/saline solution can lead to electrolyte imbalance, bronchospasm, and nausea in some patients.

Corticosteroids

Corticosteroids are anti-inflammatory drugs that relieve bronchospasm when other medications such as methylxanthine or adrenergic sympathomimetics do not produce desired relief. They are the agent of choice used to treat asthma, immunologic and allergic reactions or diseases. Typical corticosteroid medications include hydrocortisone, beclomethasone, dipropionate, prednisone, methylprednisolone, and dexamethasone. Secondary side effects include hypertension, Cushing's syndrome, bone loss, and weight gain.

Methylxanthines

Methylxanthines are bronchodilator medications. Typical medications used are theophylline and aminophylline. Secondary side effects include arrhythmias or increased heart rate, central nervous system stimulation resulting in an anxious and excitable patient, insomnia, seizures, and an increase in the production of gastric acid gastroesophageal reflux leading to indigestion or even vomiting. Due to varying metabolism and drug interaction, it is difficult to adjust the dose accurately. Monitoring blood levels is often important when these medications are used. There is much controversy over the actual beneficial effects of methylxanthines.

Anticholinergics

These are bronchodilators that function by blocking acetylcholine action. Typical examples include ipratropium (Atrovent) and atropine. Secondary side effects can include heart rate increase or tachycardia; secretion thickening; central nervous systems effects such as irritability, anxiety, pupil dilation, tremor, sleeplessness, or possible cerebral vasoconstriction, nausea, or vomiting.

Adrenergic Sympathomimetics

Beta-2 adrenergic bronchodilators are the most selective for bronchial effect (rather than cardiovascular effect). Examples include metaproterenol and albuterol. Adrenergic sympathomimetics emulate the sympathetic nervous system, increasing bronchodilatation. Typical examples include epinephrine, ephedrine, racepinephrine, isoproterenol, isoetharine, and albuterol. Secondary effects include increased blood pressure and diaphoresis (sweating). These agents are useful in the treatment of asthma; however, recent data suggest that tachyphylaxis occurs. That is, the more frequently these drugs are used, the less efficacious they become. Thus, they are best used on an as-needed basis rather than as chronic therapy.

ADDITIONAL PULMONARY REHABILITATION

Pursed Lip Breathing

Pursed lip breathing can be used only with tracheostomy or ventilator dependent patients as part of the pulmonary rehabilitation program when a speaking valve or tracheostomy tube cap or plug is in place. A patient is directed to take a normal breath through the nose while counting to two, then purse their lips and exhale slowly, and then relax to a count of four. It is helpful to initially instruct the patient to place a hand in front of the mouth to feel even exhalation airflow. This technique should be incorporated into all daily activities or exercise regimens. Pursed lip breathing is used to compensate for the exertional dyspnea in chronic obstructive lung disease and can be helpful in ventilator weaning efforts. Controlled breathing should reduce the work of breathing, improve ventilation, decrease accessory muscle use, and reduce potential air-trapping. Typically a patient will have to receive training in this technique. Many patients with chronic obstructive lung disease may become pursed lip breathers as their disease slowly progresses and the body tries to compensate for poor gas exchange. This is primarily because pursed lip breathing slows exhalation time and there is more back pressure into the lungs and a longer time for gas exchange (diffusion) to take place. Pursed lip breathing may also help to prevent airway collapse during expiration by providing a back pressure (PEEP/CPAP) effect.

Segmental Breathing

Clinical use of segmental breathing is for the treatment of decreased chest mobility or the management of retained secretions. A patient should be in a relaxed and comfortable position. Depending on the lung lobe location, the patient is instructed to place a hand on that section: (i.e. apical lobes would require placement of the hand just below the clavicle with exertion of a firm pressure at the end of exhalation). Next upon inspiration the patient should be instructed to breathe into his/her hand, then to hold that breath for 2 to 3 seconds, finally relaxing into exhalation. The technique is used to improve ventilation and increase range of motion in the chest wall in a specific area and reduce accumulation of secretions or pleural fluid. Use of this technique would be contraindicated with patients who have lung hyperinflation or air-trapping.

Diaphragmatic Breathing

Clinical indications for diaphragmatic breathing include postoperative use, the management of chronic obstructive pulmonary disease, dyspnea, and diaphragmatic weakness. A subject should be positioned comfortably. Optimally, this would be in a supine position with the head of the bed at a 30 to 40% angle. The patient should be instructed to place the dominant hand on the abdomen and the non-dominant hand on the sternum, with a gentle pressure at the end of the exhalation phase. The patient should breathe through the nose while pushing the abdomen outward. The patient should feel the abdomen rise and perceive little or no chest movement with the other hand. Exhalation should take twice as long as inspiration and be passive and relaxed with the incorporation of pursed lip breathing. This technique should be practiced with all other daily activities three to four times daily. Diaphragmatic breathing can be incorporated into ventilator use with the inspiratory cycle of the ventilator breath. The goal of this therapy is to improve ventilation, decreasing the work of breathing by the improvement of respiratory muscle coordination.

Respiratory Muscle Strengthening

Clinical indications for the use of diaphragm strengthening include patients who have less than appropriate vital capacity but fair to good diaphragm muscle strength. The goal of this rehabilitation is obviously to improve diaphragm strength, reduce the work of breathing, and increase vital capacity. The patient should be positioned supine with knees flexed. A small weight (3-5 lb) is placed across the epigastric region. Please note the weight should not rest on ribs and should be of a suitable amount for patient breathing efforts. The patient should then maintain a coordinated breathing pattern for a 15-minute period. Changes in breathing pattern could indicate fatigue, and therapy time or weights may be altered. Care should be taken that weights do not slip off the patient's abdomen and rest on hands or arms.

There is considerable research and controversy about breathing retraining and methods to increase strength and endurance. There may be more improvement in overall function than in pulmonary function tests. Breathing against resistive loads is more frequently used today than the use of weights as mentioned here. There is also concern that fatigued muscles can be harmed by too much use and exercise for many situations. More clinical research is needed on these questions.

TRENDS FOR THE FUTURE

Ventilation continues to evolve in sophistication and to provide more quantitative data to better address patient needs. In the future, optimum machinery will be able to automatically adjust to patient need due to the advancing technology of microprocessors. New monitoring systems will also continue to be developed. Due to this trend critical care personnel are constantly challenged to update their knowledge base and technical expertise. Respiratory care professionals will continue to play a crucial role in the management of the ventilator dependent population and are therefore be vital to the health care team.

REFERENCES

1. Masferrer, R., Dolan, G. K., and Ward, J. J., "History of the respiratory care profession." In *Respiratory Care, A Guide to Clinical Practice*, 3rd Edition, Philadelphia: J.B. Lippincott Co., 1991.

2. Morch, E. T., "History of mechanical ventilation." In Kirby, R.R., Banner, M.J., and Downs, J.B. (Eds.): *Clinical Applications of Ventilatory Support*, New York: Churchill Livingstone, 1990.

3. Helmholz, H. F., "Early foundations." In Smith, G.A., (Ed.): *Respiratory Care: Evolution of a Profession*, Lexena, KA: Applied Measurement Professionals, 1989; p. 15.

4. Helmholz, H. F., "Professional champions (1900-1940)." In Smith, G.A., (Ed.): *Respiratory Care: Evolution of a Profession*, Lexena, KA: Applied Measurement Professionals, 1989; p. 22.

5. Sauerbruch, Z. F., "Pathologie des offenes Pneumothorax und die Grundlagen meines ves fahrens zur seiner Aushaltung." *Mitt Greuzgeb Med Chir*, 2904; 8:399-411.

6. Shaw, L.A., and Drinker, P., "An apparatus for the prolonged administration of artificial respiration." I. A design for adults and children. *J Clin Invest*, 1929; 7:229-247.

7. Snider, G. L., "Historical perspective on mechanical ventilation: From simple life support system to ethical dilemma." *Am Rev Resp Dis*, 1989; 140:s2-7.

8. Kirby, R. R., Banner, M. J., and Downs, J. B., *Clinical Applications of Ventilatory Support*, New York: Churchill Livingstone, 1990.

BIBLIOGRAPHY

Bell, C.W., Blodgett, D., Goike, C.A., Green, M., Kieffer, J., and Smith, M.A., *Home Care and Rehabilitation in Respiratory Medicine*. Philadelphia: J.B. Lippincott Company, 1984.

California College for Health Sciences, *Technician Program Volume I*, San Diego: 1985.

Criner, G., Make, B. and Celli, B., "Respiratory muscle dysfunction secondary to chronic tracheostomy tube placement." *Chest*, 91(1): 1987; 139-141.

Daily, B.J. and Allen, M.L., "Nursing care of the mechanically ventilated patient." In Nochomovitz, M.L., and Montenegro, H.D., (Eds.), *Ventilatory Support in Respiratory Failure.* New York: Futura Publishing Co., 1987.

Eubanks, D.H. and Bone, R.C., *Comprehensive Respiratory Care*, St. Louis: The C.V. Mosby Company, 1990.

Hughes, C.W., and Popovich, J., "Uses and abuses of pressure support ventilation: PSV's value may lie in controlled weaning in special cases." *The Journal of Critical Illness*, 1989; (4): 25-32.

Johnson, D.L., Giovannoni, R.A., and Driscoll, S.A., *Ventilator-Assisted Patient Care Planning for Hospital Discharge and Home Care.* Rockville: Aspen Publishers, 1986.

Kacmarek, R.M. and Stoller, J.K., *Current Respiratory Care*, Philadelphia: B.C. Decker, Inc., 1988.

Kersten, L.D., *Comprehensive Respiratory Nursing*, Philadelphia: W.B. Saunders Company, Harcourt Brace Jovanovich, 1989.

Marini, J.J., "Mechanical ventilation: Taking the work out of breathing?" *Respiratory Care*, 1986; 31: 695-702.

McPherson, S.P. and Spearman, C.B., *Respiratory Therapy Equipment.* St. Louis: The C.V. Mosby Company, 1990.

Shapiro, B.A., Harrison, R.A., and Trout, C.A. (Eds.). *Clinical Application of Respiratory Care.* Chicago: Year Book Medical Publishers, 1979.

Wade, J.F. *Comprehensive Respiratory Care: Physiology and Technique* (3rd ed.). St. Louis: C.V. Mosby Company, 1982.

Wilkins, R.L., Sheldon, R. L., and Krider, S. J., *Clinical Assessment in Respiratory Care*, St. Louis: C. V. Mosby Co., 1990.

CHAPTER V

TRANSDISCIPLINARY TEAM CONCEPT

Marta S. Kazandjian, *M.A., C.C.C.-SLP*
Co-Director, Speech Pathology
Long Beach Memorial Hospital
Long Island, New York
Director, Speech Pathology
Village Nursing Home
New York, New York
Consultant, Silvercrest Extended Care Facility
Jamaica, New York
Executive Director
Communication Independence for Neurologically Impaired
New York, New York

Karen Dikeman, *M.A., C.C.C.-SLP*
Co-Director, Speech Pathology
Long Beach Memorial Hospital
Long Island, New York
Consultant, Silvercrest Extended Care Facility
Jamaica, New York
Consultant, Mary Manning Walsh Home
New York, New York

Edited by:

Theronne B. Singletary, *M.S., C.C.C.-SLP*
Director, Speech-Language Pathology Services
University of Tennessee Medical Center
Instructor, Department of Audiology and Speech Pathology
University of Tennessee
Knoxville, Tennessee

Ahmet Baydur, *M.D., F.A.C.P., F.C.C.P.*
Director, Chest Medicine Service
Rancho Los Amigos Medical Center
Associate Professor of Clinical Medicine
University of Southern California School of Medicine
Los Angeles, California

INTRODUCTION

Tracheostomized and ventilator dependent patients require a multifaceted treatment approach most effectively provided by the transdisciplinary team. It is the needs of these complex patients that dictate the presence of such an array of clinical professionals. The needs of the tracheostomized and ventilator dependent patients can be loosely classified into the medical, physical, communicative, psychosocial, recreational, and vocational areas. Intervention in each area, although often overlapping, will fall to specific clinical specialties. It is the intent of this chapter to illustrate that the transdisciplinary team is more than the isolated efforts of each professional, but rather a coordinated concept of care to meet the special needs of this population.

The transdisciplinary team includes a number of highly specialized professionals and clinicians commonly present in hospital and extended-care settings. Tables 5-1 and 5-2 list the individuals necessary for the management of the tracheostomized and ventilator dependent patient and the varied settings in which they work.

AREAS OF NEED FOR THE TRACHEOSTOMIZED AND VENTILATOR DEPENDENT PATIENT

Medical

Physicians

Typically, the leader of the transdisciplinary team, who coordinates the overall management of the tracheostomized and ventilator dependent patient, is the primary care physician. Depending upon the medical setting, this individual may be a pulmonologist, internist, otolaryngologist, pediatrician, neurologist, cardiologist, orthopedist, physiatrist, trauma surgeon, thoracic surgeon, neurosurgeon, intensive care or critical care physician, or perhaps a geriatrician. The primary care physician is responsible for consulting the appropriate medical and rehabilitation professionals as well as coordinating their assessment and intervention efforts with the patient. He or she then develops the timetable of treatments within the comprehensive care plan. These decisions must be communicated to the patient and his or her family in a comprehensible, nonintimidating fashion.

Medical

Primary Care Physician and Consulting Physicians may include any of the following:

Pulmonologist	Physiatrist
Internist	Trauma Surgeon
Otolaryngologist	Thoracic Surgeon
Pediatrician	Neuro Physician/Surgeon
Neurologist	Intensive Care/Critical Care
Cardiologist	Geriatrician
Orthopedist	

Medical Professionals

Respiratory/Pulmonary Therapist
Nurse Specialists (Otolaryngology, Pulmonary, Rehabilitation)
Nurse/Nurse Technician/Nurses Aide
Dietician/Nutritionist
Feeding/Swallowing Team
Pharmacist

Physical

Physical Therapist
Licensed Physical Therapist Assistant
Physical Therapy Technician
Occupational Therapist
Certified Occupational Therapist Assistant
Rehabilitation Engineer

Vocational/Recreational

Vocational Therapist
Recreational Therapist
Special Educator/Teacher

Psychosocial

Social Worker/Case Manager
Psychologist/Psychiatrist
Chaplain
Patient/Family

Communication

Audiologist
Speech-Language Pathologist

Table 5-1 Transdisciplinary Team Members.

Acute Care Facilities (Respiratory Intensive Care Unit, Surgical Intensive Care Unit, Coronary Care Unit, Trauma Unit)

Rehabilitation Units (Acute Inpatient Rehabilitation Facilities vs. Free-Standing Facilities)

Extended Care Facilities (Skilled Nursing Facilities, Specialized Ventilation Units, etc.)

Home Care

Table 5-2 Treatment Settings.

The medical setting will certainly define the role of the primary care physician. For example, in a trauma center, the critical care physician or trauma surgeon frequently places and manages the tracheostomy tube and calls in pulmonary and otolaryngology consults as needed. In the pulmonary intensive care unit (ICU), the pulmonologist functions as the patient's primary care physician. In contrast, in the long-term care setting, the internist or geriatrician provides the daily medical care. The pulmonologist in this setting is heavily involved in managing respiratory status.

As the team leader, the primary care physician provides updated information regarding a patient's medical and physical status, which will directly impact upon the type of rehabilitation provided. For example, it will be the primary care physician who clears the patient to be assessed for a one-way speaking valve by the speech-language pathologist and the respiratory/pulmonary therapist.[1] Factors such as the ability to tolerate changes in ventilatory mode and the resistance offered by placement of an external valve will impact upon his or her decision. Coordination of medications prescribed by all specialty areas will also fall to the primary care physician.

The primary care physician must have an understanding of the special skills that each team member brings to the total management of the tracheostomized and ventilator dependent patient. Beyond a recognition for skilled medical care, there should be an equally keen appreciation for the rehabilitative efforts most likely to enhance the patient's quality of life. The role of inservice education for all team members is discussed later in this chapter.

The primary care physician will contact adjunct physicians to consult with the team as appropriate. Each brings unique skills with resulting varied responsibilities to the team approach. Whatever the medical setting, the pulmonologist and otolaryngologist are usually involved with the patient throughout the course of care. These two specialty areas work closely with the speech-language pathologist.

The pulmonologist is instrumental in the decisions that determine ventilatory status and initial tracheostomy placement. The pulmonologist will order and interpret pulmonary function tests that provide information regarding O_2 saturation and CO_2 exchange. For patients with progressive respiratory diseases, such as chronic obstructive pulmonary diseases, or degenerative neuromuscular conditions, such as amyotrophic lateral sclerosis (ALS), this feedback regarding pulmonary status will guide the timetable of available treatments. Many individuals with degenerative respiratory diseases begin with O_2 delivered via nasal cannula or nasal mask, progressing to eventual tracheostomy when the pulmonologist determines that the patient can no longer maintain adequate ventilation. Pulmonary function tests will also play a major role in the weaning process for the ventilator dependent, medically stable patient.

Prior to the development of the team concept, it was more common for the pulmonologist to focus on the patient's ventilatory status, perhaps to the exclusion of other parts of the care plan, such as communication and swallowing. Feedback provided to the pulmonologist by the team is integral in total care. For example, the respiratory therapist and speech-language pathologist may actually assist in the process of weaning a patient from the ventilator. The pulmonologist approves changes that promote communication and safe swallowing, such as cuff deflation and/or changing the size of the tracheostomy tube, as well as alterations in ventilatory mode and changes in ventilatory settings. While specific changes are directed by the pulmonologist, the patient's responses to these changes are monitored by the respiratory therapist, nursing staff, and speech-language pathologist. Patient response to treatment changes must be communicated to the pulmonologist, who can then work most effectively with the "total" patient, integrating this invaluable feedback into the treatment protocol.

From the initial surgical placement of the tracheostomy tube through follow-up, the otolaryngologist (ENT) works closely with the primary care physician, pulmonologist, and other rehabilitation professionals. The ENT who is aware of the potential impact of tracheotomy will consider the impact of incision type upon speech and swallowing. Once the tracheostomy tube is in place, the ENT is often responsible for monthly tracheostomy tube changes and during these times provides input in modifying the size of the tracheostomy tube. In some facilities, depending upon the setting, this role may be taken by the thoracic or trauma surgeon, with the otolaryngologist consulted only when problems arise with decannulation.

Monitoring of the stoma site and assessment of potential airway complications are also integral to the management offered by the ENT. Problems not uncommon to the tracheostomized and ventilator dependent patient include laryngeal webs and tracheal stenosis, possible consequences of intubation trauma. Tracheoesophageal fistulas may occur as a result of overinflation of the tracheostomy tube cuff. They can be potentially life threatening due to entry of saliva or food from the esophagus into the trachea. Granulation tissue develops in many tracheostomized patients around sites of irritation, such as a fenestration in the tracheostomy tube. When granulation tissue grows into the fenestration, it anchors the tube to the tracheal wall. The ENT would be responsible for the diagnosis and surgical management of these problems.

The speech-language pathologist and ENT perform cooperative evaluations in the assessment of voice and swallowing. Vocal cord status is of primary concern to the speech-language pathologist in determining candidacy for oral communication options, such as a speaking valve or a talking tracheostomy tube. Additionally, since laryngeal valving plays a primary role in airway protection, evaluation of vocal cord status is requested by the speech-language pathologist as part of a comprehensive dysphagia evaluation. A fiber-optic endoscopic evaluation of swallowing (FEES) can be performed by the ENT and speech-language pathologist for direct visualization of the pharynx and larynx during swallowing of a controlled amount of food or liquid.[2] After joint assessment of structure and function, cooperative recommendations can then be made regarding oral intake and the need for further objective assessment (videofluoroscopy). It is through the cooperative efforts of these team members working interactively that the patient will derive the greatest benefit.

Respiratory/Pulmonary Therapist

Team interaction in decision making can be further illustrated through the role of the respiratory/pulmonary therapist. The respiratory/pulmonary therapist's involvement extends beyond the traditional, yet vital, functions of changing ventilatory tubing, monitoring biomedical equipment, adjusting ventilator settings, obtaining blood gases, suctioning, and providing respiratory treatments. The primary care physician and pulmonologist rely upon the physiological assessment performed by the respiratory/pulmonary therapist. These pulmonary function tests are interpreted by the physician and provide the basis of medical diagnoses and management. The respiratory/pulmonary therapist plays an active role in monitoring the patient's medical and respiratory status via oximetry and capnography and provides frequent updates to the entire team. This therapist identifies opportunities for retesting and determining weaning potential. Other suggestions such as modifications in ventilatory mode may also be made to the physician by the respiratory/pulmonary therapist. These recommendations are often prompted by the therapist's observations during daily interactions with the patient.

Perhaps the most recent role of the respiratory/pulmonary therapist and speech-language pathologist is their joint participation in the communicative rehabilitation of the tracheostomized and ventilator dependent patient. To maximize intervention, each specialty must develop a fundamental understanding of the principles of the other specialty. During their joint consultation, for example, the respiratory/pulmonary therapist understands that adequate oromotor and vocal cord functions are a prerequisite for oral communicative options. Alternatively, the speech-language pathologist realizes that maintenance of ventilatory volume return and the ability to clear secretions must take a priority over phonation and therefore recognizes the purpose underlying ventilator modifications. While cooperatively evaluating the patient, the respiratory/pulmonary therapist and speech-language pathologist "trouble shoot" the patient's ability to tolerate cuff deflation, changes in ventilatory settings, use of a speaking valve, or placement of a talking tracheostomy tube. For example, when placing a one-way speaking valve, the speech-language pathologist is focused upon vocal quality, while the respiratory/pulmonary therapist concentrates on the oximetry readings reflecting O_2 saturation. The end result of this team effort is the achievement of phonation with the maintenance of optimal ventilation.

Nursing Staff

Although physicians and therapists may interact with the patient on a daily basis, their focus is the delivery of specific interventions. Nurses, however, have the opportunity to review and provide feedback to all specialties throughout the day.[3] The nurse should be recognized as the informal team leader and coordinator of the patient care plan. Nursing staff is usually the first to interact with the newly admitted patient and family, and nurses obtain a case history that forms the basis for subsequent therapeutic assessments. For the tracheostomized and ventilator dependent patient, nursing staff relays objective information about ventilation, degree of secretions, suctioning needs, and status of the tracheostomy tube cuff. Patients often initially report their many anxieties related to respiratory dependence to their nurse, and they require the nurse's continued encouragement and support. Nursing facilitates daily input between the patient and the other interdisciplinary team members.

The speech-language pathologist requires nursing input in order to meet the communicative needs of the patient. The patient's communicative partners, communicative attempts, and communicative failures are best reported by a nurse who repeatedly interacts with the patient. The functional use (documenting as to actual interactive use and success) of augmentative or alternative communication systems, ranging from letter/picture boards to more sophisticated electronic devices, can be documented in varied situations. During the speech-language pathologist's clinical evaluation of swallowing, the essential team involvement of the nurse is easily illustrated. Following the initiation of the blue dye test by the speech-language pathologist, the nurse records the presence of tainted material during periodic suctioning. The nurse also reports the patient's tolerance of dietary modifications (e.g., thickened liquids). In addition, the nurse can provide information regarding the patient's cognitive status. The speech-language pathologist relies upon the nurse in many aspects of communicative intervention.

Dietician/Nutritionist

While the nurse reports the patient's daily oral or non-oral intake, the registered dietician or nutritionist is responsible for calorie counts and the actual monitoring of metabolic data via laboratory analysis. The registered dietician is also skilled in the subjective analysis of overall physical status (e.g., skin appearance) as an indicator of possible nutritional deficiencies.[4] In addition, the registered dietician makes recommendations for nutritional supplements. Ventilator dependent patents often need dietary supplements, especially during the weaning process, due to increased caloric needs. Although all tracheostomized and ventilator dependent patients do not necessarily require a specialized diet, their concomitant medical problems and unique stress factors do require particular attention. For example, a patient with a diagnosis of chronic obstructive pulmonary disease and associated cardiac problems requires a carefully controlled diet as each condition warrants different intervention. In another example, bedridden patients frequently develop decubitus ulcers, requiring the registered dietician to identify increased sources of protein. For those patients requiring tube feedings, an inability to tolerate a particular formula may pose a management challenge. The registered dietician may need to creatively alter formula type, feeding schedule and feeding method (e.g., gravity versus pump) to improve the patient's tolerance of the alternate feeding.

Parenteral nutrition may be indicated for selected tracheostomized and ventilator dependent patients. It may be used to correct severe nutritional depletion in patients unable to maintain adequate oral intake or to bypass a dysfunctional gastrointestinal tract. Some facilities utilize a team of individuals specializing in the delivery of parenteral feedings. Such a team usually includes a dietician, a pharmacist, and a nurse.

Other dietary-related problems are more specifically associated with tracheostomy and ventilator dependence. In many of these cases the registered dietician and speech-language pathologist will coordinate intervention. For some individuals, the registered dietician will relay to the speech-language pathologist a patient's complaint of bloating or fullness. These symptoms may be related to the ingestion of air during attempts to communicate orally. More seriously this bloating may exert pressure on the diaphragm and may exacerbate the symptoms of restrictive disease. The speech-language pathologist may be able to instruct the patient to use an alternate technique during phonation. Secretion management is another arena of concern for the speech-language pathologist who is attempting to provide a means of oral communication. For example, copious secretions may prevent a patient from being considered as a candidate for a speaking valve. The registered dietician may assist by eliminating foods that contribute to increased secretion production or inhibit management or control of mucus. The teamwork of the speech-language pathologist and registered dietician is crucial for the management of the dysphagic patient. The registered dietician also assists the speech-language pathologist in changing feeding schedules as the patient is weaned from an NPO (nothing per oral/mouth) to PO (per oral) status. Modification of dietary consistencies is often needed to facilitate safe swallowing in the patient with oral/pharyngeal dysphagia. The registered dietician can aid the speech-language pathologist in selecting food types that meet the patient's nutrition and hydration requirements within the recommended consistencies and in selecting supplemental feedings that adhere to consistency modifications.

Feeding/Swallowing Team

The transdisciplinary team concept is easily illustrated by the transdisciplinary "feeding/swallowing team."[5] This team is a group of professionals who collectively address the nature and cause of dysphagia as well as other potential problems that may interfere with oral feeding. The swallowing/feeding team is designed to meet the needs of all patients receiving nasogastric and gastrostomy tube feedings. The feeding/swallowing team is directed by the speech-language pathologist and consists of the physician, nurse/nurse's aide, and registered dietician. The ultimate goal of the team is to ensure that all patients are fed in the safest and most appropriate manner. This concept is easily adapted to help meet the needs of the tracheostomized and ventilator dependent patient.

Pharmacist

The team concept continues with the role of the pharmacist. Pharmacists review the applicability of specific medications for a particular patient. They also monitor possible contraindications and side effects of drug combinations and suggest possible alternatives. Pharmacological intervention for the tracheostomized and ventilator dependent patient often takes the form of daily respiratory treatments. A pharmacist, participating in transdisciplinary team conferences, may recommend particular medications to maximize the patient's performance in rehabilitation. For example, the speech-language pathologist and the physician, in an effort to reduce the potential for aspiration and improve oral communication, may consult the pharmacist in selection of medications to aid in secretion control. The pharmacist and physician would evaluate the risk-benefit ratio of such pharmacological medical intervention. The pharmacist can assist the speech-language pathologist by providing information regarding available drug mediums for dysphagic patients. For example, a particular patient with a swallowing problem may be able to tolerate a medication in liquid form versus pill form.

The complex medical needs of the tracheostomized and ventilator dependent patient require that these medical specialists and paraprofessionals work in concert with one another to provide not only skilled care but also optimal intervention.

Physical

Physical Therapist

Addressing the physical areas of need for the tracheostomized and ventilator dependent patient involve the disciplines of physical therapy, occupational therapy, and rehabilitation engineering.

The physical therapist's role incorporates more traditional therapy as well as highly specialized treatments tailored to the needs of the tracheostomized and ventilator dependent patient. These patients are often physically impaired and may be bedbound. Physical therapists, in conjunction with occupational therapists, assess bed positioning needs and potential for contractures. In addition, they assess muscle function and determine candidacy for ambulation status or, for the quadriplegic patient, provide a maintenance range-of-motion program. For a tracheostomized and ventilator dependent patient, stress testing will be conducted within the limits of the patient's pulmonary capacity. Testing is often conducted with and without a speaking valve to assess respiratory status changes under more strenuous conditions. When conveyed to the team, these results give valuable insight regarding a patient's physical and physiological status.

Physical therapists provide a specialized service in the delivery of chest physical therapy, which includes postural drainage and percussion and assessment of chest wall mobility. In some settings, this role may be assumed by the respiratory therapist. Physical therapists also work to develop respiratory musculature. In this arena, they overlap with speech-language pathologists, who focus upon breath support for phonation. Both disciplines assess breathing patterns (e.g., clavicular versus diaphragmatic) and determine candidacy for alternative breathing techniques (e.g., glossopharyngeal/frog breathing). While physical therapists evaluate the ability to coordinate respiration with movement, speech-language pathologists work to pace phonation with respiration. Another area for both specialties is cough training. Physical therapists focus upon developing the strength of the cough to expectorate secretions. Speech-language pathologists train an intermittent cough/throat clear technique to enhance airway protection during swallowing. Treatment sessions may be conducted jointly when addressing these similar goals. Once again, shared information reported at the transdisciplinary team meetings will allow for continued progress in the overall rehabilitation process.

Occupational Therapist

The occupational therapist, another member of the transdisciplinary team, is concerned with the patient's functional ability for activities of daily living. Nursing staff and other team members rely on the occupational therapist for positioning, transfer status, and equipment needs. Occupational therapists perform their initial evaluation, actively assessing the need for adaptive equipment to compensate for physical loss, such as devices to aid in mobility, dressing, eating, and writing, as well as environmental control. This assistive equipment is essential in providing some level of independence, especially for the quadriplegic ventilator dependent patient. These devices are not limited to use in the hospital setting. The ultimate goal of rehabilitation is community re-entry, therefore assistive devices are prescribed for a patient in an effort to help him/her regain a previous level of functioning.

The speech-language pathologist may request that the occupational therapist, if focusing on fine motor control, practice placement of a speaking valve or manipulation of the external port of a talking tracheostomy tube with the patient. This training benefits not only motor control but also enhances the patient's ability to communicate independently.

Occupational therapists and speech-language pathologists must coordinate their efforts in treatment of cognitive dysfunction and in the provision of alternative/augmentative communication. Given the severity of the physical injury, head-injured patients often require tracheostomy and ventilator support. For those patients whose status is post-traumatic brain injury, co-treatments target overlapping deficits. The focus of each therapy differs. The occupational therapist may be concerned with the effect of the patient's visual perceptual problems on certain environmental interactions. In contrast, the speech-language pathologist identifies the impact of the visual perceptual deficit upon reading and processing visual information. Coordination between these two disciplines as well as others is essential in the treatment of traumatic brain injury. Further coordination of treatment services is evidenced by the transdisciplinary efforts involved in augmentative/alternative communication service delivery. The patient must be able to access the communication system that has been developed by the speech-language pathologist. As a result, the specialized skills of the occupational therapist will aid in switch selection and optimal positioning to ensure that the communication system is functional in all settings (e.g., in the wheelchair, bed, during therapy sessions, etc.). In some facilities an augmentative communication clinic is utilized. Occupational therapists and speech-language pathologists work together with the patient to provide the overall evaluation and the communication system. Inservice training should follow to ensure that a nonspeaking, ventilator dependent patient can communicate with all members of the transdisciplinary team.[6]

Rehabilitation Engineer

The tracheostomized and ventilator dependent patient who requires alternative/augmentative communication (AAC) will need the services of another transdisciplinary team member, the rehabilitation engineer. The rehabilitation engineer is often consulted during the augmentative communication clinic to fabricate and adapt switches, call buzzers, and environment control equipment specified by the speech-language pathologist or occupational therapist.[7] Other team members who may consult the rehabilitation engineer include the vocational therapist and educators. These professionals may require adaptation of technology to meet the patient's particular physical, educational/vocational, recreational, and communicative needs.

Vocational/Recreational

As technological and medical advances have enabled more tracheostomized and ventilator dependent patients to return to the community and perhaps even to the workplace, the roles of the recreational and vocational therapists and educators have become clearly defined.

Vocational Therapist

The vocational therapist who intervenes with the tracheostomized and ventilator dependent individual must work with multiple factors that limit vocational options. Medical status including 24-hour ventilator dependence and need for frequent suctioning and skilled nursing care determines the setting in which the individual can work. Accessibility is an issue that the quadriplegic patient is forced to consider. However, recent legislation mandating accessibility for the disabled in all settings will create increased opportunities for the physically challenged.[8] For the patient with a degenerative neuromuscular disease, the vocational therapist must be prepared to intervene periodically as the patient's physical status changes (e.g., as ambulation or upper extremity status deteriorates). Cognitive limitations place obvious restraints on job selection. For example, the cognitively impaired patient unable to function in a regular work setting may be a candidate for a sheltered workshop program. Emotional and social issues including depression, substance abuse, the presence of a spouse and children, and premorbid work history are also factored into vocational planning. The vocational therapist working with the tracheostomized and ventilator dependent individual is challenged by these many problems. Working closely with the transdisciplinary team and incorporating information from each specialty allow a creative vocational therapist to link the patient with the world outside the medical setting.

Mainstreaming into the educational environment has also become feasible for the tracheostomized and ventilator dependent individual. The development of smaller, truly portable ventilators enables an adult or child to leave a facility to go to school. On site teaching becomes necessary for the more medically unstable patient who is yet unable to pursue educational opportunities in traditional settings. This is especially important for the pediatric patient. The special educator must modify teaching techniques to compensate for physical and medical limitations. The teacher must be prepared to work with the team and incorporate rehabilitative goals into lesson planning. Conversely, other team members should be aware of the goals that the teacher has set, especially for a child who needs continuous reinforcement.

The speech-language pathologist aids the vocational therapist and special educator in planning treatment regimens for the communicatively impaired tracheostomized and ventilator dependent patient.

Information from cognitive and linguistic assessment is valuable in judging the patient's potential for various vocational and educational programs. The treatment goals of language-impaired children are set by the speech-language pathologist but optimally are addressed in a variety of settings, including the classroom. For the nonspeaking tracheostomized and ventilator dependent patient, programming specific language to meet the communicative demands of the workplace and the needs of the classroom is an accomplishment reached through transdisciplinary effort.

The speech-language pathologist, as the swallowing specialist, may also be called upon to inservice classroom staff regarding the dysphagic patient who needs modifications of regular food (e.g., the thickening of thin liquids). Once again, information that is shared during transdisciplinary team conferences is incorporated into the intervention of each discipline.

Recreational Therapist

Recreational therapists are also challenged to modify their therapeutic techniques to meet the needs of the tracheostomized and ventilator dependent patient. Although often overlooked because of the myriad of life-threatening problems and associated complications, recreational needs must be addressed. The stress and trauma associated with tracheostomy and ventilator dependence is so overwhelming that patients themselves may lose awareness of the need for respite. However, it is the role of the recreational therapist to provide individualized activities that provide the patient with an opportunity to connect with leisure pursuits. Initially, for the medically unstable patient, therapeutic recreation may be carried out at the bedside and may take the form of low stress activities such as listening to the patient's favorite music. Outings begin as the patient is weaned onto a portable ventilator. Because the patient and therapist may be traveling far from the facility, additional portable ventilators, portable suction machines, and provisions for manual bagging are integral in the overall planning of outside events. The cooperative efforts of the team help to facilitate safe, enjoyable recreational activities. Nursing staff, for example, help to plan a modified medication schedule, while others from nursing and respiratory therapy may actually accompany the patient on the trip. Medical clearance is naturally obtained prior to including the patient on an outing. The entire team will enjoy hearing the patient's response to this normal, social activity.

The speech-language pathologist may actually co-treat during recreational activities with communicatively and swallowing-impaired patients. During an event, the speech-language pathologist may help a tracheostomized and ventilator dependent patient who is communicatively impaired to respond to a choice of activities by using an electro-larynx or a speaking valve. The speech-language pathologist may set up a specific augmentative communication system to enable a patient to interact during a specific activity. For example, the patient who has the opportunity to go to the museum can utilize a word/phrase board that was fabricated prior to the event with specific comments and questions appropriate to that setting. Any event that includes eating, such as a holiday dinner, requires that the speech-language pathologist monitor dysphagic individuals. The speech-language pathologist has the opportunity to maximize these patients' enjoyment of therapeutic recreation by facilitating or providing communication options. In addition, recreational activities are natural opportunities in which to observe carryover of communicative goals targeted in speech-language treatment.

Psychosocial

Social Worker/Case Manager

The psychosocial needs of the tracheostomized and ventilator dependent patient are therapeutically addressed by the disciplines of social work, psychology, psychiatry, and pastoral services. The family and the patients themselves are also considered valuable adjuncts to the transdisciplinary team.

The role of the social worker cannot be over estimated in the development of the comprehensive case history and in initial discharge planning. The case history includes past medical, family, social, educational, and employment information. By communicating the details obtained from the patient and family, the social worker is instrumental in introducing this patient's particular needs to the team. During the initial period of adjustment for the patient and the family, the social worker provides information on patient rights, health care proxies, right to determination, and do-not-resuscitate orders.[9] Although perhaps difficult for a family to face initially the often tenuous medical status of the patient must be acknowledged. The tracheostomized and ventilator dependent patient's status in the family has changed dramatically and therefore may require that other family members assume new responsibilities. They do so with the assistance of the social worker or case manager. Family and patients also rely upon the social worker to explain the intricacies of private and federal insurance programs and to help in coping with possible loss of income that may accompany long-term disability. When the patient is ready to be discharged to the setting previously determined (i.e., home or extended care facility), the social worker establishes a network of outside referrals and support groups. In addition, exploration of funding for modifications in the home, nursing care to assist with suctioning and gastrostomy tube feedings, and obtaining durable medical equipment may fall upon the social worker. As a member of the transdisciplinary team, the social worker routinely updates the team on the status of family dynamics and discharge planning. This information must be integrated into the treatment goals of all team members.

Psychologist/Psychiatrist

The psychologist and psychiatrist also work closely with the patient and family to help in the adjustment to a new, severe disability. Tracheostomized and ventilator dependent patients, after the initial shock of the physical limitations and change in body image, may become deeply depressed. The psychologist and psychiatrist can help these patients work through their feelings of depression, guilt, and fear of abandonment. If depression interferes drastically with rehabilitation, the psychiatrist may be called upon by the primary care physician and team to prescribe antidepressant medication. Clinical intervention may take the form of individual counseling or perhaps a support group. In these settings, tracheostomized and ventilator dependent patients can share their feelings of loss of privacy and changes in relationships with spouses (e.g., sexual interactions). When meeting with the team, the psychologist and psychiatrist can provide insight as to the patient's adjustment to his or her disability and how this may impact upon participation in the rehabilitation program.

The social worker, psychologist, and psychiatrist consult the speech-language pathologist regarding strategies to facilitate optimal communication exchanges during patient counseling sessions. Speech-language pathologists may often find themselves in the role of counselor to patients and family members. The speech-language pathologist relies upon the guidance of the psychologist and psychiatrist when counseling the patient regarding his/her potential for successful communication and oral feeding. Two examples of the transdisciplinary efforts that coordinate the skills of the speech-language pathologist, social worker, psychologist, and psychiatrist are the anarthria-psychotherapy group and the bioethical committee. An anarthria-psychotherapy group was previously co-led by one of these authors and a psychologist.[10] Nonspeaking tracheostomized and ventilator dependent patients were included in this group and were provided with a forum to express their fears and concerns regarding their disability via alternative communication systems. The bioethical committee was formed to coordinate the efforts of the medical team in dealing with determination issues: living will, right-to-die, and do-not-resuscitate (DNR) orders. As these are issues that tracheostomized and ventilator dependent patients and their families must face, they rely upon the transdisciplinary team to guide them through the moral and legal implications of such decisions. Above all, the bioethical committee was designed to protect the rights of the patient.

Chaplain

Since the patient's sense of self-worth and motivation to participate in the rehabilitation process are paramount, the supportive services of a chaplain should be incorporated into the team structure. Pastoral care is typically available across settings. It is usually free of charge and often nondenominational. Chaplains can be trained in facilitating communication with the tracheostomized and ventilator dependent patient. They can add a crucial dimension to the counseling services provided by the team.

Family and Patient

The transdisciplinary team is not complete without the involvement of the family and of course the patient. The family and/or patient will make the ultimate decision regarding placement upon discharge. For the patient to be integrated back into family life, the family must accept inservice training from appropriate team members. As spouses take on new roles and responsibilities, they may become the patient's advocate for quality care. The transdisciplinary team requires family input and cooperation when forming the patient care plan and periodically updating it according to the patient's needs. It is important for the team members to remember that the family is the ultimate caregiver.

Communication

Audiologist

Audiology plays a vital role in the communication management of tracheostomized and ventilator dependent patients. Isolation is a crucial issue for the patient who has become bedbound and unable to communicate. The additional sensory impairment of a hearing loss is often exacerbated in the noisy environment of an intensive care unit or other specialized ventilator unit. Patients may withdraw and demonstrate anger and/or depression secondary to this extreme isolation. The audiologist is responsible for assessment of conductive and sensorineural hearing losses, referrals to otolaryngology for appropriate medical management, and prescription of assistive listening devices. In addition, the audiologist will inservice the other members of the team in maximizing communication with the hearing-impaired patient.

Speech-Language Pathologist

The role of the speech-language pathologist as a member of the transdisciplinary team involves issues in the medical as well as the communicative management of the tracheostomized and ventilator dependent patient. As a member of the management team, the speech-language pathologist plays a vital role. Restoration of communication by the speech-language pathologist allows inclusion of the patient into the transdisciplinary process, facilitating optimal service delivery.

The speech-language pathologist should be involved with communicatively impaired patients on every level of hospitalization. Early intervention often starts at the bedside of intubated patients and follows them throughout the weaning process. The goal should be to ensure that the patient always has an appropriate communication system available.

As their scope of practice has broadened, speech-language pathologists routinely assess and intervene in the areas of oral and non-oral communication as well as safe swallowing. This will include a comprehensive evaluation of cognitive-linguistic status incorporating alertness, attention, memory, orientation, and behavior, as well as the presence of any aphasic component. These factors will impact upon the patient's ability to regain functional communication. Other team members must be aware of the type of communicative disability of each patient and modify their interactions accordingly.

Oral intervention begins with an assessment of the patient's mouthing ability via a comprehensive oral peripheral examination. Those patients who are orally intubated typically cannot use this modality well, while those with nasal intubation have more flexibility. To expand the use of mouthing, the speech-language pathologist can provide an alternative vibratory source (e.g., electro-larynx), eliminating the need for vocal fold vibration. For patients with inflated tracheostomy tube cuffs, assessing potential voicing via cuff deflation follows in the assessment continuum. As discussed earlier, this evaluation takes place with other transdisciplinary team members and the otolaryngologist or pulmonologist. Cuff deflation and ventilator modifications are performed after medical clearance and with the cooperative effort of the respiratory therapist. Once cuff deflation is accomplished, a speaking valve is considered for patients on or off the ventilator. Establishing a protocol that will incorporate all medical personnel will be essential to the success of these interventions. It is important, for example, that the primary care physician and consulting pulmonologist are in agreement over any changes in the patient's ventilatory status.

The maintenance of safe swallowing is very often a crucial issue for the tracheostomized and ventilator dependent patient. The speech-language pathologist understands the impact of tracheotomy upon the pharyngeal phase of swallowing. Information from the bedside swallowing evaluation, the FEES (conducted by the speech-language pathologist and an ENT), and videofluoroscopy (conducted by the speech-language pathologist and a radiologist) are incorporated into the dysphagia management program. For example, during these diagnostic procedures, a patient may be evaluated with and without a speaking valve to determine any changes in swallowing function. For the pediatric population, dysphagia management includes evaluation of oromotor responses and facilitation via neuromotor techniques such as positioning and modifying oromotor tone. Oromotor treatment should have as its goal the development of appropriate oral, respiratory, and phonatory systems. This treatment is often carried out in cooperation with the occupational and physical therapists.

For those patients unable to achieve oral communication, nonvocal intervention is initiated. Alternative/augmentative communication falls within the speech-language pathologist's scope of practice. Assessment of the tracheostomized and ventilator dependent patient's physical motor status is essential in determining the ability to activate a call buzzer or alerting system as well as evaluating for switch access. Joint involvement from each rehabilitative therapy will allow for optimal switch selection and placement. Further assessment by the speech-language pathologist regarding cognitive-linguistic status will determine potential for use of non-electronic communication systems or more sophisticated electronic devices.

As communication is the link between the patient and the rest of the team, the role of the speech-language pathologist, as the communication specialist, is to guide the team in facilitating optimal communicative interaction. Inservicing of the transdisciplinary team is essential. Conversely, inservicing *by* the transdisciplinary team is integral to the success of the overall management process. Each team member must have an appreciation of the role that others have in the rehabilitative process of the tracheostomized and ventilator dependent patient. This is not meant to reduce the independence of each clinical specialty area in their decision-making process, but allows for collaborative development of goals and avoids disciplines working in isolation.

BUDGETARY BENEFITS

As budgetary concerns have come to the forefront of service delivery in all medical facilities, the team concept has become even more important. The cooperative effort of the team facilitates timely resolution of treatment goals and overall improved service delivery. Without coordination of goals, each team member is forced to focus on his or her specific area(s), which may be duplicated by several other disciplines. Such inefficient service delivery jeopardizes patient care and is less cost effective. In actuality, the goals of each individual team member cannot be achieved without joint effort. One example is placement of the speaking valve with speech-language pathology and respiratory therapy, an intervention that could not be achieved in isolation. When the transdisciplinary team concept is proposed to an uninformed and therefore unenthusiastic administrator, he or she may tend to focus solely on staffing issues. However, the same administrator must be educated in the budgetary benefits that arise from collaborative treatment. As the patient's overall rehabilitative program progresses, the need for skilled care decreases proportionately. In addition, as medical condition dictates length of stay, the patient who has benefited from transdisciplinary intervention is much less likely to overstay the allotted reimbursable time frame.

It is the transdisciplinary team concept that allows the tracheostomized and ventilator dependent patient to achieve maximum rehabilitative benefit. As the skills of the speech-language pathologist in the management of these challenging patients have evolved, the role of the speech-language pathologist on the team has become recognized. In cooperation with fellow team members, the speech-language pathologist, as facilitator of communication and swallowing specialist, completes the circle of quality care for the tracheostomized and ventilator dependent patient.

CASE STUDIES

The following case studies illustrate the transdisciplinary team concept in the management of the tracheostomized and ventilator dependent patient.

Case 1

A.B. was a 35-year-old man with a diagnosis of amyotrophic lateral sclerosis (ALS), respiratory insufficiency, 24-hour ventilator dependence, and quadriplegia. This case illustrates rehabilitation with a patient in an extended care facility. Upon admission, the patient was evaluated by the transdisciplinary team on the respiratory rehabilitation unit.

Medical and pulmonary assessment determined that weaning potential was poor secondary to the degenerative condition. Around the clock nursing care was necessary due to the need for frequent suctioning. Pharmacological intervention was attempted to reduce copious secretions. At this time the patient was tolerating an oral diet. Due to the patient's quadriplegia, physical therapy was limited to bed positioning, passive range of motion, and chest physical therapy. Occupational therapy provided A.B. with a mouthstick to assist in environmental control. He was then able to access his television and tape recorder. Recreation therapy intervened with favorite music and talking books at the bedside. The speech-language pathologist and respiratory therapist initially worked with cuff deflation and ventilatory modifications to allow the patient to achieve voice. The patient was also provided with a letter board that he accessed with his mouthstick, usually at night when the cuff was inflated and phonation could not be achieved. Within several months, vocal options were not possible as A.B.'s condition progressed and he became anarthric, aphonic, and dysphagic. When the patient became unable to utilize the mouthstick and letter board, an eyegaze communication system was developed. All team members were inserviced in the use of this alternative communication system.

Psychosocial needs were predominant with this patient and occupied much of the team's intervention. A.B. was married, with young children. With the support of the social worker and psychologist, he and his family established a living will and requested a do-not-resuscitate order. The living will included a provision refusing alternative feedings. As the patient's oromotor function declined, he became severely dysphagic. The speech-language pathologist and dietician could no longer provide compensatory strategies and dietary modifications to facilitate safe swallowing. Nonetheless, the patient refused either a nasogastric or gastrostomy tube. This was especially difficult for nursing and dietary staff who could not provide adequate and safe PO intake. These issues were discussed during the weekly team meeting. The primary care physician and speech-language pathologist suggested a vocal cord suture to eliminate aspiration. This procedure was performed by the consulting otolaryngologist at an affiliated hospital. Unfortunately, this procedure was unsuccessful in preventing aspiration during oral feeding.

At this point the bioethical committee met to discuss A.B.'s case. As A.B. was nonspeaking and relied on alternative methods of communication, the speech-language pathologist served as translator for the patient and the rest of the team. As A.B.'s physical status continued to deteriorate, he eventually accepted a gastrostomy tube. He requested other revisions of his living will via the speech-language pathologist. A.B. passed away in the extended care facility not long after the placement of the feeding tube. A.B. was one of the more emotionally draining cases for the transdisciplinary team members. The role of each individual was vital, however, in ensuring some quality of life for this young man. The speech-language pathologist provided A.B. with a means of communication through the end stages of the disease, maintaining his ability to make choices and to express his needs and sustaining his link with the team.

Case 2

B.C. is a 7-year-old boy with a diagnosis of Werdnig-Hoffman's disease, respiratory insufficiency, 24-hour ventilator dependence, and quadriplegia. The patient was admitted to an extended care facility for long-term rehabilitation.

Medical and pulmonary assessment revealed poor weaning potential from mechanical ventilation; however, the patient was considered a candidate for cuff deflation and placement on a portable ventilator. B.C. had been residing in hospital settings for a major portion of his life. In the absence of an active family, nursing staff had functioned as his primary caregivers. B.C. was tolerating a regular diet at the time of admission. Physical and occupational therapies provided intensive intervention in the form of chest physical therapy, bed positioning, motorized wheelchair access, adaptive slings to enhance upper extremity function, and environmental controls for games, television, and radio. This intervention was coordinated with the inhouse special educator and the recreational therapist who also requested adaptation of educational materials. B.C.'s initial language status, despite his chronological age, was 5 years 5 months. Speech-language pathology's long-term plan included microcomputer-assisted language treatment to address the language delay. Restoration of voice was coordinated with respiratory therapy via cuff deflation, ventilatory modifications, and use of a ventilator speaking valve (Passy-Muir). Preservation of speech and swallowing was also focused upon.

The team was forced to make many of the treatment decisions in the absence of family input. The social worker and psychologist remained closely involved as different medical, financial, and educational issues arose. These professionals along with nursing staff were also integral in the disciplinary needs of a growing boy.

Over the course of two years, the patient continues to be ventilator dependent and communicates orally with functional speech and voice. B.C. was eventually mainstreamed into the public school system with an accompanying nurse and portable ventilatory and suctioning equipment. He continues to be followed by the team as his disease progresses and his chronological age advances.

APPENDIX

WORKING WITH THE TEAM:

WHERE TO START AND WHAT TO ASK

Medical

What is the diagnosis and the neurological condition?

Was the patient in coma? How long?

Did the patient have any surgery?

Are there any cardiac or other precautions related to the patient's diagnosis?

What are the results of the radiological tests?

What medication is the patient receiving?

What are the patient's vital signs? Have they been relatively stable or do they fluctuate significantly?

Was the tracheostomized patient ever intubated? How long?

What is the type and size of the tracheostomy tube?

Is there a cuff? If so, is it inflated? Can it be deflated?

What is the patient's ventilator schedule?

What are the ventilator settings? Tidal volume? FIO_2? Mode? PEEP?

What are the results of the blood gas analysis?

What are the patient's secretions like?

What is the weaning protocol for this patient, as determined by pulmonary function tests?

What is the status of the pharynx and larynx including vocal fold function, as determined by nasopharyngolaryngoscopy?

Is there a history of aspiration pneumonia?

How is the patient currently receiving nutrition and hydration? If NPO, why were alternate feedings initiated (e.g., dysphagia vs. inadequate oral intake?)

How is the patient tolerating tube feedings?

Is there a history of any dysphagia: oral, pharyngeal, esophageal, (effects of tube feedings, positioning, tube feeding rate, etc.)?

Physical

What is the degree of physical ability at this time? Is it subject to improvement or deterioration?

Is fatigue an issue in the patient's treatment day?

What is the activities of daily living (ADL) status?

Can the movements that the patient has available be used for communication? For example, can the patient write if speech is unavailable?

If not, what movement can we use as a response mode?
Is the patient bedbound or on bed rest (temporary restrictive status vs. "bound")?

How long can the patient tolerate sitting in the chair?

Does the patient have a productive cough?

Does the patient coordinate respiration with other motor movements?

Vocational/Recreational

What is the patient's potential for return to previous employment?

Is the patient considered a candidate for mainstreaming into the educational setting?

What are the patient's previous leisure interests?

Psychosocial

What are the discharge plans?

Is there family support?

Is there funding, (i.e., for electronic communication systems?)

What is the patient's social history, including education, employment, potential for community re-entry?

Has the patient established a living will, advance directives, and/or DNR orders?

What is the patient's emotional status? Is there a history of depression? Is there any current situational depression?

Communication

Does the patient have a history of or signs of an acute hearing loss?

Can the patient understand and follow simple directions?

Does the patient attempt to communicate in any way?

Can the patient mouth words?

If the patient has a cuffed tracheostomy tube, can he/she produce any leak speech? Can the patient tolerate cuff deflation?

What level of mobility does this patient have (i.e., head movements, limited extremity movement, eye-blinks only?)

If vocal strategies are not an option, what non-vocal communication methods are most appropriate?

If able to use a vocal method of communication, will a back-up nonvocal system need to be made available to the patient?

What training is needed for staff, patient, and family to facilitate consistent carryover of the communication system being utilized?

REFERENCES

1. Frey, J.A., and Wood, S., "Weaning from mechanical ventilation augmented by the Passy-Muir speaking valve." Presented at American Lung Association/American Thoracic Society International Conference, Anaheim, California, 1991.

2. Langmore, S., Schatz, K., and Olson, N., "Endoscopic and videofluoroscopic evaluations of swallowing and aspiration." *Annals of Otology, Rhinology and Laryngology*, 1991; 100: 678-681.

3. Make, B., Gilmartin, M., Brody, J.S., and Snider, J.L., "Rehabilitation of ventilator-dependent subjects with lung disease." *Chest*, 1984; 86(3): 358-365.

4. Curran, J., "Nutrition assessment and intervention." Presented at the Fourth Multidisciplinary Symposium on Dysphagia, Baltimore, Maryland, 1992.

5. Kazandjian, M., and Schwartz-Cohen, A., "Team approach to dysphagia essential in long-term care approach to dysphagia." *Advance*, 1993; 3, 9, 8.

6. Fried-Oken, M., Howard, J.M., and Stewart, S.R., "Feedback of AAC intervention from adults who are temporarily unable to speak." *Augmentative and Alternative Communication*, 1991; 7: 43-50.

7. Levine, S.P., Koester, D.J., and Kett, R.L., "Independently activated talking tracheostomy systems for quadriplegic patients." *Archives of Physical Medicine and Rehabilitation*, 1987; 68: 571-573.

8. American Disabilities Act (ADA), PL 101-336, July 26, 1990.

9. Maynard, F.M., and Muth, J.D., "The choice to end life as a ventilator-dependent quadriplegic." *Archives of Physical Medicine and Rehabilitation*, 1987; 68: 862-864.

10. Kazandjian, M., and Christopher, F., Personal communication, 1992.

CHAPTER VI

NONVOCAL TREATMENTS FOR SHORT AND LONG-TERM VENTILATOR PATIENTS

***LISA ADAMS**, M.A., C.C.C.-SLP*
Clinical Supervisor
Queens College of the City
University of New York
New York, New York

***MARIA A. CONNOLLY**, D.N.Sc., R.N., C.C.R.N.*
Assistant Professor of Nursing
Department of Medical-Surgical Nursing
Niehoff School of Nursing
Loyola University of Chicago
Chicago, Illinois

Edited by:
***Carole Oglesby**, M.S., C.C.C.-SLP*
University Speech Pathology Associates
Louisville, Kentucky

***Mary F. Mason**, M.S., C.C.C.-SLP*

INTRODUCTION

This chapter is written in two parts: the first part addresses the immediate communication needs of the short-term critically ill, often unstable, nonvocal patient in the intensive care unit (ICU), and the second part addresses, the more stable, long-term, often tracheostomized patient who may be in an ICU, a step-down unit, respiratory unit, long-term care facility, or at home.

As nursing is usually the first service to meet and begin caring for the patient in the ICU, Part 1 of this chapter is written by Maria A. Connolly from the nursing perspective. The second part of this chapter is written by Lisa Adams from the speech-language pathologist's perspective.

The goal for optimum patient care is to have a speech-language pathologist consult requested for the ICU patient as soon as the patient attempts to communicate and his or her cognitive status permits. The transdisciplinary team approach to patient care for tracheostomized and ventilator dependent patients is becoming the standard level of care in many institutions today. This is providing the opportunity for earlier intervention by the speech-language pathologist with the ICU patient and improving communication options for the patients, staff, and patients' family members.

PART 1

***MARIA A. CONNOLLY**, D.N.Sc., R.N., C.C.R.N.*

KEY WORDS

Aided: Symbols that require some type of external assistance, aid, or device for production of a message (e.g., paper and pencil, alphabet board, Magic Slate).

Unaided: Symbols that do not require any aid for production other than manipulation of a body part (e.g., hand movements, eye blinking, mouthing words).

Ventilator: A machine that connects to an endotracheal or tracheostomy tube in the patient and is designed to assist with breathing. The ventilator (older term: respirator) can do all the work of breathing or partially assist with breathing.

Short-Term Ventilator Dependent Patient: A patient who is intubated with an endotracheal tube and placed on a ventilator for 10 to 14 days or less. Usually, the short-term ventilator dependent patient is acutely ill and often in an intensive care unit of the hospital. The majority of these patients do not have any pathology involving organs of speech.

Long-Term Ventilator Dependent Patient: A patient who is intubated with either an endotracheal or tracheostomy tube and placed on a ventilator for 14 days or longer, even for months or years. Usually, the long-term ventilator dependent patient may be either acutely or chronically ill but generally is stable. These patients can be in the intensive care unit, a respiratory step-down unit, an acute or chronic respiratory facility, or at home.

Weaning: A process whereby ventilator dependent patients become less dependent on the mechanical ventilator and eventually are able to breathe on their own without the aid of the machine.

NONVOCAL TREATMENTS FOR VENTILATOR DEPENDENT PATIENTS

One major psychosocial problem of mechanically ventilated patients in the intensive care unit (ICU) is their inability to speak because of the cuffed endotracheal or tracheostomy tube obstructing the larynx and airflow.[1] The inability to speak is frustrating for the patients, the nurses, and all members of the health care team. Impaired communication related to intubation and mechanical ventilation of a patient results in anxiety, frustration, and fear that can have deleterious effects on the patient's emotional and physical condition. Early assessment of communication abilities of these patients by the nurse and speech-language pathologist can result in effective communication essential for patients' self-esteem and quality of life.

The purpose of this section is to identify nonvocal treatment interventions that can be utilized to facilitate communication for the intubated ventilator dependent patient. Nonvocal treatments usually give ventilator dependent patients immediate success in their communication interactions. Readers are cautioned that the nonvocal treatments described in the following discussion are representative of some (not all) of the methods and types of communication devices available.

DESCRIPTION OF THE TEMPORARILY NONVOCAL VENTILATOR DEPENDENT PATIENT

Nonvocal short-term ventilator dependent patients in ICUs are quite unlike medically stable, nonvocal patients who are ventilator dependent for months and who can be taught more complex methods of communicating. First, ICU ventilator dependent patients are critically ill and unable to participate in lengthy teaching sessions with communication methods and devices. Second, these patients are often medically unstable, leading to frequent changes in their cognitive and motor capabilities. Third, these patients and their nurses have busy schedules that require that communication intervention plans be extremely flexible. Last, the communication needs of these critically ill patients are immediate and often require quick and decisive nursing intervention.

SHORT-TERM VENTILATOR DEPENDENT PATIENTS

The short-term ventilator dependent patient is usually only temporarily nonvocal. Generally, the ventilator dependent patient has intact organs of speech, and when the physical condition improves the endotracheal or tracheostomy tube can be removed. After extubation of the endotracheal or tracheostomy tube, most patients will be able to speak and communicate much as they did prior to their illness or injury.

Due to the nature of the patient's diagnosis, disease, surgical interventions, trauma, or injuries, the respiratory system is compromised and the patient needs assistance with breathing. If an endotracheal tube is passed through the patient's nose or mouth into the trachea, obstruction of the larynx occurs (Figure 6-1). This obstruction results in the inability to speak. To date, no known effective method is available for patients with endotracheal tubes in place to vocalize or speak. Therefore, patients with endotracheal tubes must rely on nonvocal methods of communication.

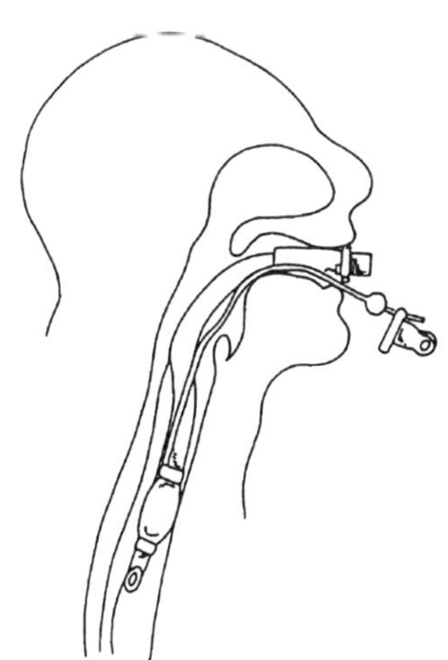

Figure 6-1 An endotracheal tube in place. (From Beukelman, D.R., and Mirenda, P., Augmentative and Alternative Communication: Management of Severe Communication Disorders in Children and Adults, *pg. 359, Figure 19.1, Paul H. Brookes Publishing Co., P.O. Box 10624, Baltimore, MD 21285-0624.)*

ASSESSMENT OF COMMUNICATION ABILITIES

Most short-term ventilator dependent patients are critically ill and in an ICU. Other characteristics of ventilator dependent patients may include changes in their level of consciousness, cognitive abilities, physical and mental strength, motor coordination and dexterity, and cultural influences.[2] These changes can alter any or all of the nonvocal approaches to effective communication.

A thorough assessment of the patient's communication abilities can be performed by both the ICU nurse and the speech-language pathologist by reviewing the ICU bedside chart, which usually includes an hourly update of both physical and mental status. Level of orientation is usually assessed by the nurse using some form of the Glasgow Coma Scale.[3] This scored scale is based on evaluation of three categories: best eye opening, best verbal response, and best motor response (Table 6-1). Possible scores range from 3 to 15, with a score of 15 indicating an alert and oriented patient, while a score of 8 or less usually indicates coma. Although the best verbal response is not applicable in the intubated ventilator dependent patient, questions addressing orientation to person, time, and place can be evaluated by asking patients to use "yes" or "no" gestures.

Another assessment tool developed by Dowden, Honsinger, and Beukelman, entitled the "Initial Cognitive-Linguistic Screening Tasks,"[2] evaluates the patient's ability to pay attention to questions, follow single-step commands, and answer three "yes" or "no" questions assessing level of orientation. Failure to complete at least two of these tasks is taken as evidence that the patient is not alert enough to communicate nonverbally (Table 6-2). This is a very quick and easy method of assessment, which can take less than three to four minutes to execute.

After ICU patients successfully pass a preliminary screening tasks, such as the Glasgow Coma Scale and the Initial Cognitive-Linguistic Screening Tasks, a more extensive assessment of communication capabilities should be done. Beukelman and Mirenda[4] discuss a flowchart developed by Mitsuda to guide the decision making process in providing ICU patients with the appropriate alternative communication interventions (Figure 6-2). Patients are evaluated for either voicing or writing options.

Category	Score	Response
Eye opening	4	Spontaneous—eyes open spontaneously without stimulation
	3	To speech—eyes open with verbal stimulation but not necessarily to command
	2	To pain—eyes open with noxious stimuli
	1	None—no eye opening regardless of stimulation
Verbal response	5	Oriented—accurate information about person, place, time, reason for hospitalization, and personal data
	4	Confused—answers not appropriate to question, but correct use of language
	3	Inappropriate words—disorganized, random speech; no sustained conversation
	2	Incomprehensible sounds—moans, groans, and mumbles incomprehensibly
	1	None—no verbalization despite stimulation
Best motor response	6	Obeys commands—performs simple tasks on command; able to repeat performance
	5	Localizes to pain—organized attempt to localize and remove painful stimuli
	4	Withdraws from pain—withdraws extremity from source of painful stimuli
	3	Abnormal flexion—decorticate posturing spontaneously or in response to noxious stimuli
	2	Extension—decerebrate posturing spontaneously or in response to noxious stimuli
	1	None—no response to noxious stimuli; flaccid

Table 6-1 Glasgow Coma Scale. (With permission from Hogstel, M., and Keen-Payne, R., Practical Guide to Health Assessment Through the Lifespan, *Philadelphia: F.A. Davis Co.; 1993, p. 23.)*

Attending behaviors:

Attends to spoken name	yes	no
Attends to "Look at me"?	yes	no

Orientation questions:

"Is your name ______?"	yes	no
"Is the current year ___?"	yes	no
"Is ___ your home town?"	yes	no

Single step commands:

"Close your mouth."	yes	no
"Open your mouth."	yes	no

Failure to complete at least two of these tasks is taken as evidence that the patient is not alert enough to communicate nonverbally.

Table 6-2 Initial Cognitive-Linguistic Screening Tasks. (With permission from Dowden, P., Honsinger, M., and Beukelman, D., "Serving nonspeaking patients in acute care settings: An intervention approach." Augmentative and Alternative Communication, *Seattle: University of Washington; 1986; 25-33.)*

UNAIDED AND AIDED NONVOCAL TREATMENTS

It is appropriate to use nonvocal, easy-to-use (portable), and inexpensive methods of communication with ventilator dependent patients who are going to be voiceless for less than a few weeks. These nonvocal treatments can be further divided into two categories: unaided and aided. Examples of unaided nonvocal treatments are described as symbols that do not require any aid for production other than manipulating body parts.[5,6]

According to Lloyd[6] in his Augmentative and Alternative Communication Model (AAC), unaided nonvocal communication is typically instantaneous through auditory, visual, and/or tactile senses. "Yes" or "no" questions and answers, sign language, gestures of head and hand, mouthing of words/lip reading, eye blinking, facial expressions (mime), physical touch, pointing with head and extremities, writing symbols or words on the nurse's hand, hand grasps, and display of emotions such as crying or withdrawing are some examples of unaided communication methods.

Aided nonvocal communication is defined by Lloyd as symbols that require some type of external assistance, aid, or device for production of a message (paper and pencil, alphabet or picture board)[6] (Table 6-3).

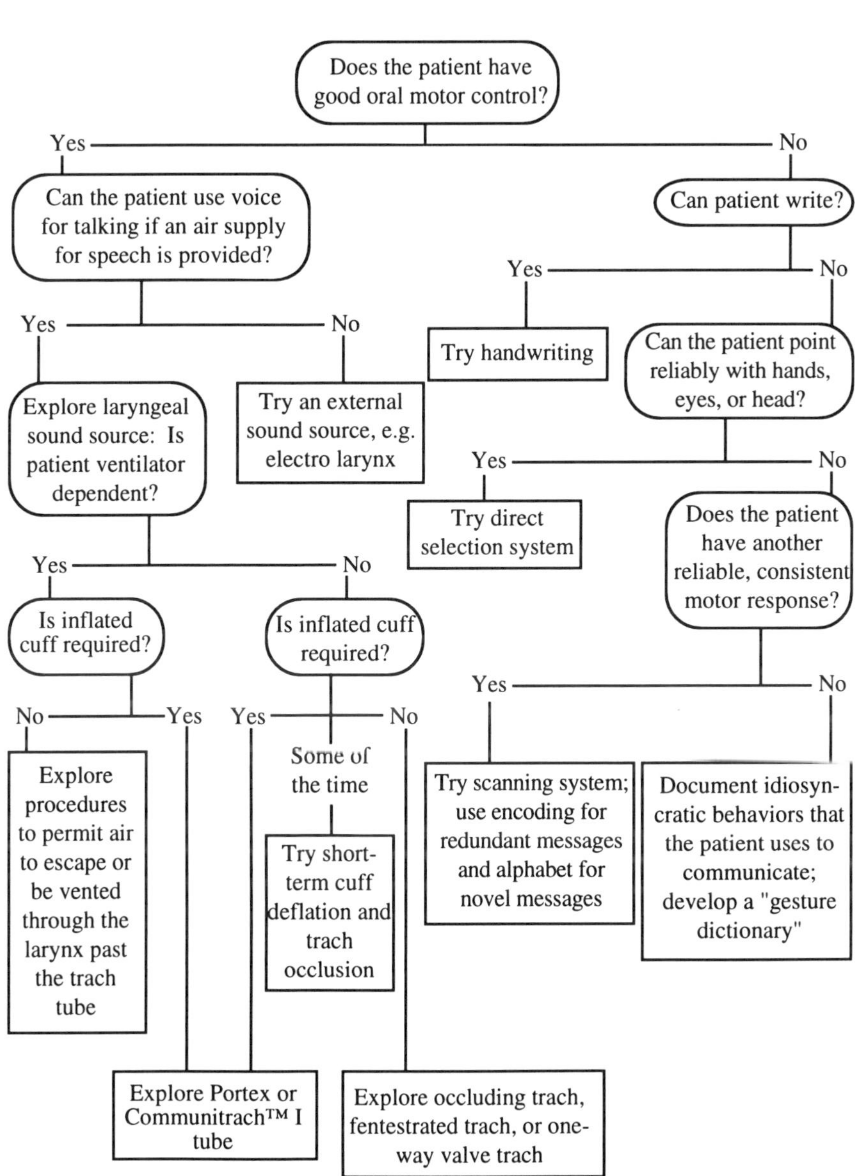

Figure 6-2 AAC intervention planning flowchart for intensive care unit applications. (From Paul H. Brookes Publishing Co., P.O. Box 10624, Baltimore, MD 21285-0624. Adapted from Mitsuda, Baarslag-Benson, Hazel and Therriault, 1992.)

Unaided Treatments

Unaided communications are those that rely heavily on the use of gesture. Beukelman[5] states that gestural communication varies along a number of dimensions. How meaningful a gesture can be relies on the level of symbolism. Some gestures are generally well understood by most people in the United States, while other gestures can be highly symbolic and designed for a community of users, like the deaf and their partners.

Category 1: Verbal/Nonverbal Language

"Yes" or "no" questions and answers
Sign language
Gestures (hand and head movements)
Lip reading, mouthing words
Physical touch
Pointing with head and extremities
Facial expressions (mime)
Writing symbols or words on nurse's hand
Hand-grasp/eye blinking
Emotions (crying, withdrawing, etc.)

Category 2: Assist Devices for Short-term Ventilator Patients

Pencil and paper (chalk and board)
Magic Slate
Magnetic plastic letters and board
Alphabet board
Picture board
Symbol board
Speak & Spell electronic game
Flash cards
Flip charts

Category 3: Assist Devices for Long-Term Ventilator Patients

Electric typewriter
Computers (word processor)
Passy-Muir tracheostomy speaking valve
Olympic Trach Talk
COMMUNItrach™I
Electro larynx
Portex Trach-Talk

Table 6-3 Identification of Communication Methods. (From Connolly, M., and Shekleton, M., "Communicating with ventilator dependent patients." Dimensions in Critical Care Nursing, *Philadelphia: J.B. Lippencott Co.;1991; 10:115-122.)*

According to Skelly,[7] a gestural system for use in a clinical setting is Amer-Ind, which is based on American Indian Hand Talk. Skelly's six criteria for this gestural system include:

1. Low level of symbolism plus a concrete referent base for gesture
2. Ease of acquisition by the nonvocal patient
3. Ease of interpretation by the viewers (nurses and families)
4. Flexibility in the encoding of concepts (acutely ill ventilator dependent patients usually have neither the physical stamina nor the mental alertness for dealing with syntactic structure and grammatical rules)
5. Adaptability to existing gestures; the gestures should be field-tested for their usefulness
6. Potential speed of execution; the gestural system must exceed that of aided written communication in the conversational setting[7]

Skelly's Amer-Ind has been tested in the clinical setting with severely communicatively impaired adults and children, particularly mentally retarded ones. To use Amer-Ind a patient must have essentially normal neuromuscular functioning of at least one upper extremity. While Amer-Ind signs normally require two hands, many of the gestures can be encoded with one hand.[7] This is particularly desirable with ventilator dependent patients because they usually have one hand that is restrained with a soft wrist cuff to limit arm movement and potential disruption of intravenous lines and radial arterial catheters for monitoring direct blood pressures.

The potential exists for the short-term ventilator dependent patient to learn Amer-Ind quickly as many of the gestures are intelligible to most untrained observers. It must be kept in mind that patients in the ICU have basic physical needs. Therefore, most messages the patients will need to communicate lie within a narrow range: "pain," "suction me," "I'm hot," "water," and "sleep." Connolly[1] found that short-term ventilator dependent patients usually perform gestures that are a form of Amer-Ind and address basic needs and activities of daily living (Table 6-4).

McNeill[8] describes gestures that occur with speech and those that do not occur with speech. According to McNeill[8] those persons without the ability to speak will use pantomime or emblems. Emblems require no speech to communicate meaning. Each emblem has an exact meaning, which is consciously directed to a specific receiver. The following is an example of an emblematic gesture for "time": the person uses his index finger and touches his opposite wrist area, which ordinarily is where a watch would be worn. Most observers would interpret that gesture to mean that the person wanted to know the time.

Pantomimes can be used with or without speech and consist of complex actions and sequential movements that substitute for a verbal utterance. These gestures are creative representations of meaning and are not as easily understood by the observer.[8] Therefore, short-term ventilator dependent patients generally may not be as successful in communicating in this "charade"-like manner because they have limitations of movement and are often "too sick" to concentrate.

Other gestural strategies

Many manual shorthand gestural systems have been developed for a variety of patients. Earlier, Goldstein and Cameron[9] devised a set of 20 self-care hand signals. They reproduced a chart that was given to each patient (Figure 6-3). This was a gestural system devised for basic needs for aphasic, dysarthric, and dysphonic patients. All gestures in this system could be done with one hand. Eagleston, Vaughn, and Knudson[10] in 1970 developed a manual communication system for expressive aphasics who had right hemiplegia (Figure 6-4).

These two gestural strategies require time and training for both the staff and the patients. The short-term ventilator dependent patient may be nonvocal for only a brief period of time (e.g., 1 to 14 days);

1. Drink*	10. Breathe*
2. Eat*	11. Write*
3. Hot*	12. Numbers*
4. Pain shot*	13. Suction
5. Pray*	14. Drive*
6. Telephone*	15. Kiss
7. Time*	16. Sleep*
8. Towel/Wash*	17. Zipper
9. Walk*	18. Wheelchair

*Skelly's Amer-Ind

Table 6-4 Examples of Gestures for Needs of Short-Term Ventilator Patients. (From Connolly, M.A., Temporarily Nonvocal Trauma Patients and Their Gestures: A Descriptive Study, *[unpublished dissertation] University Microfilm International-Dissertation Abstracts, September, 1992.)*

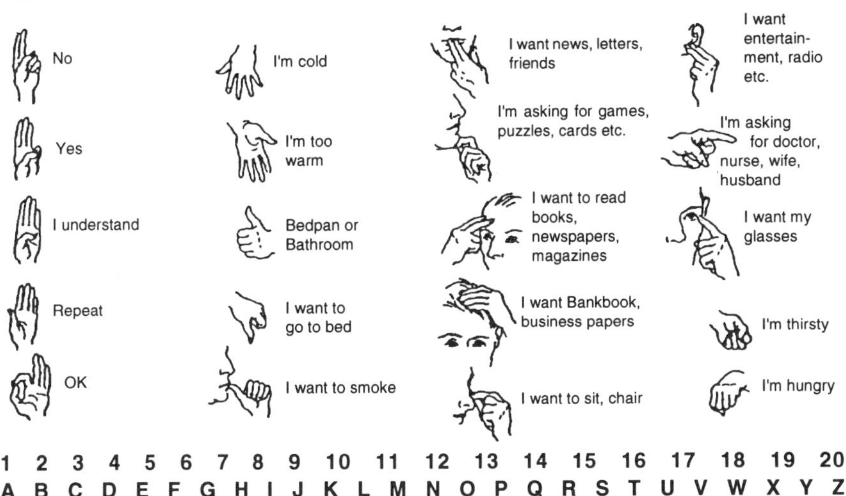

Figure 6-3 Hand talking chart. The sign language in the designs speaks for itself. The figures and letters across the bottom are independent of the designs. By pointing with pencil or finger to the letters or figures needed to further a conversation, communication between patient and friend can be amplified even to the "dictation" of a letter by the patient who otherwise would remain completely inarticulate. (From Goldstein, H., and Cameron, H., Arizona Medicine, *1952. Courtesy of Arizona Medical Association.)*

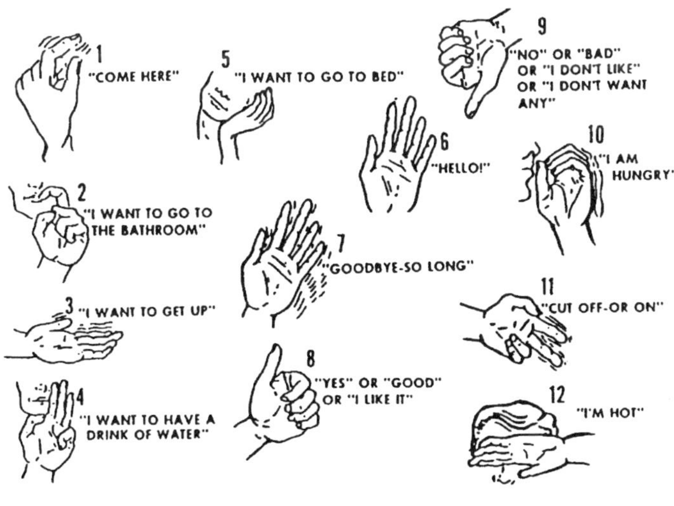

Figure 6-4 Manual self-care signals. (From Eagleston, Vaughn, 1970.)

therefore, a gestural system must be easily acquired with a low level of symbolism for ease of interpretation by both the nonvocal patient and staff.

For patients with extensive neurological injuries or disease, eye movements are the only locus of control. For communication with this particular group of ventilator dependent patients, an eye-blink encoding strategy can be developed. In 1966, Adams[11] developed a specific number of eye blinks that would signal a particular basic need. For example:

Number of Eye blinks	Meaning
1	No
2	Yes
3	I want to use the bedpan.

Using this coded eye-blinking system may only be appropriate for ICU patients who are physically stable and able to concentrate on learning.

Aided Nonvocal Treatments

A convenience sample of 17 critical care nurses attending a critical care continuing education program were asked what method of communication they used most frequently with nonvocal patients in the ICU. Of the 15 methods listed, the most commonly selected forms of communication in this sample were: (1) paper and pencil, (2) alphabet/picture boards (Figure 6-5), and (3) lip reading.[1]

It is not surprising that critical care nurses prefer to use those familiar methods that are easily implemented with nonvocal ventilator dependent patients. However, patients have reported in other studies that paper and pencil were difficult to use and often not as effective as mouthing words, lip reading, or gestures. Understandably, it is quite difficult to write supine, often without an adequate hard writing surface, limited visual fields, and hand restraints (e.g., injured writing hand, restraints, arm boards, intravenous tubing [IVs], arterial lines, etc.).

The use of paper and pen can be made more effective if the patient has a firm surface on which to write, like a clipboard, and uses a felt-tipped pen that will write in any position. If the patient is able to wear eye glasses and have one hand free of restraints, this will also improve the legibility of the writing. Some patients prefer to write on a tablet and save messages, so that they can begin to construct their own communication booklet.[4] Rather than write the same thing over and over again, the patient will just flip back to the previously written message.

Many patients prefer the Magic Slate so they can erase messages when they are finished writing and thus maintain their privacy.[4] Similar to the Magic Slate is yet another toy, the Magna Doodle, which allows the patient to write on a larger lightweight plastic screen and erase the message with a lever at the bottom of the doodle board. Both the Magic Slate and the Magna Doodle are inexpensive and can be purchased at any local department or toy store.

Many nonelectronic boards have been developed using the alphabet, numbers, pictures, and short phrases addressing basic needs and concerns of most patients (Figure 6-5). It is important to note that many of these boards are the invention of necessity, designed by nurses, and families of nonvocal patients. One board called the Silent Speaker was invented by two ICU nurses who experienced the daily frustration of their patients' inability to communicate (Figure 6-6). While some patients find these boards very useful, many complain that they just didn't have the patience or the mental stamina to spell out words. Patients had difficulty focusing their eyes to read the boards. Many of the boards have very crowded messages with small letters, which, in some cases, makes their usefulness questionable in the ICU.

Flash cards have provided some limited value as another method of communication, but like the picture boards, patience on both the part of the patient and the nurse is required to "sort through" various possible needs of the patient.

CHALLENGES IN INTEGRATION OF NONVOCAL OPTIONS IN THE INTENSIVE CARE UNIT

The ICU presents many learning constraints. Clearly, optimal teaching and learning opportunities are minimal. Patients and fami-

A	B	C	D	E	F
G	H	I	J	K	L
M	N	O	P	Q	R
S	T	U	V	W	X
		Y	Z		

0 1 2 3 4 5 6 7 8 9

PleaseTurn On/Off	I'm Thirsty/Nauseated
TV Radio Lights	I'm Hungry
Please Elevate/Lower	Eyeglasses
My Head My Legs	Mouth Care
Please Bring/Empty	Please Let Me Sleep
Bedpan, Urinal, Blanket	Bring Sleeping Pill
Please Turn Me	Need Pain Medication
Please Straighten Bed	Pain Level:
YES NO	1 2 3 4 5 6 7 8 9 10
Room:	I want to see my Doctor
Too Warm Too Cold	Thank you

Figure 6-5 Alphabet/numeric board.

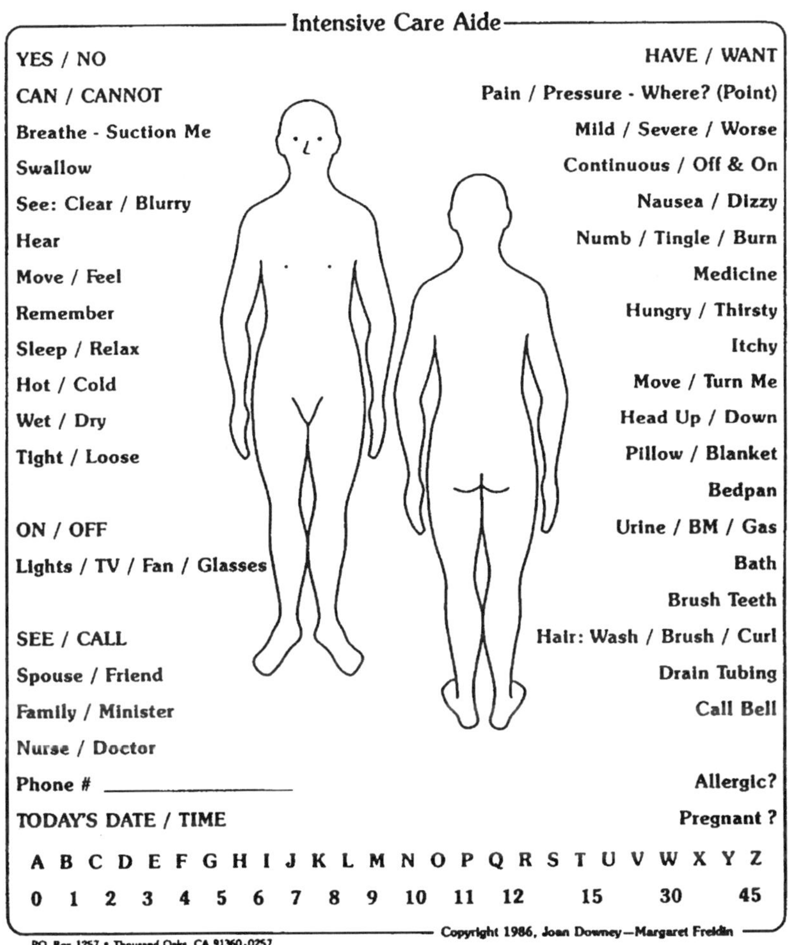

Intensive Care Aide

YES / NO
CAN / CANNOT
Breathe - Suction Me
Swallow
See: Clear / Blurry
Hear
Move / Feel
Remember
Sleep / Relax
Hot / Cold
Wet / Dry
Tight / Loose

ON / OFF
Lights / TV / Fan / Glasses

SEE / CALL
Spouse / Friend
Family / Minister
Nurse / Doctor
Phone # ________
TODAY'S DATE / TIME

HAVE / WANT
Pain / Pressure - Where? (Point)
Mild / Severe / Worse
Continuous / Off & On
Nausea / Dizzy
Numb / Tingle / Burn
Medicine
Hungry / Thirsty
Itchy
Move / Turn Me
Head Up / Down
Pillow / Blanket
Bedpan
Urine / BM / Gas
Bath
Brush Teeth
Hair: Wash / Brush / Curl
Drain Tubing
Call Bell

Allergic?
Pregnant ?

A B C D E F G H I J K L M N O P Q R S T U V W X Y Z
0 1 2 3 4 5 6 7 8 9 10 11 12 15 30 45

P.O. Box 1257 • Thousand Oaks, CA 91360-0257
Copyright 1986, Joan Downey—Margaret Freidin

Figure 6-6 The Silent Speaker. (Courtesy of Trademark Corp., Fenton, MO.)

lies are under a considerable amount of stress and demonstrate little, if any, tolerance for learning. Yet many patients and families are very willing to learn as much as possible in order to communicate with their loved ones. The integration of nonvocal options for these patients requires a creative plan supported by all staff members.

Barriers to Overcome in the Intensive Care Unit

Knowledge of the ICU policies and procedures may reveal unit protocol that may limit some nonvocal options for the patients. For instance, some ICUs require all patients with endotracheal or tracheostomy tubes in place to have both hands in soft restraints to protect the patient from accidental self-extubation. These restraints can limit gesturing, ability to hold a pad and pen, or other writing devices.

Experienced critical care nurses, respiratory therapists, and physicians have learned various ways to communicate with nonvocal patients. Some of these methods may need modifying. For instance, nurses may know the basic needs of these patients and often approach the patients with a standard "twenty questions" routine, which can be overwhelming to the patients. Patients interviewed after their experience in the ICU often stated that these questions would confuse them, only to remember what they wanted after the nurse left the room.[12]

IMPLEMENTATION OF NONVOCAL STRATEGIES

Nurses, speech-language pathologists, and other members of the health care team working in specialty units (ICUs) should identify the common needs and characteristics of their patient populations. For example, similarities exist in surgical trauma units where patients are typically younger and in relatively good health until the time of their accident or injury. Methods of communication may include a lexicon of gestures reflecting basic needs along with aided nonvocal methods like a pen and paper on a clipboard.

If a patient has a language barrier, often a picture board is an appropriate device for communicating along with gestures. Language cards that contain common ICU words and phrases in foreign languages, such as Spanish or Italian, can be made or purchased.[13]

Once the most suitable communication method have been identified for a particular patient, it should be integrated into the written plan of care. In a very busy intensive care environment, it is easy to forget about the patient's need for communication. Having continuity among the health care professionals in their approach to communication with these nonvocal patients will improve the quality of care and decrease the frustrations of their patients.

REIMBURSEMENT ISSUES

Communication devices such as alphabet boards, flash cards, picture boards, or pad and pen are relatively inexpensive. Some of these aided devices can be obtained free from various medical suppliers. Nurse managers would find the placement of these items at each bedside cost-effective and a time-saving device for the ICU nurses.

Funding for augmentative and alternative communication services is usually provided by the same funding sources responsible for the hospitalization.[4] Education of the ICU's medical, nursing, and other members of the health care team in the use of unaided and aided options is essential for effective communication with the nonvocal patient.

RESEARCH IMPLICATIONS

The majority of the nonvocal treatments addressed in this section have not been sufficiently tested with the ventilator dependent population in intensive care units. The efficacy of many of these methods remains speculative and their usefulness relies on trial and error. Research on communication with ventilator dependent patients needs to be done. Current research questions that need to be investigated include:

What communication methods are most successful with nonvocal ICU patients?

What methods work best with short-term ventilator dependent patients?

What methods work best with long-term ventilator dependent patients?

REFERENCES

1. Connolly, M.A., and Shekleton, M., "Communicating with ventilator dependent patients." *Dimensions of Critical Care Nursing*, Philadelphia: J.B. Lippencott Company; 1991; 10(2):115-122.

2. Dowden, P.A., Honsinger, M.J., and Beukelman, D.R., "Serving nonspeaking patients in acute care settings: An intervention approach." *Augmentative and Alternative Communication*, Seattle: University of Washington; 1986; 25-33.

3. Teasdale, G., and Jennett, W., "Assessment of coma and impaired consciousness; a practical scale." *Lancet,* 1974; 2:81.

4. Beukelman, D.R., and Mirenda, P., "AAC in intensive and acute care settings." In: *Augmentative and Alternative Communication: Management of Severe Communication Disorders in Children and Adults*, 1992; Baltimore: Paul H. Brookes Publishing Co., 1992; Chapter 19, pp. 357-370.

5. Beukelman, D.R., Yorkston, K.R., and Dowden, P.A., *Communication Augmentation: A Casebook of Clinical Management*, San Diego: College-Hill Press, 1985.

6. Lloyd, L.L., Quist, R. W., and Windsor, J., "A proposed augmentative and alternative communication model." *Augmentative and Alternative Communication*, 1990; Spring:172-181.

7. Skelly, *Amer-Ind Gestural Code Based on Universal American Indian Hand Talk*, New York: Elsevier North Holland, Inc., 1979: 4-15.

8. McNeill, D., *Hand & Mind: What Gestures Reveal about Thought.* Chicago: University of Chicago Press, 1992.

9. Goldstein, H., and Cameron, H., "New Method of Communicating for the Aphasic Patient." *Arizona Medicine*, 1952; 8:17-21.

10. Eagleston, H., Vaughn, G., and Knudson, A., "Hand Signals for Dysphasia." *Archives of Physical Medicine and Rehabilitation*, 1970; 51:111-113.

11. Adams, M.R., "Communication Aids for Patients with Amyotrophc Lateral Sclerosis." *Journal of Speech and Hearing Disorder*, 1966; 31: 274-275.

12. Connolly, M.A., *Temporarily Nonvocal Trauma Patients and Their Gestures: A Descriptive Study,* Chicago: Rush University, 1992; Unpublished Dissertation.

13. Lawless, C.A., "Helping Patients with Endotracheal and Tracheostomy Tubes Communicate." *American Journal of Nursing*, 1975; 75: 2151-2158.

PART 2

***Lisa Adams**, M.A., C.C.C.-SLP*

KEY WORDS

Long-Term Tracheostomy: Tracheostomy that extends past the 7-to-10 day acute care phase. In long-term tracheostomy, aphonia may be present part or all of the day secondary to cuff inflation. Oral-motor weakness may or may not be present; however, there is a strong likelihood of eventual decannulation. Population may include spinal cord injury, cerebrovascular accident.[4]

Permanent Tracheostomy: The placement of a tracheostomy tube for extended periods of time, often with no plan for decannulation. Aphonia may be present part or all of the day secondary to cuff inflation. Oral motor weakness may or may not be present. Population may include neuromuscular disease patients (e.g., amyotrophic lateral sclerosis), end-stage pulmonary/respiratory disorders (e.g., chronic obstructive pulmonary disease).[4]

Access Method: The physical method by which the user will indicate items on the communication system. This may be directly (e.g., pointing) or indirectly (e.g., stopping a cursor on a desired letter).

Direct Selection: Technique in which the message sender indicates elements of his message by directly pointing to them in some manner.[5]

Scanning: Technique in which message elements or groups of elements are presented one at a time to the message sender who signals the desired element.[5]

Coded Systems: A pattern or code of signals that indicates the message elements.[5]

EXTENDED COMMUNICATION MANAGEMENT

Although the special communication needs of the ICU patient are often met by the critical care nurse, extended communication management is the responsibility of the speech-language pathologist. Once the patient has reached a point of medical stability, the speech-language pathologist, with other members of the rehabilitation team, can assess the amount of time that the patient will require tracheostomy. Many factors play into this decision, including the patient's diagnosis, respiratory/pulmonary status, and swallowing ability. The speech-language pathologist must have a thorough understanding of these factors and, most importantly, of the patient's diagnosis, in order to provide appropriate communication management.

LONG-TERM TRACHEOSTOMY

Long-term tracheostomy use is defined as a tracheostomy that extends past the 7 to 10 day acute care range. There is, however, an eventual plan for removal of the tracheostomy tube (decannulation). The use of long-term tracheostomy may be necessary for patients in certain etiological groups whose respiratory, pulmonary, or swallowing system has been compromised. However, in this etiological group, respiratory/pulmonary function and/or swallowing is expected to improve over the course of long-term rehabilitation.[4] Possible populations may include high spinal cord injury or cerebrovascular accident.

Long-term tracheostomy may alter the communication ability of the patient by interfering with voice use. The long-term tracheostomy patient may experience periods of aphonia, during which voice is not available through part or all of the day secondary to cuff inflation. Additionally, these patients may or may not have weakness of the lips, tongue, pharynx, and larynx, which adds to communication difficulty. Weakness in the oral, pharyngeal, and laryngeal areas, known as *dysarthria*, will make mouthing words difficult, if not impossible.

PERMANENT TRACHEOSTOMY

Other etiological groups, including patients with progressive neuromuscular disease or end-stage pulmonary disease, deteriorate to a point at which tracheostomy and/or mechanical ventilation is required constantly. Once this point is reached, decannulation is not considered feasible due to the progressive deterioration of the system. These patients may be considered permanent tracheostomy users.[4]

Achieving a thorough understanding of the patient's status as a short-term, long-term, or permanent tracheostomy user allows the speech-language pathologist to outline communication options for the patient with both the present and the future in mind. It also allows the speech-language pathologist to formulate a plan for a communication system that addresses communication needs both vocally and nonvocally, dependent upon that patient's unique medical plan.

CHOOSING NONVOCAL COMMUNICATION

As the patient reaches a point of medical stability, cognitive awareness and orientation often improve markedly. With this awareness may come a renewed desire to communicate with family and staff. The patient's messages may become less focused on directing medical care and meeting activities of daily living (ADL) needs and more oriented toward inquiring about family members, children, business, and so forth. Although the patient may have a renewed desire to communicate, the presence of the tracheostomy tube and/or the presence of dysarthria may prevent him from engaging in a communicative exchange. Inability to communicate results in feelings of frustration, anger, anxiety, and powerlessness.[3]

When a desire to communicate is present but communication cannot be accomplished vocally, then nonvocal communication options must be available. Nonvocal communication options are methods of communication that do not require speech. Language is represented through a nonspoken mode, by writing or by pointing to letters or symbols. Nonvocal communication options may be considered as augmentative or alternative. Augmentative communication options are designed to "build up" the existing communication skills of the patient. For example, a patient may have speech, but it may not be understandable. An augmentative system acts as a supplement to or as a "backup" for speech, so that unintelligible letters or words can be understood. Alternative communication options are designed to take the place of speech completely.

Augmentative and alternative communication options are offered when speech is unavailable. For some patients, speech may be unavailable for only small portions of the day. This may be a patient with respiratory quadriplegia who can use speech during the day, but requires an inflated tracheostomy tube cuff and ventilatory support for 12 hours each night. This patient would use a nonvocal communication system only as needed in the evening.

For other patients, speech may be permanently unavailable. This may be a patient who suffered a cerebrovascular accident in the brain stem, resulting in paralysis of the speech musculature.

Progressive neuromuscular disease patients will progress to the permanent tracheostomy stage. As the respiratory system fails, these patients will also demonstrate concurrent weakening of the speech musculature. Aphonia and severe dysarthria will exist in this patient group, making nonvocal communication techniques a necessity. These patients accomplish all communication by using a nonvocal system.

The decision to utilize a nonvocal means of communication is usually made together with the patient, family members, the speech-language pathologist and other members of the medical and rehabilitation team. Once the decision is made, the speech-language pathologist performs a full diagnostic assessment that is specially designed for nonvocal communication users.

AREAS OF ASSESSMENT

The diagnostic procedure for considering nonvocal communication options is performed by the speech-language pathologist. The goal of the assessment is to achieve an understanding of the patient's residual strengths and weaknesses, so that a prescription for a communication system can be formulated. The speech-language pathologist examines several areas of patient functioning before making a recommendation, including speech and vocal capability, expressive and receptive language ability, cognitive skill, physical-motor functioning, vision, and hearing. At times, tests need to be altered, such as cutting out materials, and placing them on an eyegaze board to achieve an optimal assessment.

Speech and Vocal Capability

It is essential to incorporate all of the patient's residual skills into the communication system, including any speech or vocal ability the patient may have. The speech-language pathologist must assess oral-motor and laryngeal functioning as well as articulatory ability. This examination will yield information about the quality and consistency of speech in order to determine its effectiveness as part of the patient's communication.

Speech may be relatively unchanged in some patient groups, and voicing options may be available for part or all of the day. The diagnostic assessment should include an accurate schedule of the patient's "free time" during which he is off the ventilator and has available voice use.

Another patient may be unable to utilize voice but may have good articulatory control that allows him to mouth words. These are important findings. If mouthing is available, vocal augmentation in the form of an electro-larynx may be considered.

Other patients may not demonstrate the ability to mouth or use voice. If there is evidence of dysarthria (oral-motor weakness), speech intelligibility may be compromised to a greater or lesser degree. The patient's speech may be understandable to family members but not to busy medical staff. The speech-language pathologist assists the patient in deciding whether speech is an option and provides the patient with guidance in choosing the optimal times to use speech or nonvocal communication.

Expressive and Receptive Language

The job of assessing receptive and expressive language with physically disabled, ventilator dependent patients becomes complicated because the normal methods of responding to test stimuli are altered. This means that the patient may not be able to generate responses vocally. Additionally, he or she may not be able to point to pictured objects or written responses due to physical limitations.

When possible, the speech-language pathologist should conduct testing sessions when voice use is available. For patients who do not have any vocal ability due to dysphonia, alternative response modes must be developed. These alternative response modes must be within the patient's range of physical ability and must be consistent and easy to use. If these criteria are not met, the test results could be faulty. Optimally, the patient should have a highly consistent yes/no response. With a consistent yes/no response, the speech-language pathologist can gather a great deal of information about the patient's receptive language. It is helpful to have a strong clinical impression of the patient's receptive language before going on to expressive language tasks. Good receptive language skills may be a sign that the patient's overall language ability is intact.

Assessing expressive language may be quite challenging if the patient has severe physical limitations. The patient may have no hand function or pointing ability. In that case, the speech-language pathologist should choose a motor response that the patient can utilize consistently and reliably (e.g., upward eyegaze, lifting a finger, raising eyebrows). Once this response is identified, the speech-language pathologist can present stimuli to the patient one item at a time, thereby allowing the patient to signal a choice with the motor response. This may make the language testing extremely time consuming; however, it is a necessary step in the assessment process. Informal or formal language testing should be utilized and should include an assessment of the patient's ability to use alphabet spelling. The findings of this testing will strongly influence how the speech-language pathologist proceeds in developing a communication system. Some patient groups, such as those with amyotrophic lateral sclerosis, show no change in linguistic function. Other patient groups may show marked changes, such as closed head injuries or cerebrovascular accident (CVA) patients. It is also important to note that a full medical history is recommended in order to uncover old neurological injuries that may be affecting the patient's present performance. It is also important to note the patient's native language and the degree of literacy achieved in that language. A previously illiterate patient will require special problem solving, since written language cannot be used as an alternative communication system.

Cognition

The speech-language pathologist will face challenges in assessing cognition if the patient's natural modes of responding are altered. A reliable yes/no response mode will allow the tester to assess the patient's general orientation to person, place, and time. Before administering any formal cognitive testing, the speech-language pathologist can gather information informally on the patient's general state of awareness and desire to communicate from family members and medical staff. Sometimes informal data gathering is enough to make a decision about cognitive function. Formal testing may be conducted using a standardized instrument; however, the method of presentation must be altered for physically disabled patients so that choices can be made with a single motor response.

Certain patient groups may be more likely to demonstrate cognitive changes, including closed head injury or CVA patients. Some progressive neuromuscular diseases result in definite cognitive changes (e.g., Huntington's chorea), while others may or may not yield such changes (e.g., multiple sclerosis). It is important to note any medications that might be inducing lethargy or cognitive fluctuation (e.g., seizure medications). Patients who are treated with multiple medications may also appear cognitively impaired, as will some geriatric patients who may simply be agitated and confused. The presence of a cognitive impairment will not necessarily preclude the use of an alternative communication system. It may, however, influence the speech-language pathologist's choice in terms of the sophistication of that system.

Physical Motor Functioning

In some respects, the physical motor assessment is the key area of assessment because it allows the speech-language pathologist to "tap into" the language and cognitive functioning of the nonvocal, physically disabled patient. Without a means of saying yes/no or making choices, there is no way to know the patient's abilities. Unfortunately, this is the area that most speech-language pathologists know the least about, since it is not a required part of speech- language pathology training.

Therefore, the speech-language pathologist is assisted in this area by an occupational therapist (OT) and/or physical therapist (PT) to establish a consistent movement to respond or answer yes/no. The OT or PT is invaluable in identifying functional movement patterns and can also influence movement patterns by altering aspects of the patient's positioning. Appropriate positioning in or out of the wheelchair is essential for patients who are going to utilize an alternative method of communication. The OT or PT will work with the speech-language pathologist in deciding what part of the body the patient will use to operate the communication system. This could be a finger, a fist, an eyebrow, or a foot. The OT or PT then designs the positioning so that these movement patterns are optimized. OT and/or PT goals can be readily combined with speech-language goals so that the patient's communicative independence is achieved.

Vision

Although we do not need vision to use speech, the nonspeaking client will most likely be relying on letters, symbols, or photos on a board or computer to communicate. Therefore, vision becomes an essential part of communication for some nonvocal patients. The speech-language pathologist should recognize that visual changes can occur following stroke, head injury, or various disease processes. This does not mean that blindness will be the end result. It does mean that visual changes can be present, including diplopia (double vision), nystagmus (involuntary eye movements), or field cuts. Before presenting visual information to your patient, it is best to assess visual status. Materials that are presented outside of the patient's range of vision will not be seen. Although the patient may understand the information, he may not respond correctly if he cannot see it.

An understanding of the diagnosis will assist the speech-language pathologist in gathering information in this area. Discussions with family and medical staff will also help. The opinion of an ophthalmologist, especially one specializing in brain injury, may also be warranted. A communication system that meets the visual needs of this patient, such as one with large size graphics, should be a strong consideration.

Hearing

Hearing is also essential to the patient using an alternative system of communication. This is especially true for patients who are severely visually impaired or blind. For these patients, information may be presented auditorily instead of visually. However, even those patients who are not blind will require hearing in order to respond to questions and conversation. Information on the patient's hearing may be readily available from family members. However, previously normal hearing may have been affected by neurological injury. A quick hearing screening performed by an audiologist will usually alert the speech-language pathologist to further hearing problems and the need for follow-up and management.

DETERMINATION OF COMMUNICATION NEEDS

The communication needs of patients are highly variable. Some patients will require a nonvocal system for only a few hours a day, while others will need their system around the clock. Some patients will be able to generate lengthy, sophisticated messages, while others may communicate only basic needs. The speech-language pathologist is instrumental in identifying the communication needs of the patient and developing a communication system that will meet those needs. The *Communication Needs Assessment*, formulated by Dowden, Honsinger, and Beukelman, assists the speech-language pathologist in generating a "list of specific communication requirements for each patient, with specific information regarding environments for communication, the partners and their needs, the output required, and the message flexibility requirements."[1] For example, the *Communication Needs Assessment* identifies all the possible message receivers (e.g., children, hearing-impaired people), the means in which the message must be sent (e.g., synthesized speech, writing), and the possible locations and positions from which the message sender may want to communicate (e.g., while in bed, over the phone). Optimally, the needs assessment should be completed with the assistance of the patient, his or her family, and the caregivers, so that communication needs are examined from a variety of perspectives. The speech-language pathologist must also take into consideration the patient's diagnosis and the probable length of time that the patient will be nonvocal. Some long-term tracheostomy users, such as the high spinal cord injured patient, recover speech fairly rapidly. A simple, low-technology system, such as a mouthstick and alphabet chart, may meet the communication needs until speech is recovered. In other patient groups, oral-motor weakness will progress until the speech musculature is paralyzed. The patient with amyotrophic lateral sclerosis may initially present with periods of aphonia and no oral-motor weakness. As the musculature deteriorates, the patient begins to rely on nonvocal communication techniques more frequently. End-stage amyotrophic lateral sclerosis patients have no speech or vocalization and accomplish all communication nonvocally. These patients' communication needs may not be met as simply.

The completion of the needs assessment enables the speech-language pathologist to choose or develop a communication system that has the sophistication and flexibility required by the patient. It may appear that the speech-language pathologist must choose between a simple, low-technology system or a high-technology, computer-based system. This is not necessarily the case. The speech-language pathologist should keep in mind that communication is a system, with many parts working together. Communication needs are often most successfully met when a variety of communication options are available, with the quickest and most convenient mode being selected as needed by the patient.[2,3] This usually means that both low-tech and high-tech systems are developed and made available in order to meet a variety of communication needs.

INTERVENTION

Upon completion of the diagnostic assessment, the speech-language pathologist should be able to answer the following questions:[4]

Voice/Speech

1. Is voice a usable mode of communication now?
2. Are there limitations on voice use (e.g., a free time schedule)?
3. Is there dysarthria (oral-motor weakness) that will interfere with voice use?
4. Will there be oral-motor weakness in the future?

Language

1. Does the patient have sufficient language ability to freely generate messages using alphabet?
2. If not, can the patient use other means of representing language such as symbols or photographs?
3. Has receptive language been affected? If so, to what degree? How will this influence use of a nonvocal system?

Cognition

1. Has cognitive function changed? To what degree?
2. How will this influence the selection of a nonvocal system and the use of this system?

Physical Motor

1. What is the patient's optimal motor response mode?
2. Is this movement reliable and consistent?[3] Is positioning optimal?

Vision

1. Has vision changed?
2. How is it affecting use of the communication system?
3. How can visual problems be circumvented?

Hearing

1. Has hearing changed?
2. How is it affecting use of the communication system?

ALERTING SYSTEMS

When enough information has been collected to answer these questions, intervention techniques can be considered.

The establishment of an alerting system is the first and most essential area for intervention with a population that will be aphonic for any portion of the day. The speech-language pathologist cannot assume that the patient can activate the standard nursing call buzzer that is provided on the medical unit. Limited upper extremity strength may interfere with the pressure needed to "ring in" when an emergency occurs. Although most medical units offer a small variety of call buzzers, they may not be designed to fit the unique physical needs of more disabled patients. The speech-language pathologist or occupational therapist will often have a range of switches that can be easily altered to fit the existing call system. The occupational therapist may be called upon to assist the speech-language pathologist in identifying a reliable motor movement that will allow the patient to activate this call buzzer consistently and reliably when alone. For example, the patient may be able to roll his or her head onto a soft "pillow" type switch or sip on a pneumatic (air-activated) switch.

COMMUNICATION SYSTEMS

Once an alerting system has been established, the speech-language pathologist can begin to formulate a communication system that will provide the patient with the ability to produce more complex messages. The complexity of the message will be influenced by the patient's level of linguistic functioning. Therefore, the speech-language pathologist must know the language level at which the patient can work (e.g., alphabet, symbols, pictures, photographs).

This information has been ascertained during the diagnostic assessment. Additionally, information about the patient's physical motor status is available so that the speech-language pathologist can concentrate on finding a method of "access." The term *access* refers to the method in which the patient will act upon the communication system. Choice of an access method is dictated by the amount of physical ability that the patient has retained.

The OT or PT assists the speech-language pathologist in identifying residual movements. These movements are assessed for reliability and consistency. If these criteria are achieved, the patient may be able to use the movement as an input signal for controlling a communication system.

It is important to note that a patient with a progressive neuromuscular disease will demonstrate a deterioration in physical motor ability. Early in the disease, this patient may be able to use his fingers to point to letters. Over time, this movement may be lost due to the disease process. Once this has occurred, another movement pattern, such as upward eyegaze, must be considered. The likelihood of deterioration must be considered when choosing an access method.

Access Methods

The following are access methods that may be considered when designing a nonvocal communication system:

Pencil and Paper Writing

Patients with movement of at least one upper extremity may utilize writing as the most convenient form of nonvocal communication. Writing may be easily combined with vocal approaches, as a supplement to voice for communication breakdowns, or as an alternative to voice during periods of cuff inflation. Positioning adaptations may be required as the patient should have a lap board or bed table to lean on for support or a built-up pen to write with.

Direct Selection

Direct selection is an access technique in which the message sender indicates elements of the message by directly pointing to them in some manner.[5] The patient does not have to have movement of the fingers or hands to be a direct selector. Patients with direct selection capability can also choose items using a mouth stick, a head stick, or a light pointer. In this case, the residual motor movements would be in the head (Figure 6-7).

This technique does require that the message sender have good control over the portion of the body that is being used for selection. If the control is poor, the message sender will not be accurate in choosing an item and the message will not be understood. Direct selection can be used with alphabet, symbols, pictures, or photographs. Some message senders may also have some residual speech function and may elect to point to the initial letter of each word while simultaneously saying or mouthing the word. This technique may significantly improve the intelligibility of the speech or mouthing.

Scanning

Patients without direct selection capability can use a scanning display. Scanning is a technique in which message elements or groups of elements are presented one at a time to the message sender. The message sender signals the desired element in some way.[5] The signal given by the message sender need only be a single, consistent motor response, such as upward eyegaze, head nodding, or finger flexion. Scanning is an access technique that is usually utilized by individuals with minimal motor movement or very uncontrolled motor movement.

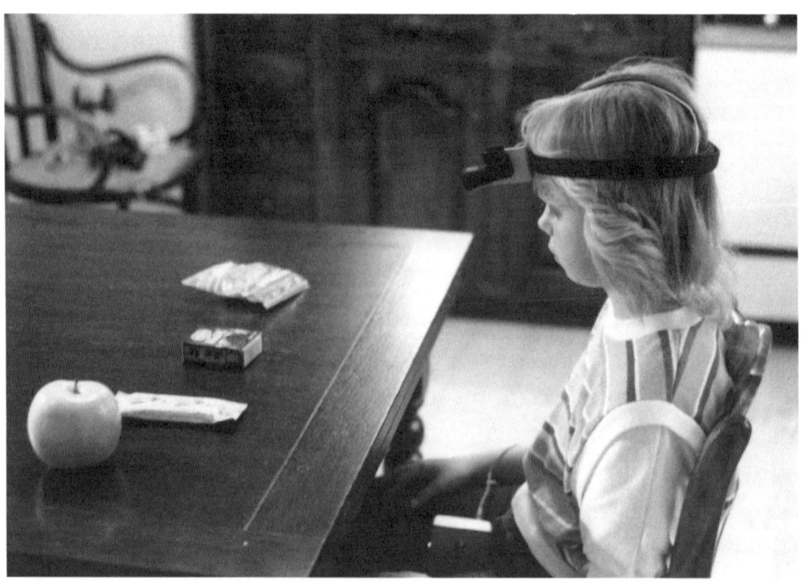

Figure 6-7 Viewpoint Optical Indicator. (Courtesy of Prentke Romich Co., Wooster, OH.)

Eyegaze Systems

Eyegaze is considered to be a form of direct selection in that the eyes are responsible for pointing to an item. However, eyegaze is not always readily considered and its usefulness may be overlooked. This type of system is particularly useful for alert, intact patients who have excellent control over eye movement but severely limited movement in other parts of the body, for example, a patient with advanced amyotrophic lateral sclerosis. Eyegaze systems are usually designed to preserve face-to-face communication and are created using clear materials such as plexiglass. Eyegaze systems can carry alphabet displays and/or carry pictures and symbols for nonspellers or more linguistically impaired patients. Eyegaze systems require time and patience to learn but can be an excellent alternative to a slower scanning-type of system. Examples of eyegaze systems include the E-Tran or Eye-Link.

An E-Tran design utilizes a cutout square. Language items are placed along the perimeter and in the corners of the square. The square is held so that the message sender and the message receiver are face to face. The sender directs his or her gaze to either a corner or some designated spot along the periphery. The receiver looks in that spot to determine the item chosen (Figure 6-8).

An Eye-Link system works in much the same way; however, there are language items on the entire board. The message sender looks at the desired item and the message receiver moves the board until the message receiver's eyes "link" with the message sender's eyes. The desired item is then determined.

Coded Systems

A coded system is selected when the user wants to say several things but doesn't have the motor control to point to all the desired items. In order to give the user more language in the system, the items (alphabet, symbols, or pictures) are coded using a series of numbers. A combination of numbers or colors stands for a letter or symbol (e.g., the patient looks at or points to numbers 1 and 4; this means letter "D"). Coded systems require that both the user and the listener

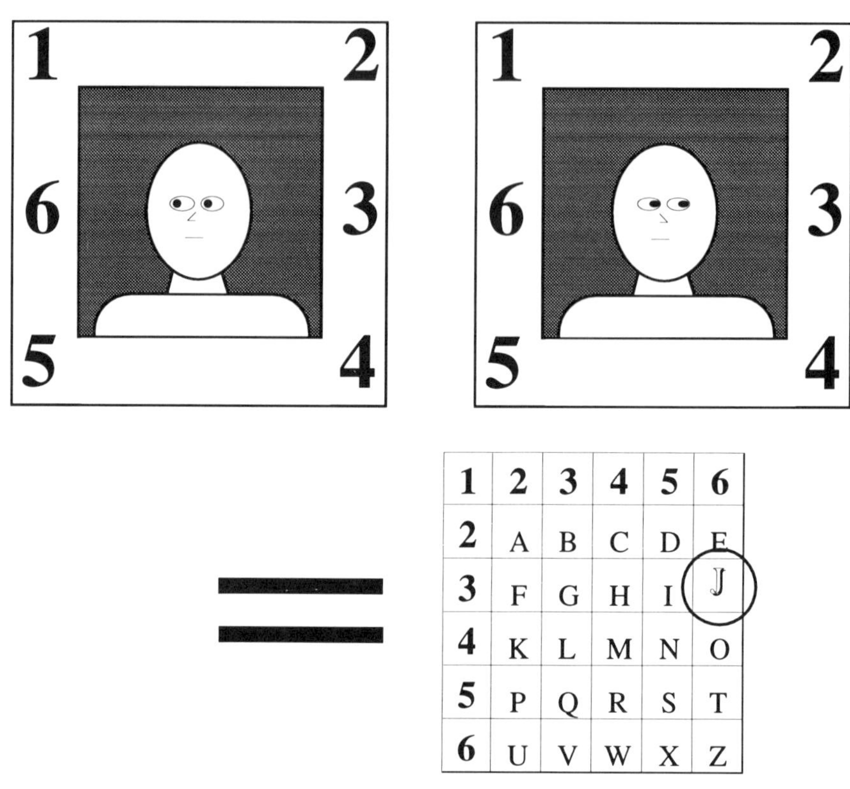

Figure 6-8 Use of an E-Tran number chart to indicate code elements with the eyes.

understand the code in order to decipher the message. Morse code is a form of communication in which the patient operates a single or multiple switches. The code is sent by manipulating the length of the switch beep to form dots and dashes. A combination of dots and dashes stands for a letter.

Nonelectronic Communication Systems

Nonelectronic communication systems have the advantage of being inexpensive, readily available, highly portable, and resistant to breakage. A nonelectronic communication system can take almost any form including a Magic Slate toy for writing; an A to Z alphabet board; sound letter cueing; a picture, word, or phrase board; a plexiglass E-Tran or Eye-Link; or a simple wallet with photos and words. The system is custom designed and highly tailored to the user. Any access technique is usable with a nonelectronic system. One patient may use scanning, while another uses direct selection through eyegaze (Figure 6-9).

Although there are many advantages, there are communication needs that cannot be met with a nonelectronic system. A nonelectronic system requires that the message receiver be in close proximity to the message sender, or the message will not be transmitted. Some non-electronic systems require that the message receiver participate in deciphering the message by scanning through items and waiting for the sender's signal. This creates a situation of dependence that speaking people do not have to endure. Additionally, few non-electronic systems allow for a written or hard copy message. This means that the message cannot be preserved and referred to at a later date.

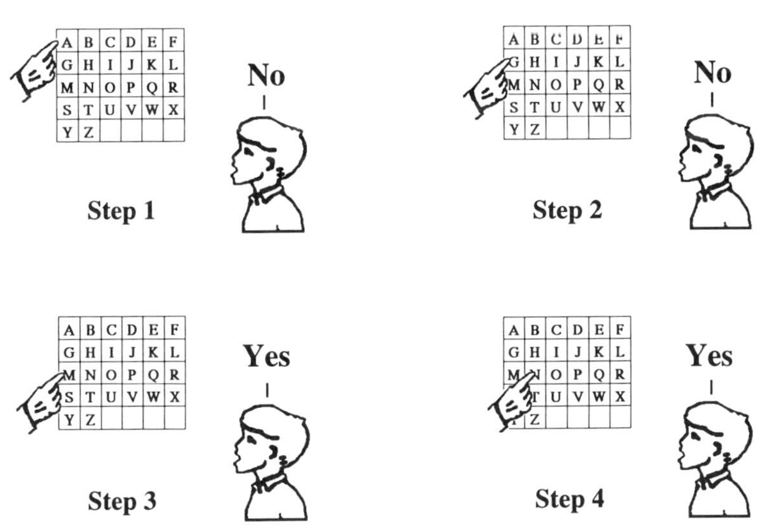

Figure 6-9 An example of row-column scanning with a non-electronic communication aid. Message sender (patient) responds with yes/no signal.

Electronic Communication Systems

Electronic communication systems can offer the nonvocal user increased independence and message flexibility in a variety of ways. Aside from getting "set up," the electronic communication system can be operated with no assistance, thereby providing the user with independence in communication. The provision of synthetic voice and written output allows the user to "speak" or "write" messages, thereby increasing his degree of control over the environment. This type of system may also provide increased speed of communication through keystroke-saving software programs such as those offering word prediction or abbreviation-expansion capabilities.

There are also electronic systems that are less technologically advanced. These "lower tech" systems may meet the needs of certain patients. For example, a patient may have voice for periods throughout the day. However, at night the patient may want to compose a note to a family member but is unable to do this due to physical limitations. A simple electronic system may be utilized that allows the patient to print a message but that has no synthetic speech (Figure 6-10). However, with the features offered by electronic systems, the user will also discover considerable headaches, such as difficulty learning to operate the system, difficulty storing vocabulary, computer breakdowns, power failures, and lack of portability. Successful integration of technology into the life of the user requires that the speech-language pathologist teach not only the user how to communicate with this system, but everyone involved with the user as well. The time commitment and level of sophistication required to operate such a system make its use impractical for short-term tracheostomy users.[3]

If a recommendation has been made for a sophisticated, electronic communication system, the speech-language pathologist's role is extended to include interfacing the patient with the system, programming the vocabulary, and teaching the patient how to use the system and to communicate successfully (Figure 6-11). Interfacing the client with the communication system means that an access technique must be chosen. It does not have to be the same access technique used for the nonelectronic system. However, it must be consistent, reliable, and easy to use. The occupational therapist is

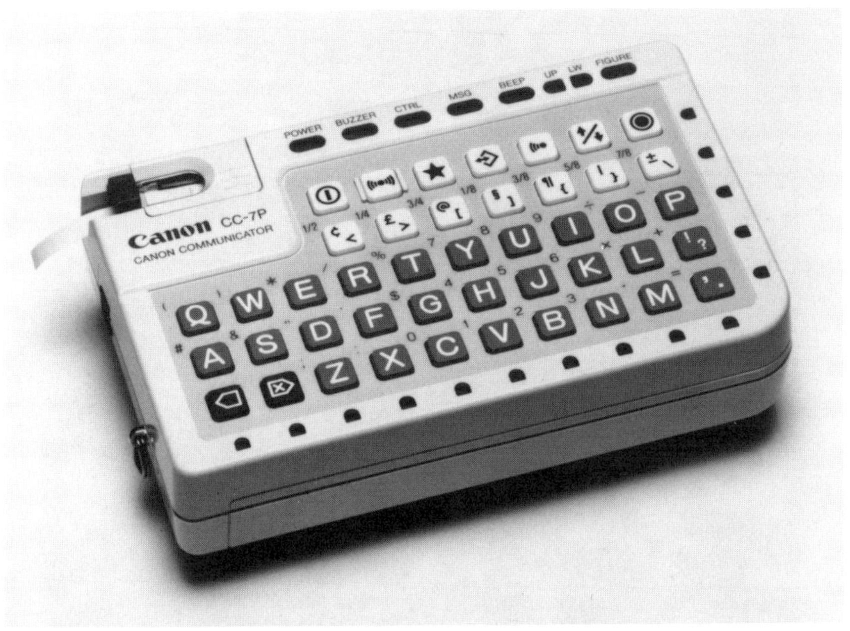

Figure 6-10 The Canon Communicator, an electronic aid that is activated by exerting pressure on its keys. (Courtesy of Canon U.S.A. Inc., Lake Success, NY.)

again highly instrumental in identifying a movement pattern that will allow the patient to operate the system.

Although some electronic communication systems have only one or two modes of access, other electronic communication systems have multiple modes of access, including direct selection, scanning, or Morse code input. Direct selection access means that the patient can use his hands, a mouth stick, a head stick, or a light pointer.

Patients who use a scanning or coding technique will operate the system through one or two motor responses. These responses allow the patient to touch one or more switches to send a control signal to the communication system. There are a vast number of switches available. Individual switches are manufactured to work with the patient's existing movement patterns and have a range of sensitivity. Some switches are sturdily built for patients whose motor movements are uncontrolled. Other switches are highly sensitive and will respond to minute movements. Infrared switches do not have to be touched at

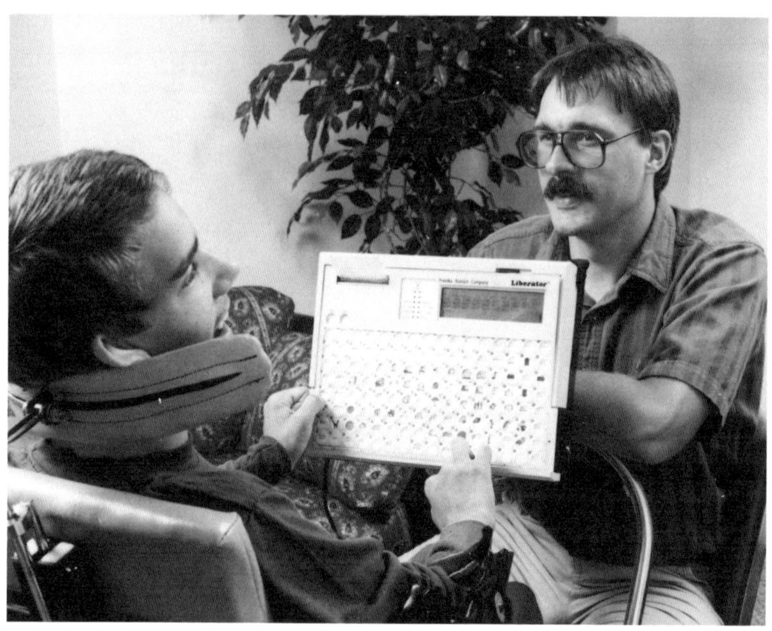

Figure 6-11 The Liberator™ is a sophisticated programmable speech synthesizer. (Courtesy of Prentke Romich Co., Wooster, OH.)

all and respond to any small movement, including an eye blink. This type of switch is often used to interface end-stage amyotrophic lateral sclerosis patients with their electronic communication systems.

There are constant advances in the development of electronic communication systems. As technology advances, so do the communication options for physically disabled, nonvocal patients.

CONCLUSION

In many etiological groups, the loss of speech is combined with a serious medical illness that compromises breathing. The patient is unable to call for help, ask questions, direct his care, or voice his concerns. In her 1986 study, Fried-Oken cites fear as the primary reaction of patients with severe expressive communication disabilities.[3] This fear can be alleviated by addressing even a brief or temporary loss of speech through the provision of a nonvocal communication system. Rapid intervention can be accomplished through the development of a simple, nonelectronic mode of communication, such as a scanning alphabet board or Eye-Link. This allows family members and medical staff to intervene smoothly and also allows the patient to ask questions and receive information.

Once communication has been re-established, the speech-language pathologist can focus on the long-term communication needs of the patient. Identifying the length of time that the patient will be nonvocal is of primary importance. Strong consideration must also be given to the communication needs of the patient before making a decision about the provision of an electronic communication system.

The role of the speech-language pathologist extends past the recommendation of such a system to the training and integration of the system into the patient's life. Nonvocal communication intervention may be arduous and time consuming. However, communication must be considered the patient's lifeline to the medical staff. The speech-language pathologist must consider the job of re-establishing communication to be of utmost importance to the entire rehabilitation team.

PRODUCT MANUFACTURERS

Adaptive Communication Systems, Inc.
354 Hookstown Grade Road
Clinton, PA 15206
Electronic communication aids, mounts, alternative keyboards

Canon U.S.A., Inc.
One Canon Plaza
Lake Success, NY 11042-1113
Communication aids

Crestwood Company
6625 N. Sidney Place
Milwaukee, WI 53209
Communication aids, nonelectronic communication aids, symbols, photos

Don Johnston Developmental Equipment, Inc.
P.O. Box 639
1000 N. Rand Road, Bldg. 115
Wauconda, IL 60084
Communication software, switches, alternative keyboards

IBM Special Needs Division
Referral Center
P.O. Box 2150
Atlanta, GA 30301-2150
Communication software, adaptive equipment

Innocomp
26210 Emery Road, Suite 302
Warrensville Heights, OH 44128
Communication aids

Mayer-Johnson Company
P.O. Box 1579
Solana Beach, CA 92507-1579
Communication symbols, software and folders

Phonic Ear, Inc.
3880 Cypress Drive
Petaluma, CA 94954-7600
Communication aids

Prentke Romich Company
1022 Heyl Road
Wooster, OH 44691
Communication aids, mounts, switches

Sentient Systems Technology, Inc.
2100 Wharton Street, Suite 630
Pittsburgh, PA 15203
Communication aids

TASH, Inc.
Unit 1, 91 Station Street
Ajax, Ontario, Canada LlS3H2
(416) 686-4129
FAX (416) 686-6895
Switches

Words+
P.O. Box 1229
Lancaster, CA 93584
Communication aids, mounts

Zygo Industries, Inc.
P.O. Box 1008
Portland, OR 97207-1008
Communication aids, switches, mounts

An extensive vendor and technology list can also be found in *The Handbook of Assistive Technology*. (1992), Church, G., and Glennen, S., Singular Publishing Group, Inc., San Diego, CA.

RESOURCES

International Society of Augmentative and Alternative Communication (ISAAC)
P.O. Box 1762, Station R
Toronto, Ontario, Canada M494A3

United States Society of Augmentative and Alternative Communication (USAAC)
C/O California School for the Blind
500 Walnut Avenue
Fremont, CA 94536

Rehabilitation Engineering Society of North America (RESNA)
1101 Connecticut Ave., NW, Suite 700
Washington, DC 20036

Communication Aid Manufacturers Association (CAMA)
518-26 Davis St., Suites 211 - 212
Evanston, IL 60201

REFERENCES

1. Dowden, P.A., Honsinger, M.J., and Beukelman, D.R., "Serving nonspeaking patients in acute care settings: An intervention approach." *Augmentative and Alternative Communication*, 1986; 25-33.

2. Dowden, P., Beukelman, D.R., and Lossing, C., "Serving non-speaking patients in acute care settings: Intervention outcomes." *Augmentative and Alternative Communication,* 1986; 38-44.

3. Fried-Oken, M., Howard, J.M., and Stewart, S.R., "Feedback on AAC intervention from adults who are temporarily unable to speak." *Augmentative and Alternative Communication*, 1991; 43-50.

4. Kazandjian, M., Dikeman, K. and Adams, L., "Communication management of the tracheostomized and ventilator dependent patient." Presented at the American Speech Language Hearing Association Annual Convention, Atlanta, November 25, 1991.

5. Vanderheiden, G., and Lloyd, L., "Communication systems and their components." In S. Blackstone and D. Bruskin (Eds.), *Augmentative Communication: An Introduction*, Rockville, MD: 1986.

BIBLIOGRAPHY

Beukelman, D.R., Yorkston, K.M., Dowden, P.A., Mitsuda, P.A., and Lossing, C., *Communication Augmentation: A Casebook of Clinical Management,* San Diego: College Hill Press, 1985.

Dowden, P., Beukelman, D.R., and Lossing, C. "Serving nonspeaking patients in acute care settings: Intervention outcomes." *Augmentative and Alternative Communication*, 1986; 38-44.

Fishman, Iris, *Electronic Communication Aids: Selection and Use*, Boston: Little, Brown & Company, 1987.

Musselwhite, C.R., and St. Louis, K.W., *Communication Programming for the Severely Handicapped: Vocal and Non- vocal Strategies,* San Diego, CA: College Hill Press, 1982.

CHAPTER VII

VOCAL TREATMENT STRATEGIES

***Mary F. Mason**, M.S., C.C.C.-SLP*

Edited by:

***Kris Ward**, M.S., C.C.C.-SLP*
Pulmonary Rehabilitation Program
Tustin Rehabilitation Hospital
Tustin, California

***Roxann Diez Gross**, M.A., C.C.C.-SLP*
The Eye and Ear Institute
Department of Otolaryngology
University of Pittsburgh Medical Center
Pittsburgh, Pennsylvania

INTRODUCTION

"If all my possessions were taken from me with one exception, I would choose to keep the power of communication, for by it I would soon regain all the rest." Daniel Webster

The power of communication has been written about many times. It is through communication that a person is able to interface with others, share ideas, and display human emotions. Communication allows a means to demonstrate creativity, intellect, and the human spirit. Every individual has a unique personality that is expressed through communication. The ability to communicate is taken for granted until it is compromised. The inability to communicate affects our identity, independence, and spirit. When we can't communicate, we experience anxiety, fear, frustration, and isolation.

The focus of this discussion is the patient who no longer communicates verbally because of dependency on an artificial airway and/or mechanical ventilation. The ability to interface with others and express thoughts normally is sometimes affected by these life support procedures. Intervention to establish a means of expression is essential for the overall recovery process of patients. The inability to communicate creates a great amount of anxiety and fear in patients and is detrimental to the healing process and delivery of medical care. A study conducted in Sweden, by Bergbom-Enberg and Haljamae,[1] with tracheostomized and ventilator dependent patients reported that patients' primary concern during the period they were unable to communicate was that it created feelings of insecurity, anxiety, fear, and even of agony and panic. They also noted in this study that the inability to communicate corresponded directly to the patient's inability to obtain restful sleep. The lack of restful sleep affects the overall medical recovery of the patient. The emphasis on the importance of communication with staff and family is vital for the patient's physical and psychological recovery. When patients utilize energy in attempts to communicate and are unsuccessful, they exhaust energy they could have contributed toward their recovery. According to Levine, Kiester, and Ket,[2] "Communication is critical to patients' overall medical care, psychological functioning, and social interactions." Sparker, et al.

state, "When communication breaks down between the patient and the health care professionals, the patient's ability to participate meaningfully in the health care plan is greatly restricted."[3]

The loss of verbal/vocal communication can be devastating to adult patients who have lost their ability to interact as they have previously done. The inability of an infant or child to vocalize can be traumatic to his/her development, as cognitive and social development can be delayed. The absence of verbalization can be difficult for the child as well as for the care-giving parents who must gauge the needs of this child. Verbal communication is important in the development and functioning of every individual, regardless of age or prior abilities. Communication is the tool that enables each person to participate in his or her own care, environment, development, and rehabilitation process.

NONVOCAL SYSTEMS FOR TRACHEOSTOMIZED PATIENTS

Although verbal expression is optimal in the interaction of one's thoughts, needs, and desires, nonvocal communication can facilitate the expression of basic needs and wants to family, friends, and caregivers. Nonvocal communication systems are essential to relieve the immediate frustrations of patients. A nonvocal system should always be established immediately after verbal expression is lost. If voicing is not achieved early in the rehabilitation process due to complications, the nonvocal communication system becomes imperative. Complications that may limit vocalizations can include vocal cord damage, severe dysarthria of speech, severe airway obstruction, or other laryngeal obstructions.

The nonvocal communication system selected for the immediate communication needs of the patient is identified and implemented by members of the transdisciplinary team who interface with the nonvocal individual. Educating the family and caregivers of the patient as to the use of this system is critical for success. The potential for use of a vocal communication system can then be discussed and selected with the patient providing input, via use of his or her nonvocal system. Nonvocal options are delineated in Chapter 6.

APHONIC ANATOMY OF THE TRACHEOSTOMIZED PATIENT

A means to establish immediate vocalization should be identified as soon as possible. Prior to investigation and implementation of a vocal communication system, a level of understanding of the aphonic anatomy should be reviewed with the patient. In many cases, patient education on the anatomical alteration of a tracheostomy has not been provided in detail or has been reviewed quickly by medical personnel. It is important to emphasize to the patient that his/her vocal cords are functional (if that is the case). Information overload, anxiety, and denial may play a part in the patient needing several explanations or detailed descriptions to understand the anatomical and physiological changes that have taken place. The use of diagrams of the upper and lower airway can be useful in facilitating the patient's understanding of his or her aphonic status. It is important to explain that the aphonic condition is due to a lack of airflow through the larynx because air exchange has been diverted from the upper airway and is now taking place through the tracheostomy tube.

An illustration can be utilized to show that the upper airway is being bypassed by the placement of the tracheostomy tube and that the purpose of the tracheostomy tube is to provide direct access to the lower airway, assisting in ease of ventilation and gas exchange (Figure 7-1). Each patient will have a different diagnosis that led to the need for tracheostomy tube placement, and specific information should also be shared and described appropriately to the staff.

PHYSIOLOGICAL FUNCTIONS AFFECTED BY A TRACHEOSTOMY

Placement of a tracheostomy tube causes a reduction in airflow above the level of the tracheostomy tube. This airflow reduction affects several physiological functions.

Speech/Voice Production

With the absence of airflow through the vocal cords, the most significant alteration is the lack of vocalization for effective communication.

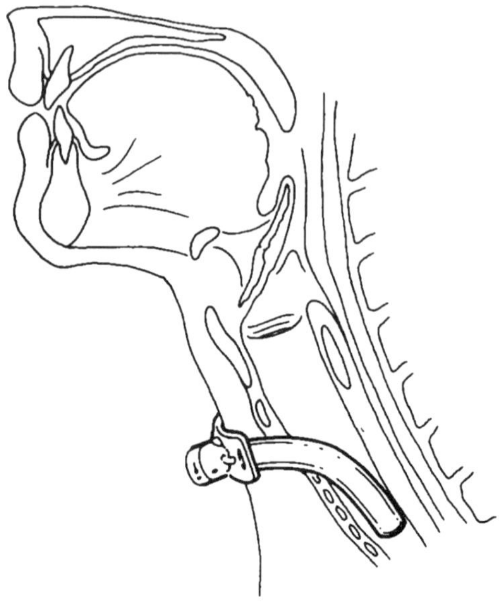

Figure 7-1 Anatomical placement of tracheostomy tube in the airway.

Olfaction and Gustation

The patient's ability to smell and taste is altered due to the lack of airflow in the oral/nasal chambers. This alteration affects appetite and the patient's ability to maintain appropriate body weight.

Secretions

The natural processes of evaporation and filtration through the mucosal tissue passages in the upper airway are not available because the upper airway is bypassed. Consequently, the amount of tracheal secretions present will increase. In addition, the body reacts to the presence of a tracheostomy tube as a foreign body by producing increased secretions.

Cough

The patient's ability to produce adequate velocity of air movement and pressures needed for coughing is compromised by the presence of the tracheostomy tube.

Infection

A tracheostomy tube presents an increased risk of infection due to the direct access to the lower airway and the bypassing of upper airway filtration that it creates. Bacterial colonization flourishes in wet, and warm places due to unfiltered air and the contamination caused by finger occlusion of the tracheostomy tube and stoma hygiene.

Swallow

Swallow function can be altered with the placement of a tracheostomy tube. With no airflow in the upper airway, oral/pharyngeal sensation is decreased, which adversely affects the ability to clear the throat or activate additional swallows to clear food particles from the pharynx. Pressure gradients needed for bolus propulsion in the oropharynx are also altered as the patient no longer has a closed physiology.

Oxygenation

Normal gas exchange may be decreased due to normal intrapulmonary pressures bleeding through the tracheostomy tube. Molecular changes of diffusion at the alveolar level may be altered, which in turn can affect oxygenation and result in the patient experiencing a diminished energy level.

Defecation

Defecation may become difficult due to the presence of a tracheostomy tube because of changes that occur in the subglottic and intrathoracic airflow pressures needed in this physiological function.

PATIENT EDUCATION ON VOCAL OPTIONS

It is important for the speech-language pathologist to determine when the appropriate time is to provide patient education as well as what depth of information to provide. Some patients may have difficulty handling the information whereas others may appreciate being given in-depth details concerning their status. The speech-language pathologist should initiate education regarding all vocal options available and should assure the patient that his or her vocal function can be restored with tracheal plugging, use of a talking tracheostomy tube or a speaking valve device, or decannulation (removal of the tracheostomy tube).

When providing patient education and subsequent assessment for vocal options, it is important to keep in mind that many patients will react with considerable anxiety and even panic. Most patients who are tracheostomized or ventilator dependent are understandably very apprehensive of and sensitive to any activity or procedure involving their airway. Consequently, the clinician needs to be patient and empathetic and should attempt to utilize any motivational techniques that appear appropriate.

Some patients are motivated by being able to visit with their family and friends, by having more control over their daily activities, by the hope of going back to work, or even by the possibility of weaning and/or being suctioned less frequently.

VOCAL OPTIONS

Prior to assessing a patient for vocal communication options, a complete history and physical review should be completed. It is necessary to know why the tracheostomy tube was placed so that the appropriate intervention strategy can be identified. Not every tracheostomized patient can vocalize immediately with ease, and some patients can achieve voicing only with extensive intervention.

Some anatomical conditions may result in permanent aphonia. These include severe vocal cord paralysis, vocal cord fixation, severe glottal obstruction, severe tracheal stenosis, and severe upper airway obstruction. Other patients may have a compounding diagnosis or physiological conditions that may prevent successful verbal expression. Neuromuscular involvement, glossectomy, and craniofacial anomalies are some of the conditions that can affect oral motor movement and speech production. In these cases, even if voicing is achieved, communication may not be optimal as coordinated vocal and articulatory movements cannot be achieved. Nonetheless, it is important to consider that, for some patients, output of less than optimal communication through verbalization is an important expressive achievement. In these cases, a communication system of sounds can be developed to meet basic needs. It is necessary to recognize that even sounds of laughter and crying are functional and meaningful forms of communication.

Most tracheostomized and/or ventilator dependent patients will have excess secretions. The critical aspect of secretions is their manageability for each particular patient. Overabundance, viscosity, or ongoing infection can interfere with secretion manageability. Some patients can manage more and/or different secretion viscosities than other patients. The use of various vocal options, especially fenestrated tracheostomy tubes, talking tracheostomy tubes, and tracheostomy speaking valves, may be limited or temporarily suspended until secretions can be controlled. Clinicians can recommend treatment for secretion management to better control secretion levels. Such treatments include humidification, medications, bronchial hygiene regimen, and suctioning schedules.

Before discussion of the vocal options for tracheostomized and/or ventilator dependent patients, a brief discussion about tracheostomy tube cuff deflation is warranted as this is an important consideration in the determination of the most appropriate vocal option.

It is important to know that not every patient who has a cuffed tracheostomy tube or who is ventilator dependent with a cuffed tube requires cuff inflation at all times. Many respiratory therapists and/or pulmonologists falsely believe that patients cannot be adequately ventilated with cuff deflation; however, a majority of tracheostomized patients with severe respiratory insufficiency and reasonably competent oropharyngeal muscles can be safely and adequately mechanically ventilated up to 24 hours a day with their cuffs deflated or with cuffless tracheostomy tubes.[5] *Adjustments of ventilator volume settings, breath rate, back-up rate, sensitivity settings for assisted breaths, oxygen levels (FIO$_2$) and the inspiratory/expiratory ratio are needed to achieve safe and adequate ventilation. Continuous pulse oximetry can ensure patient safety when the cuff is deflated for initial assessment. Additional discussion on cuff deflation relating to dysphagia can be found in Chapter 10.*

Vocal communication options available for patients who are tracheostomized and/or dependent on mechanical ventilation can be divided into four categories:

1. Pneumatic and electrical devices
2. Fenestrated tracheostomy tubes
3. Talking tracheostomy tubes
4. Tracheostomy speaking valves

The speech-language pathologist should endeavor to identify the most optimal method of vocalization available for each patient. Some methods may be more desirable than others, as some utilize the patient's own vocal production system versus options in which mechanical airflow and vibration produce pseudovoicing for expression.

Pneumatic and Electrical Devices

Pneumatic and electrical communication devices are utilized when it is not possible to achieve vocalization with the patient's natural voice. Operation of these devices is generated by a battery-operated vibratory source that the patient uses while articulating words and sentences. These devices provide verbal/vocal expression without using the patient's own air source or vocal cords and were originally developed for laryngectomized individuals. These devices are placed in the patient's oral cavity or against the patient's neck area and are conspicuous for the user. The sound created is robotic and mechanical in nature. When used by tracheostomized and/or ventilator dependent patients, it can be difficult for the listener to hear them over the oxygen flow from the ventilator and other environmental noises present. Some of these devices are costly and can pose reimbursement challenges. Appropriateness of their use is with the patient who cannot achieve success with the other vocal options available. This could be the patient with vocal cord closure problems, an inability to tolerate cuff deflation, or other compliance issues needed for natural voice production. Some of these devices include electrolarynges, such as the Servox which is commonly used via placement on the neck or cheek and the Cooper Rand which is an intra-oral electrolaryngeal device (Figure 7-2).

Fenestrated Tracheostomy Tubes

The fenestrated tracheostomy tube was designed primarily to reintroduce airflow to the upper airway for weaning purposes and is available from several manufacturers in both cuffed and cuffless tube designs. With a fenestrated tube, air flows through the fenestration(s)

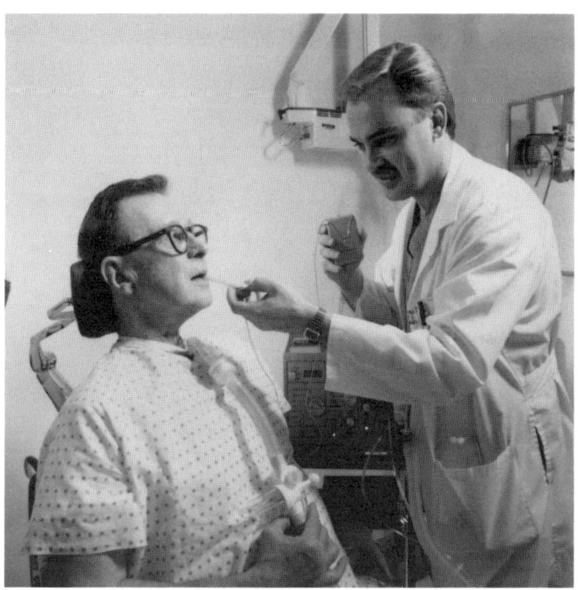

Figure 7-2 Artificial larynx product: The Cooper Rand. (Courtesy of Luminaud, Inc., Mentor, OH.)

(a small hole or group of small holes depending on the manufacturer and style of the tube). Fenestration(s) are on the curved part of the body of the outer cannula of the tracheostomy tube. When the inner cannula is removed, the inhaled and exhaled air is allowed to flow through the fenestration(s) past the vocal cords and exhaled out of the mouth and nose. Patients can achieve voicing with fenestrated tracheostomy tubes if they have sufficient airflow. To accomplish this, the inner cannula of the tracheostomy tube must be removed as the patient cannot breathe through the fenestration when it is blocked by the inner cannula. Complications from the use of fenestrated tracheostomy tubes include growth of granuloma tissue into the fenestration, which can create a tracheal obstruction;[4] blockage of the fenestration with secretions and/or improper positioning of the fenestration in the trachea, causing blockage against the tracheal lumen. Most tracheostomy tube manufacturers have developed fenestrated tubes (Figures 7-3 and 7-4). Although these tubes are a viable option for vocal production in tracheostomized patients, use of these tubes to provide voicing should be considered in conjunction with the awareness of the complications that can develop. These tubes are described further in Chapter 3.

Mallinckrodt, the manufacturer of Shiley tracheostomy tubes, is

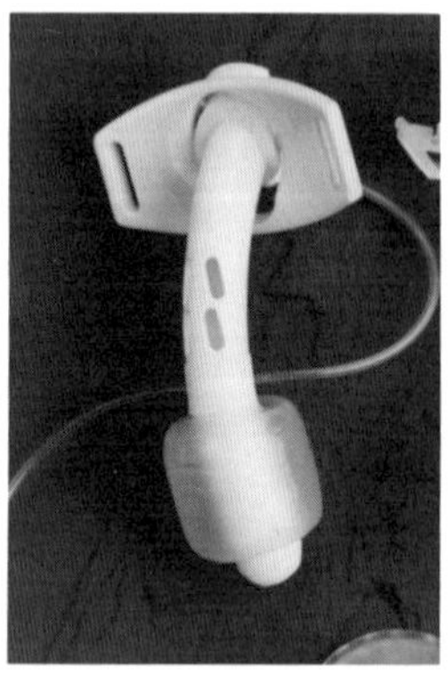

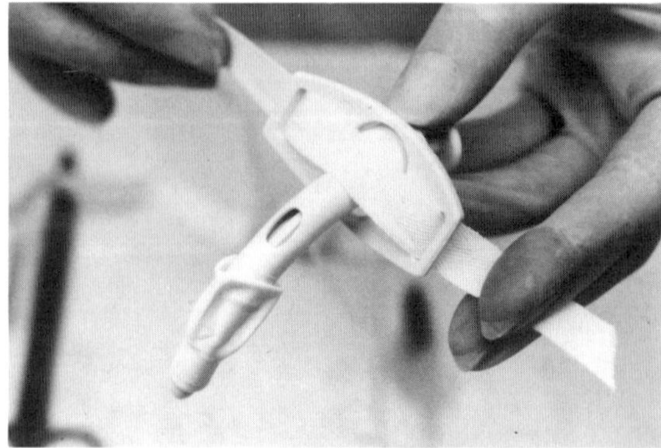

Figure 7-3 Shiley fenestrated cuffed tracheostomy tubes. (Courtesy of Mallinckrodt Medical TPI, Inc. Irvine, CA.)

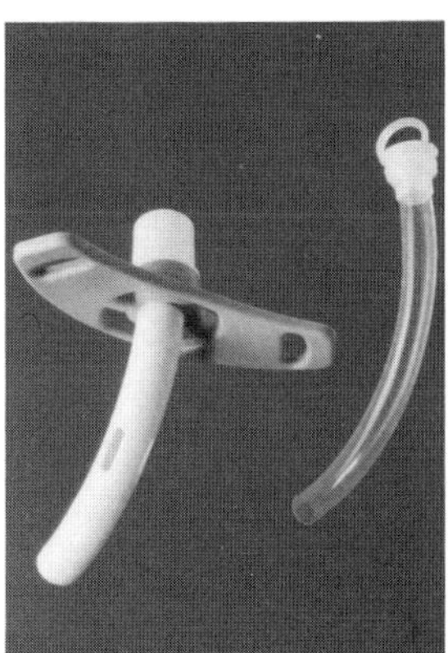

Figure 7-4 Concord/Portex fenestrated tracheostomy tube. (Courtesy of Concord/ Portex, division of Smiths Industries Medical Systems, Keene, NH.)

presently developing a double fenestrated tracheostomy tube. This design will provide a fenestration in both the outer and inner cannulas of the tracheostomy tube. This will allow the fenestration to be used with the inner cannula still in place for hygiene purposes. In addition, this tube will provide a 15 mm hub attachment, which will allow it to be used in conjunction with a tracheostomy speaking valve (a vocal option discussed later in this chapter).

Tucker Tracheostomy Inner Cannula

The Tucker tracheostomy tube has been available for many years and is different from the other fenestrated tracheostomy tubes. This inner cannula is available for use with a sterling silver Jackson or Tucker tracheostomy tube and has a leaflet that closes upon exhalation to redirect airflow to be exhaled from the mouth and nose. The inner cannula needs to be removed to clean secretions that accumulate in the leaflet. This tracheostomy tube does not have a 15 mm hub, is cuffless, and cannot be used with ventilator dependent patients (Figure 7-5).

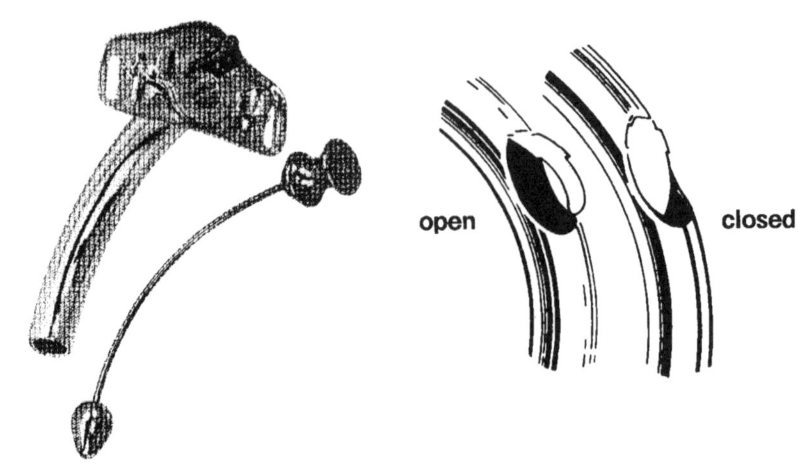

Figure 7-5 Tucker inner cannula. (Courtesy of Pilling Co., Fort Washington, PA.)

Talking Tracheostomy Tubes

Types of Talking Tracheostomy Tubes

Talking tracheostomy tubes are standard cuffed tracheostomy tubes designed with modifications to provide a means of verbal communication for tracheostomized and ventilator dependent patients who, after assessment, cannot tolerate cuff deflation. Speech/voice production is supported by an independent air source that creates voicing as air flows through an airflow line to fenestrations or conduits just above the tracheostomy tube cuff. This air flows through the patient's glottis, and voice is achieved as air flows over the vocal cords. A patient's ventilatory system remains closed and controlled because the tracheostomy tube cuff remains inflated. A closed ventilatory system can be vital in achieving successful ventilation for patients who cannot tolerate any air leakage or who have severe aspiration problems and require cuff inflation at all times.

The three most widely available talking tracheostomy tubes are the COMMUNItrach™ I, the Portex "Talk" Tracheostomy Tube, and a foam-filled† talking tracheostomy tube.

†This manufacturer refused permission to reference or to reprint photographs of these products.

The COMMUNItrach™ I

The COMMUNItrach™ I (Implant Technologies, Inc./Spectrum Medical of California) (Figures 7-6 and 7-7) is a low-pressure, high-volume, single-cuffed, double-cannula talking tracheostomy tube. This device creates airflow through the vocal cords from a compressed air source. The airflow is directed through the air supply tubing, via eight fenestrated holes inferior to the vocal folds. The position of the air-flow tubing at the six o'clock position can cause kinking and air leakage between the inner and outer cannulas.[6] This

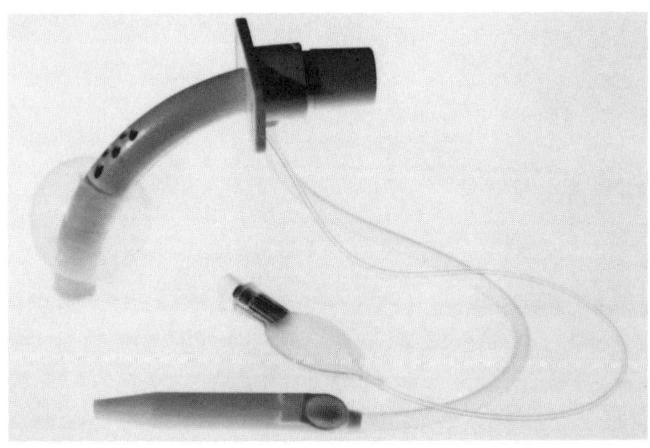

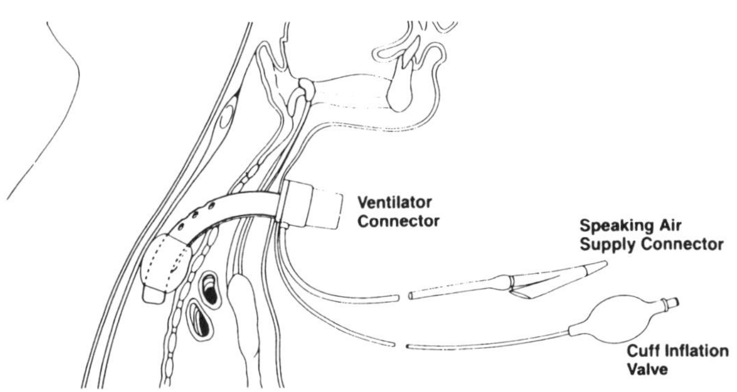

7-6 COMMUNItrach™ I products. (Formerly Implant Technologies, courtesy of Spectrum Medical, Irvine, CA.)

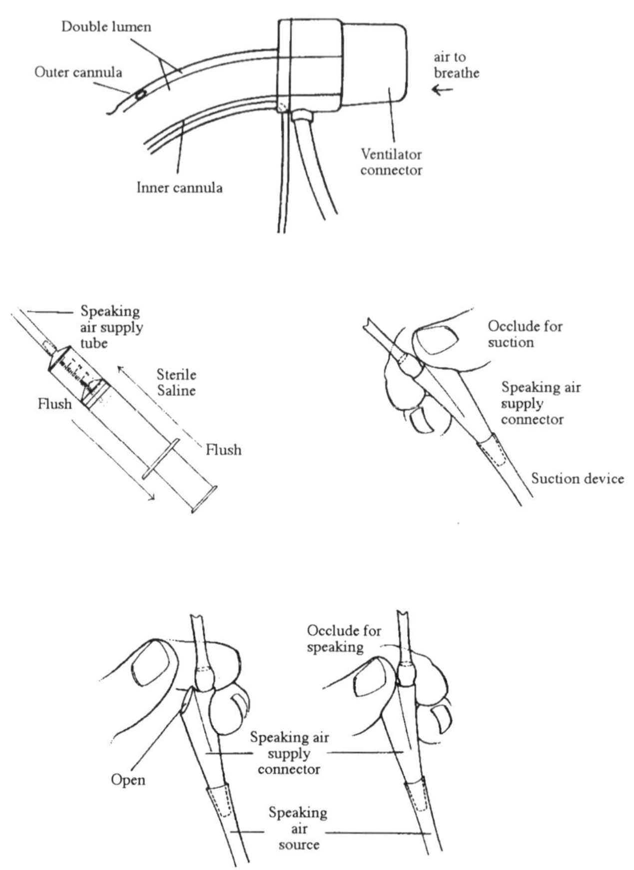

Figure 7-7 COMMUNItrach™ I. (Formerly Implant Technologies, courtesy of Spectrum Medical, Irvine, CA.)

tracheostomy tube is available in adult sizes 7, 8, and 9. There is a mechanism to flush and suction the airflow line to clear secretions and food particles, which may sit above the tracheal cuff. This feature assists in tracheostomy care and management. (Figures 7-6 and 7-7).

The Portex "Talk" Tracheostomy Tube

The Portex "Talk" tracheostomy tube (Concord/Portex, Inc.) is a double-cannula, single-cuffed tracheostomy tube that provides a means for vocalization. This tube has a narrow slit along its convex surface that terminates above the inflatable cuff. The external end of this slit can be connected to a source of compressed air, and the airflow is regulated by means of a thumb port on the catheter tubing. When this port is occluded, air travels through the airflow line, then exits through a slit superior to the cuff and continues through the glottis and vocal tract, allowing for speech. Inserting the tube at the nine o'clock position may prevent kinking and the elimination of air between the inner and outer cannula."[6] This tube is available in adult sizes 6, 7, and 8 (Figure 7-8).

The Foam-Filled Talking Tracheostomy Tube

This tube allows air to flow through an air port, directing air through the larynx to promote voicing. This tracheostomy tube is different from the other talking tracheostomy tubes because the cuff is silicone foam-filled, rather than air-filled. The foam cuff is designed to eliminate the potential for overinflation and permit the maintenance of a lower cuff pressure. The self-limiting expansion of the foam cuff can reduce the incidence of tracheal dilation, which may

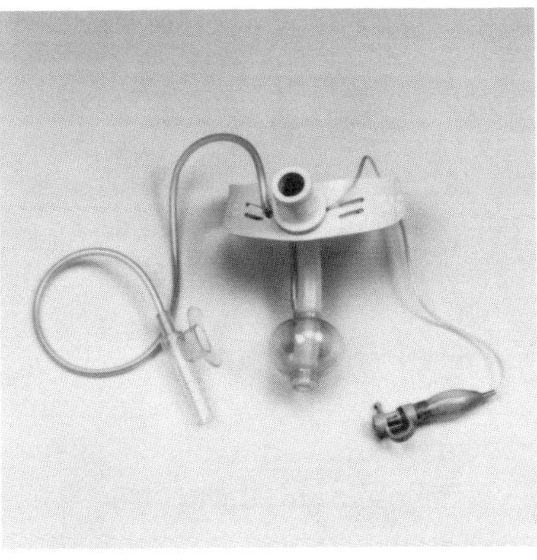

Figure 7-8 "Trach-Talk." (Courtesy of Concord/Portex, division of Smiths Industries Medical Systems, Keene, NH.)

be an important consideration if the trachea has suffered primary damage, as with burn injuries.[7]

A decrease in elasticity of the foam filling the cuff can cause the seal to loosen, which will create an air leak. Sizing this tube to the patient's trachea is more critical and difficult than with air-inflated cuffed tubes.[7] Manufacturer's recommendations for sizing should be reviewed.[†]

Talking Tracheostomy Tube Considerations

Consideration of these devices should include a review of the particular characteristics of these tubes, including the necessity of an additional air source, level of hygiene care needed, manual dexterity required, and voice quality produced. Because the outside air source used is not humidified, the mucosal tissue in the trachea can become dried and irritated. This may cause discomfort for the patient, and humidification will need to be addressed. Secretions can plug the fenestration or air port needed for airflow through the vocal cords, therefore, diligent cleaning and flushing are necessary to ensure optimum performance. To operate this device to produce voicing, the patient must shunt the tubing connected to the outside air source with his or her finger or thumb to direct airflow up through the fenestration(s) in the tube and then through the vocal cords. This may not be possible for a patient who has paralysis, paresis, or any type of neuromuscular involvement that prohibits upper extremity movement. Family and staff can be trained to digitally occlude this tubing if the patient is unable to do so; however, this makes the patient dependent on someone else to enable him or her to vocalize.

The patient's voice quality when using these devices is often a breathy or hoarse whisper or wet and gurgly, rather than normal voicing. With appropriate therapeutic intervention provided by a speech-language pathologist, this voice quality can improve.

Talking tracheostomy tubes are available in most common adult sizes. If a patient must maintain cuff inflation at all times for adequate ventilation, then the talking tracheostomy tubes are the recommended option for vocal communication.

[†]This manufacturer refused permission to reference or to reprint photographs of these products.

Tracheostomy Speaking Valves

This category of devices offers appropriate patients the optimal method of verbal communication, because patients are able to utilize their own breathing for natural voicing. As explained previously, with an open tracheostomy tube air is inhaled and exhaled through the tracheostomy tube, thereby bypassing the upper airway. Use of a tracheostomy speaking valve forces exhaled air through the upper airway (Figure 7-9). The flow of air goes through the vocal cords and is exhaled through the mouth and nose, thus allowing the production of natural voice and speech. These devices are one-way valves that were designed to create normal voicing for optimal verbal communication. Most of these devices fit on the end of the standard 15 mm hub of a tracheostomy tube and are simple to place and utilize. Use of a tracheostomy speaking valve allows patients to have the benefit of inhalation and ventilation through the tracheostomy tube but exhaled air is redirected through the upper airway and out the oral and nasal cavities.

A thorough assessment of upper airway patency (clearance) and pulmonary status is necessary and should be ongoing when considering use of these devices. Due to the positioning of the speaking valve on the tracheostomy tube, the air inhaled through the tracheostomy

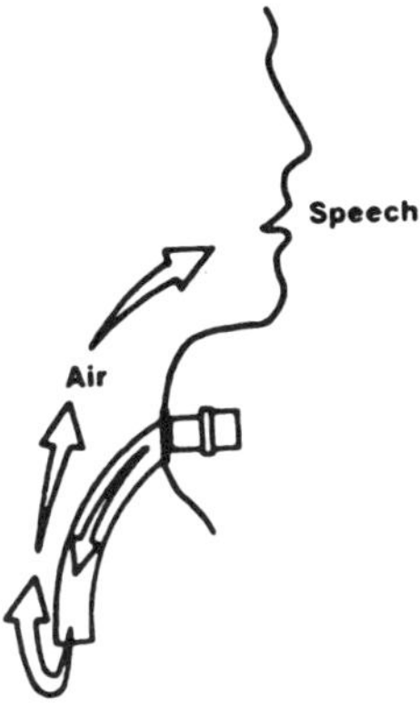

Figure 7-9 The tracheostomy speaking valve enables speech by redirecting exhaled air around the tracheostomy tube and through the nose and mouth.

tube also passes through the speaking valve. However, with the one-way speaking valve in place the air will not be exhaled through the tube and speaking valve but will instead be redirected upward around the tracheostomy tube and out the mouth and nose as in normal exhalation. Consequently, it is imperative that the clinician assess the patient for both upper airway patency and lower airway pulmonary function. When a speaking valve is in place, the patient must have enough airway clearance around the tracheostomy tube and deflated cuff (if the patient has a cuffed tube) to exhale the same amount of air that was inspired. The patient will also need sufficient pulmonary (lung) function to push the air up through the upper airway to exhale out the mouth and nose. Patients with end-stage disease of the lungs should be assessed carefully to ensure that adequate function exists to exhale without causing air-trapping. The majority of tracheostomy and ventilator dependent patients will have sufficient upper airway patency and pulmonary function to use a tracheostomy speaking valve; however, this cannot be assumed and careful assessment is critical to the successful use of this type of device.

PHYSIOLOGICAL FUNCTIONS REESTABLISHED WITH USE OF TRACHEOSTOMY SPEAKING VALVES

Speech

Tracheostomy speaking valves redirect air flow through the vocal cords for uninterrupted phonation. Patients have increased length of utterance and normal speech pattern. Although all speaking valves can be used with tracheostomized patients, the Passy-Muir positive closure speaking valve is the only valve that is FDA registered for use with ventilator dependent patients.[8-18] Use of this valve by ventilator dependent patients allows them to form sentences naturally and does not limit them to one or two syllables that can be produced with each ventilator cycle (termed "leak speech"). In addition, the vocal intensity produced is louder and can be more easily heard over the ventilator and other environmental noise.

Secretion Management

Secretions are often reduced and easier to manage in conjunction with use of a speaking valve device because air is redirected up through the oral and nasal cavities, thus reestablishing the evaporation process of fluids in these chambers. This reduces the amount of secretions present in the hypopharynx. Research has shown that a speaking valve device may facilitate cough, swallow, and oral expectoration of upper airway and lower lung secretions, which subsequently can result in less suctioning and improved pulmonary hygiene.[7-12,16,17]

Olfaction and Gustation

Because air is inspired and expired through the tracheostomy tube, bypassing the upper airway and nasal and oral chambers, tracheostomized patients often complain that they cannot smell or taste. This loss of smell and taste affects the appetite. Use of a tracheostomy speaking valve allows inspired air to be redirected to the nasal chamber, thus restoring the sense of smell.[8,9,11-13,16,17] Restored olfaction along with the presence of airflow in the oral cavity enhances gustation and ultimately improves appetite and facilitates nutritional intake which is vital to medical recovery.

Infection

Use of a tracheostomy speaking valve eliminates the need for digital or finger occlusion, which is a source of contamination. In addition, the valve may act as a filter, catching some of the airborne particulates in the inspired air, which assists in preventing contamination of the tracheobronchial passages. With a positive closure speaking valve, research has shown that a patient is able to cough and expectorate orally, which prevents secretions from being coughed out the tracheostomy tube, thus reducing contamination risk to others in the patient's environment.[9-13,17,18]

Swallow

The placement of a tracheostomy tube between the second and third cartilaginous rings anchors the laryngeal structure. The open-ended tube that exists with a tracheostomy in place depletes pressures in the pharyngeal and pulmonary areas. This can be compared to an open-ended cylinder of air where there is equal pressure on both ends of the cylinder. If one end of this cylindrical tube is capped, there would be a build-up of air pressure behind the cap. Similarly, when a "positive closure" type of valve is placed on the hub of the patient's tracheostomy tube, a positive back pressure is created in the tube. This pressure increases the pharyngeal pressures that are needed to move the food bolus down the pharynx and into the esophagus. Speech-language pathologists have reported viewing improvement in patients' swallowing function during videofluoroscopy assessments when a positive closure speaking valve is utilized. This may not be true of other speaking valves because they are designed to remain in an open position except on exhalation and thus do not establish a closed system for the patient.[10-12,17,18,19]

Physiological PEEP

The enhancement of physiologic positive end expiratory pressure, sometimes referred to as (Auto) PEEP, may be a benefit of a positive closure speaking valve. Valves that do not have a positive closure design may not be able to provide PEEP as they are always in the open position and allow air leakage. A speaking valve that provides positive closure can restore back pressure (also known as expiratory retard). Expiratory retard refers to the natural back pressure accumulation into the lungs that occurs when we breathe against our upper airway structures. A speaking valve with positive closure simulates a normally closed tracheobronchial system and can result in improved alveolar patency and more normal pulmonary exchange (gas diffusion). This can at times be observed clinically as improvement in the patient's blood oxygen level as indicated by oximetry readings. Auto PEEP provided with the use of a positive closure speaking valve is thought to be of benefit in the weaning process.[10,12,15,17,18]

Decannulation

Physicians utilize different methods of decannulation (removal of the tracheostomy tube). One-way speaking valves can offer a transitioning method to help prepare the patient and assist the physician in the decannulation process.[9,15,20]

The following are specific reasons why speaking valves can facilitate decannulation of a tracheostomized patient:

1. Easier to tolerate than capping or plugging of the tracheostomy tube.

Prior to capping or plugging the tracheostomy tube, the valve can be used to gain access to the upper airway during exhalation. The inspiratory and expiratory effort of breathing around a tracheostomy tube can be difficult for any patient to tolerate because of the size of the tracheostomy tube. The work of breathing will be much easier with a speaking valve in place rather than with a cap or plug because the valve allows the patient to inspire through the tracheostomy site as well as the upper airway.

2. Airway patency assessment.

Use of a valve can assist in airway patency assessment as airflow is reintroduced for the exhalation part of the breathing cycle. Exhalation flows can once again be measured orally.

3. Building patient confidence and reducing anxiety.

Patient confidence builds as exhalation is felt and tolerated. The patient is reoriented to the upper airway functions of speech, secretion management, expectoration, and more normal swallowing process. Anxiety in response to decannulation can be reduced dramatically if valve usage is incorporated as soon as possible after the tracheostomy placement.

4. Expediting the decannulation process.

Aten and Light[20] report that mean time saved with a positive closure speaking valve was an average of five days in decannulation of chronic tracheostomized patients.

5. Improved oxygenation.

Improvement in oxygenation may be facilitated by the back pressure (Auto PEEP) produced with a positive closure valve.[9,15]

ASSESSMENT ISSUES WITH TRACHEOSTOMY SPEAKING VALVES

Upper Airway Assessment

When assessing patency of the upper airway (Table 7-1), the patient's complete history should always be reviewed, including the details and events leading to tracheostomy tube placement, previous airway diagnostics performed (e.g., bronchoscopy), and intubation history. Specific information on upper airway obstructions such as tumors, stenosis, and granulomas should be obtained as well as how these obstructions will be managed or reduced. If necessary, the patient's upper airway should be assessed clinically. Bronchoscopy and laryngoscopy are procedures performed by the physician that can confirm airway patency. These procedures are optical exams of the upper airway in which an endoscope is passed through the oral cavity, nasal cavities, or tracheostomy tube, allowing visualization of the trachea, internal larynx, and bronchi. Fiberoptic scopes are often utilized. They enhance visualization due to the flexibility of the scope during the exam.

A bedside assessment of upper airway patency can be performed by the clinician via tracheal occlusion when the tracheostomy tube

1. Complete history reviewed
2. Tracheostomy tube history
3. Previous airway diagnostics performed
4. Intubation history
5. Presence and management of upper airway obstructions

Table 7-1 Assessment Issues.

cuff (if present) is fully deflated. In this technique a gloved finger is utilized to cover the tracheostomy tube while listening and observing for exhaled air through the oral and nasal cavities (Table 7-2). Subjective observation of performance activities such as sound production, cotton ball and feather blowing, or mirror condensation while the tracheostomy tube is being occluded can confirm upper airway patency. A more accurate assessment of exhaled air can be made using spirometry. With this technique, the patient is instructed to take a full inspiratory breath through the tracheostomy site. The clinician then occludes the tracheostomy tube with a gloved finger while the patient blows into a spirometer. A reading of exhaled tidal volume is recorded by the spirometer. Appropriateness of these measurements will vary depending on age, body weight, and disease process. (This same measurement can be made with a ventilator dependent patient but only when a speaking valve approved for in-line ventilator use is utilized.) The valve is placed in-line for the ventilator circuitry and the patient is able to accept inhaled ventilation through the tracheal stoma site; however, exhaled air is redirected through the mouth and nose. Like the tracheostomized, nonventilator dependent patient, the mechanically ventilated patient can then blow exhaled tidal volumes through the upper airway and into the spirometer. This measurement provides information on upper airway patency because the exhaled volumes can then be compared to the inspiratory volumes being delivered to the patient by the ventilator. If the exhaled volumes measured are significantly smaller than the inspiratory volumes delivered, further investigation regarding upper airway patency is warranted.

---

1. Tracheal occlusion
2. Subjective observation of sound production
3. Spirometry readings
5. Size of the tracheostomy tube

Table 7-2 Exhalation Assessment.

Upper Airway Treatment Strategies

If assessment reveals that adequate airway patency is not being achieved, an evaluation of the size of the tracheostomy tube should be pursued. Many physicians size the tube to be approximately two-thirds the size of the tracheal lumen (opening). A tracheostomy tube should not be any larger than necessary to provide ventilation and should allow enough room in the trachea for airflow around the tracheostomy tube and out the upper airway. A suggestion to the patient's primary physician to "downsize" (replace with a smaller tube) a tracheostomy tube may be necessary to provide adequate airway patency. An endoscopy can be performed by the physician if, following the tracheostomy tube downsizing, airway patency is not achieved.

Lower Airway Assessment

Pulmonary assessment is an evaluation of the patient's ability to mobilize airflow and oxygenate adequately. Measurement of this breathing capacity reflects the ability to perform necessary exhalation to utilize a tracheostomy speaking valve for vocalization. Measurement of exhaled tidal volume will be objectively revealed through spirometry assessment. As previously mentioned in conjunction with upper airway patency assessment, this procedure can be performed at bedside with both tracheostomized and mechanically ventilated patients.

Appropriate ventilation can be assessed through good clinical observation and assessment of vital signs. Any increased work of breathing, obvious fatigue, or skin discoloration are signs of intolerance and may limit time and usage of a tracheostomy speaking valve. Compensation strategies to assist patients in the use of a tracheostomy speaking valve should be attempted by authorized personnel. Such strategies would include adjusting breath rate and/or increasing tidal volume on ventilator dependent patients or providing higher levels of supplemental oxygen usage to tracheostomized patients. Blood gas monitoring via oximetry also provides objective data. This is a technique for measuring oxygen and saturation of hemoglobin in the

1. Assessment of vital signs
2. Increased work of breathing
3. Compensation strategies
4. Blood gas monitoring through oximetry

Table 7-3 Lower Airway Monitoring.

quick, and noninvasive monitoring but should not replace comprehensive blood gas analysis, which provides a more complete assessment of oxygenation and adequacy of ventilation as reflected by PCO_2 levels.

Air-Trapping/Stacking

The presence of air-trapping or the inability to properly exhale and mobilize air is a result of airway obstruction or inadequate pulmonary function. Air-trapping occurs when the patient is not able to exhale all the inspired air, causing a sensation of fullness and distress to the patient, which can sometimes lead to barotrauma. Air-trapping or stacking can result from the presence of an upper airway obstruction that blocks air outflow. The patient may report that he cannot breathe in; however, this sensation is actually caused by the inability to exhale completely, thus air becomes "trapped" and stacks up in the lungs.

Lower Airway Treatment Strategies

Air-trapping can sometimes be remedied by correcting the upper airway obstruction or reducing the resistance by decreasing tracheostomy tube size or replacing a cuffed tracheostomy tube with a cuffless tracheostomy tube. There will be some cases in which a certain amount of air-trapping while utilizing a tracheostomy speaking valve may be tolerated. Patients with inadequate pulmonary function and ventilation who have a significant need to communicate and patients who have experienced severe trauma, severe burns or who are dying, may need to communicate to discuss vital matters and have closure on personal issues before they die. To accomplish this closure, these patients need to be able to communicate and interact with family and friends. **Consequently, for some critically ill and medically unstable patients, oxygen desaturation and decreased pulmonary function may be acceptable for brief periods of time to allow necessary communicative expression to take place.**

Precautions with Using the Speaking Valves

A speaking valve should not be used when a severe upper airway obstruction is present because air cannot move up around the tracheostomy tube to be exhaled out the oral and nasal cavities. Speaking valves should not be used with pulmonary secretions that are too tenacious and may obstruct the upper airway that leads to the oral and nasal cavities.

Some speaking valves can be used with the Portex fenestrated tracheostomy tube only when the cuff is completely deflated and the inner cannula is removed. The Portex disposable inner cannula tracheostomy tube can be used with tracheostomy speaking valves; however, caution is advised as this type of inner cannula has a ring that protrudes and can block the valve. Therefore, the inner cannula should be removed to prevent possible occlusion. Shiley fenestrated tubes require the inner cannula to be in place for use with a speaking valve. The inner cannula is needed to provide the 15 mm hub to which the speaking valve is connected. With the inner cannula in place, however, the fenestration is blocked; therefore, if a tracheostomy tube cuff is present, it must be deflated while using a speaking valve to allow exhalation through the upper airway. Metal tracheostomy tubes do not have an inner cannula 15 mm hub to which a speaking valve can be attached. With metal tubes an endotracheal tube adapter can be used to establish a 15 mm connection. Tracheostomy speaking valves cannot be used with foam cuff tracheostomy tubes because the cuffs do not deflate adequately and reinflate spontaneously (Table 7-4).

Tracheostomy speaking valves are not voice prostheses and should not be confused with a voice prosthesis (e.g., Blom-Singer), which is a device designed for laryngectomized patients. Speaking valves should be used with caution in patients with end-stage pulmo-

1. Do not use with a severe airway obstruction
2. Use with caution with increased or thick pulmonary secretions
3. Cannot be used with an inflated tracheostomy cuff
4. Cannot be used with a foam-cuffed tracheostomy tube
5. Not a voice prosthesis (cannot be used with laryngectomized patients)
6. Caution with use on patients who have end stage pulmonary obstructive diseases

Table 7-4 Precautions in Use of Speaking Valves.

nary obstructive diseases associated with decreased pulmonary elastic recoil and variable airway resistance because ventilator settings necessary for adequate ventilation may be highly variable and can fluctuate from one hour to the next or from day to day.

TYPES OF TRACHEOSTOMY SPEAKING VALVES

There are five types of tracheostomy speaking valves described in this section. These valves include the Olympic Trach Talk, the Montgomery Speaking Valve, the Kistner Speaking Valve, the Hood Speaking Valve, and the Passy-Muir Speaking Valves. Although these devices are all referred to as speaking valves, in design and function they are quite different from one another.

The Olympic Trach Talk

This device attaches to the end of any standard 15 mm tracheostomy tube (Figure 7-10). The valve mechanism is designed as a one-way valve held in an open position by a stainless steel spring. The valve remains open except when the patient exhales, at which time the force of the exhaled breath closes the valve and diverts air through the larynx, enabling vocalization. This valve is not indicated for use with patients being mechanically ventilated. It is always in the open position until exhalation pressures force it closed. It has air leak in both directions. Suctioning (by authorized medical personnel) without removal of the valve is possible and it can be connected to a

T-piece to provide oxygen blow-by for weaning. The spring mechanism may accumulate mucus and should be closely monitored and taken apart to be cleaned. This valve is considerably larger and heavier than the other valves. This valve does free a patient from unsanitary and conspicuous finger occlusion. It cannot be utilized with an inflated tracheostomy cuff, with severe upper airway obstruction, or with stenosis. Use with pediatric patients is not reported.

The Montgomery Speaking Valve

The Montgomery Speaking Valve provides one-way airflow using a thin silicone hinged diaphragm that is designed to stay in the open position and closes upon expiration, eliminating the need for finger occlusion. The valve has a cough release feature designed to prevent the valve from being blown off when the patient coughs. When the patient coughs, the diaphragm pops out and is then tucked back to its normal position with a fingertip following the coughing episode. This cough-resistant feature of the valve may be sensitive to coughing or heavy breathing and may require frequent repositioning of the diaphragm in the valve by the patient. Secretions can sometimes be coughed through the valve and can potentially affect the diaphragm's movement. This device is not intended for use with a patient on a ventilator (Figure 7-11).

The valve's function should eliminate the need for finger occlusion; however, the patient does need to utilize his or her finger to

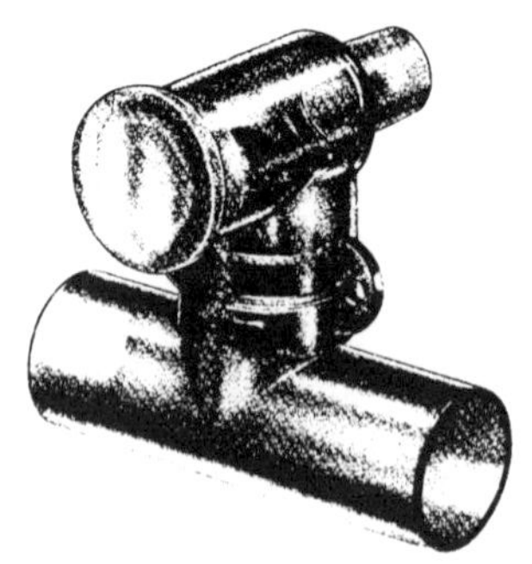

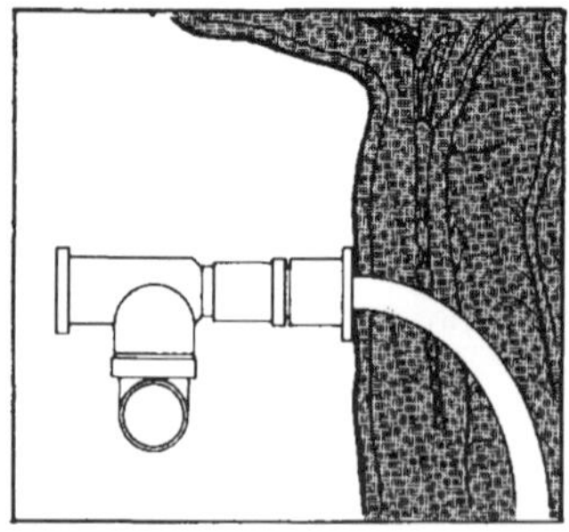

Figure 7-10 Trach Talk™. (Courtesy of Olympic Medical, Seattle, WA.)

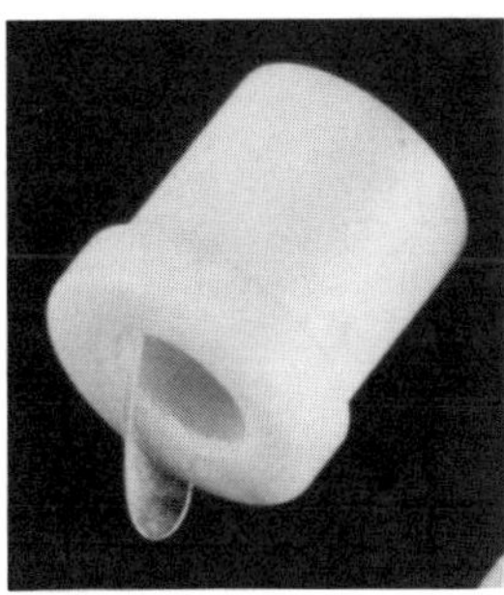

Figure 7-11 Montgomery speaking valve. (Courtesy of Boston Medical Products, Inc., Waltham, MA.)

replace the diaphragm after the cough is released. As with all tracheostomy speaking valves, the Montgomery Speaking Valve cannot be used with an inflated tracheostomy cuff or with patients who have severe upper airway obstruction or stenosis. Data on the utilization of this valve with pediatric patients is not available.

The Hood Speaking Valve

The Hood Speaking Valve provides one-way airflow using a tiny ball enclosed in a chamber (Figure 7-12). The ball moves to open and close the chamber based on expiratory and inspiratory forces. The Hood valve was originally designed to fit the Hood Stoma Stent. Recently, it has been adapted with a 15 mm connector. This valve is not indicated for use during mechanical ventilation. The Hood Speaking Valve is in an open position and therefore will allow some air leakage in both directions until exhalation forces move the ball to a closed position. The diameter of the airflow chamber of the Hood Speaking Valve is much smaller than that of other speaking valves, which will affect inspiratory effort in some patients. There are no reported uses of this valve with pediatric patients.

The Kistner One-Way Valve

The Kistner Speaking Valve is in the open position and closes upon exhalation. This valve was one of the earliest valves available

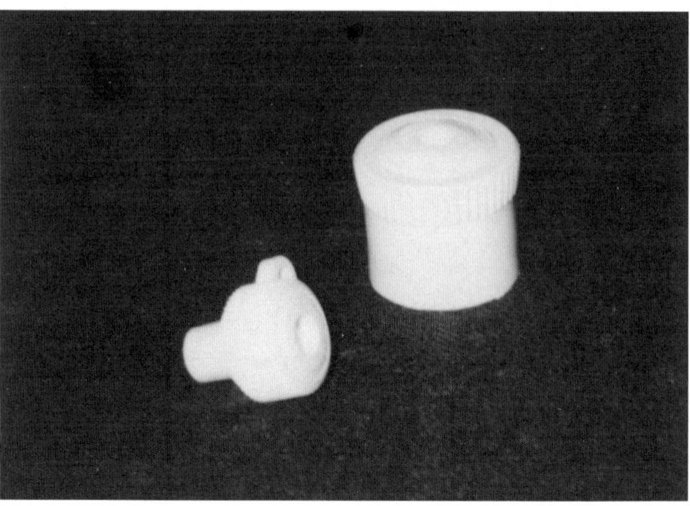

Figure 7-12 Hood Stoma Stent speaking valve and Hood speaking valve. (15 mm tracheostomy tube connection) (Courtesy of Hood Laboratories, Pembroke, MA.)

and the diaphragm in the valve is made of more rigid plastic and is smaller in diameter. This creates more inspiratory resistance and can cause a clicking noise when it seals with exhalation. This valve is designed to snap onto the Jackson Tracheostomy Tube or the Kistner Plastic Tracheostomy Tube and cannot be used with other standard tracheostomy tubes. There is no reported pediatric use of this valve in the literature. As with all speaking valves, it cannot be used with an inflated tracheostomy cuff, severe upper airway obstruction or stenosis (Figure 7-13).

Passy-Muir Tracheostomy Speaking Valves

The Passy-Muir Tracheostomy Speaking Valves are different from other one-way valves because of their "positive closure" design and their ability to be used with a ventilator (Figure 7-14). Historically, concerns with the use of other one-way valves have included occlusion problems, high resistance levels, size, adaptability, reduced air volume, safety, and durability. David Muir, a quadriplegic muscular dystrophy patient, invented the Passy-Muir Tracheostomy Speak-

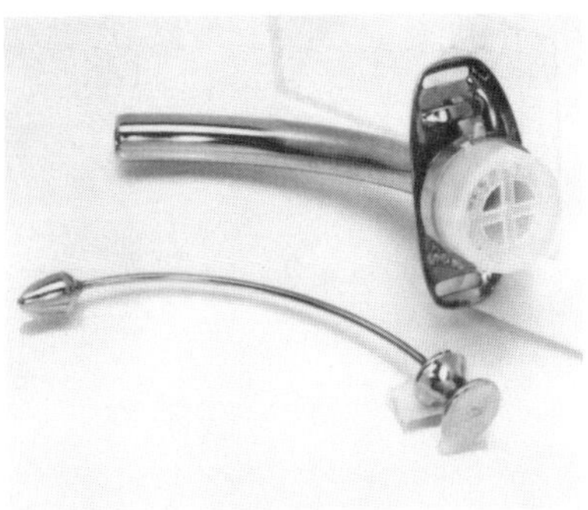

A

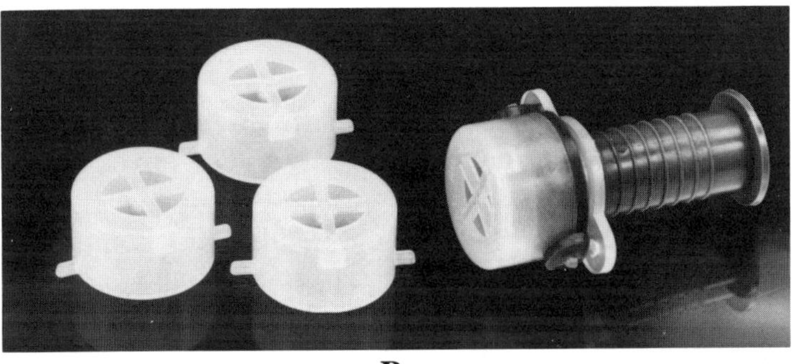

B

Figure 7-13 **A**, *Jackson metal tracheostomy tube with Kistner speaking valves.* **B**, *Kistner tracheostomy tube with Kistner speaking valves. (Courtesy of Pilling Co., Fort Washington, PA.)*

ing Valve for his own use and was able to overcome these problems with his positive closure design. David Muir's story is delineated in Chapter 9. There are several significant differences in the Passy-Muir Tracheostomy Speaking Valve design from other one-way speaking valves. The following is an explanation of these differences and their effects on the physiology of the tracheostomized and ventilator dependent patient.

Positive Closure Design

The Passy-Muir valve is always closed because it is biased (or positioned) to stay in the closed position and opens only on inspira-

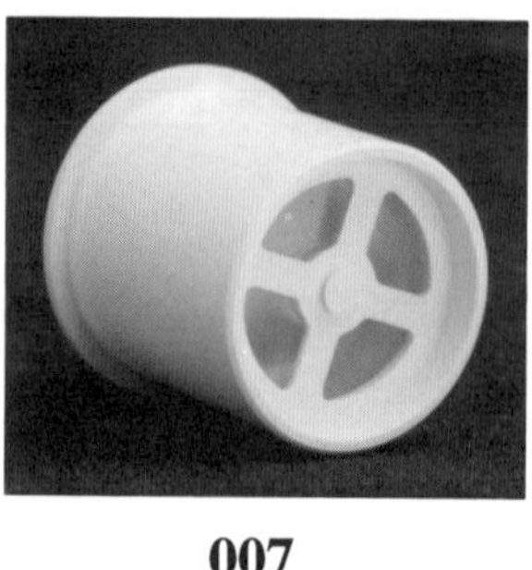

007

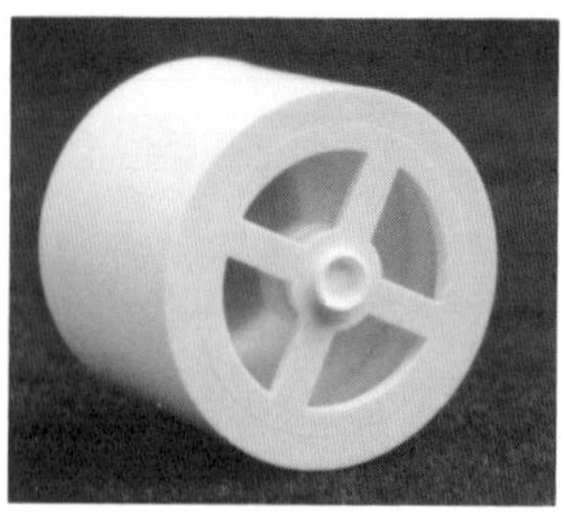

005

Figure 7-14 #007 Passy-Muir ventilator speaking valve (Aqua) and #005 Passy-Muir tracheostomy speaking valve (White). (Courtesy of Passy-Muir, Inc., Irvine, CA.)

tion. With this positive bias, the valve actually closes automatically before the end of the inspiratory cycle. With the valve always being closed except when the patient inspires, air is trapped in the valve and in the tracheostomy tube, which theoretically acts as a buffer to resist secretions coming up the tube. This air buffer and the restoration of the ability to cough and redirect secretions to be expectorated orally, thus inhibiting the secretions from accumulating in the tube and the valve.[7,16] This concept can be demonstrated with a glass inverted and then placed in water. A column of air is trapped in the glass, and when immersed in water the air will remain in the glass, preventing water from entering the glass. This is the theory of the positive closure mechanism of the Passy-Muir valve. The positive closure design provides a patient with a closed system and more normal physiology of the body, affecting secretion management and pulmonary function (Figure 7-15).

Other tracheostomy speaking valves are in an open position until expiration pressure reaches a level to close the valve. Consequently, there is some air leakage around these valves upon exhalation, which may allow for the encroachment of secretions.

VENTILATOR APPLICATION OF THE PASSY-MUIR TRACHEOSTOMY SPEAKING VALVE

The Passy-Muir Tracheostomy Speaking Valves can be incorporated into ventilator weaning or rehabilitation processes as an effec-

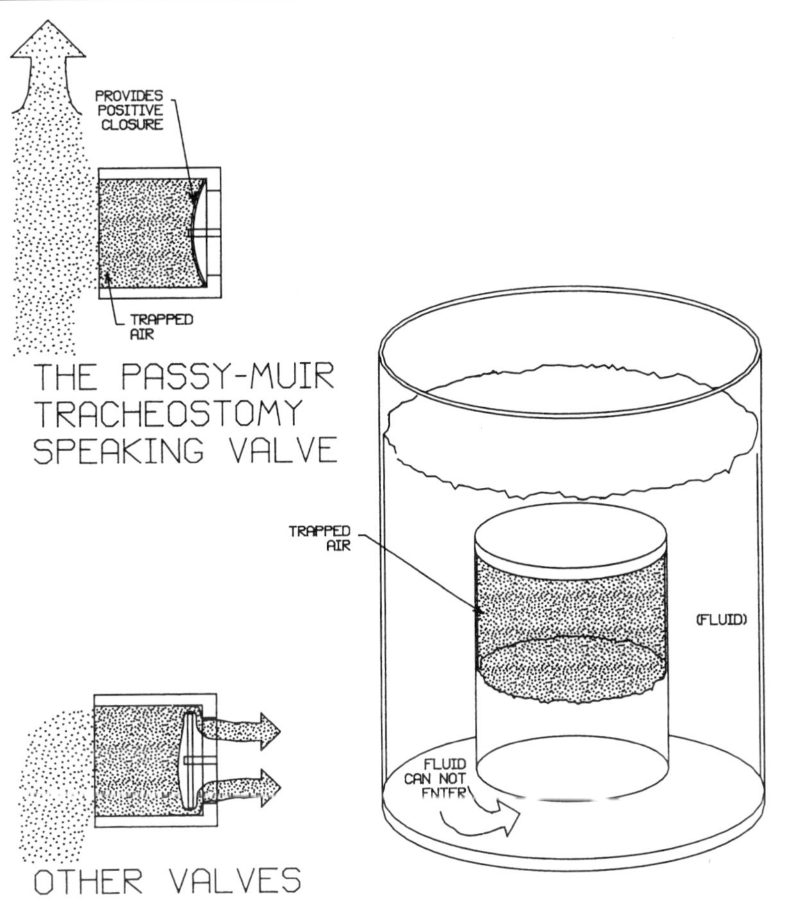

Figure 7-15 Positive closure design concept of the Passy-Muir valves. (Courtesy of Passy-Muir, Inc., Irvine, CA.)

tive communication option for both adult and pediatric ventilator dependent patients.[8-10,12-17] At this time, the Passy-Muir Valves are the only speaking valves designed and FDA registered for in-line ventilator use (Figure 7-16).

With severe upper airway obstruction or stenosis, individual assessment is critical as the use of the valve is dependent upon the degree of obstruction. The patient must have enough airway around the tracheostomy tube and cuff (if it is a cuffed tube) to exhale the inspired breaths. The Passy-Muir Valve cannot be utilized with an inflated tracheostomy cuff or a foam-cuffed tracheostomy tube.

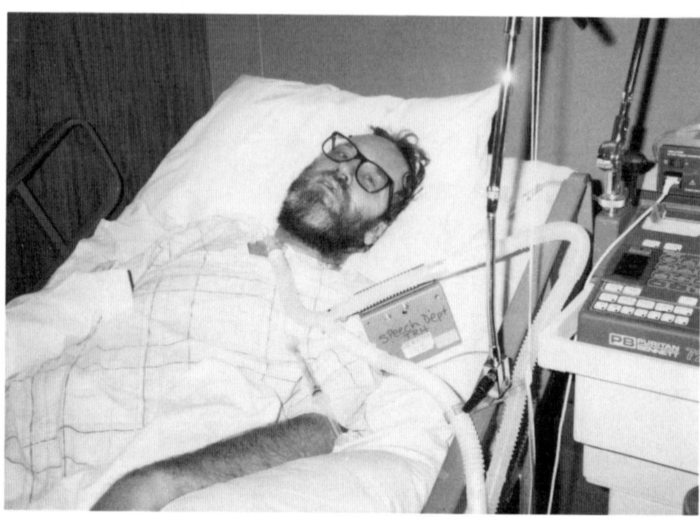

Figure 7-16 Passy-Muir Ventilator speaking valve in-line. (Courtesy of Passy-Muir, Inc., Irvine, CA.)

These valves should be used with caution on ventilator dependent patients with "end-stage" pulmonary obstructive disease (COPD). With advanced COPD, the lungs lose their elasticity, and adequate pulmonary function cannot be achieved; thus the patient cannot exhale air. Each patient needs to be evaluated individually to determine if an adequate degree of compliance is present to allow use of the valve.

Cuff Deflation Assessment

Respiratory professionals working with ventilator dependent patients are usually concerned with being able to ventilate these patients adequately if the tracheostomy tube cuff deflated. Patients can be ventilated with the cuff deflated according to a study by Bach and Alba[5]. Of 104 patients of differing diagnoses, "The study indicated that the vast majority of tracheostomized patients with severe respiratory insufficiency and reasonably competent oropharyngeal muscles can be safely and adequately ventilated up to 24 hours a day with their cuffs deflated or removed (preferably cuffless tube)."[5] However, when a ventilator dependent patient is medically stable and alert, can tolerate air leakage, and has some spontaneous breathing, the patient should be considered ready to be evaluated for use of the valve. A patient who is comatose, has an airway infection, or is at the very end stage of lung disease (can't passively exhale air up to the oral/ nasal chamber) may be able to use a speaking valve on a limited basis with careful monitoring.

Leak Speech vs. Speech Using The Passy-Muir Valve

With the Passy-Muir Valve in-line in the ventilator circuitry, patients can speak in complete sentences, with more volume that allows them to speak conversationally over room noise and on the phone.

Some patients may achieve intermittent vocalization with cuff deflation. This type of speech (termed *leak speech*) is limited to one or two words per ventilator breath; however, it increases the patient's work of breathing. With valve placement, a patient should be able to speak in sentences, with a louder voice and clearer speech. Many patients will be able to control voice volume and length of utterance immediately, but some patients may take some time to acclimate to a more normal pattern of speech. It is the role of the speech-language pathologist to help the patient's transition through this process. Patient participation is important as any attempt to converse will allow a patient to gain confidence in speech patterning. One of the best techniques is merely to distract the patient so he or she is not trying too hard to coordinate speech. The valve will provide airflow on exhalation and will act as a control mechanism to allow the patient to voice on demand. Thus some ventilator dependent patients can speak nonstop on inspiration and expiration.

Ventilator Adjustments

Safety alarms on the ventilator will still be active, including low-pressure disconnect alarms, parameter alarms, and high-pressure obstruction alarms. All pressure alarm levels should be checked with valve placement because the new airflow pattern may require settings to be adjusted higher or lower. The valve can be used during pressure support, CPAP, SIMV, IMV, CMV, and all ventilator modes. Ventilator modes are described in Chapter 4 of this text. After initial placement and patient adjustment, back pressures generated by valve use may affect initial compensation settings, allowing them to be reduced.

Humidification

Humidity levels may need to be addressed as heat-moisture-exchange (HME) filter devices may be less effective when exhalation is no longer passed through the filter to provide airflow to collect moisture. A secondary humidification system such as a reservoir device may be needed (Table 7-5).

TRANSITIONING ISSUES WITH VENTILATOR DEPENDENT PATIENTS

Ventilator dependent patients who have been on a ventilator for an extended period of time sometimes react with anxiety to the initial placement of a ventilator speaking valve. It is important to have the speech-language pathologist involved with this treatment to assist in transitioning these patients to successful usage. The speech-language pathologist can help the patient become accustomed to the feeling of

1. Exhale volume alarm becomes invalid because measurement not available
2. Reduce or eliminate PEEP requirement
3. Adjust rate for work of breathing (WOB)
4. Tidal volume increase based on exhaled volume return values (as confirmed by spirometry)
5. Increase in supplemental oxygen for transition purposes
6. Recheck low pressure/disconnect settings or alarms
7. Check humidification system-Heat moisture exchanger (HME)

Table 7-5 Ventilator Adjustments and Compensation.

airflow in the oral/nasal cavities, learn to swallow, cough, blow the nose, and expectorate secretions orally.

The Passy-Muir Speaking Valve can serve as an intermediate step to facilitate weaning from the ventilator as it can improve oxygenation, patient confidence, and motivation. Frey and Wood[15] report improved oxygenation with valve use in a study of ventilator dependent patients.

PEDIATRIC VOCAL TREATMENT OPTIONS

Vocal treatment options with the tracheostomized or ventilator dependent pediatric population are extremely limited. Talking tracheostomy tubes are not available in pediatric sizes and use of electronic devices, discussed earlier, is not an effective vocal option with this population. With the exception of all but one of the speaking valves described in this chapter, data on use of these devices are not available. The only speaking valve currently being utilized with tracheostomized and ventilator dependent children is the Passy-Muir Speaking Valve.[13,16] Consequently, the following information on pediatric vocal options discusses issues surrounding use of this particular valve (Figure 7-17).

It is important to remember that tracheostomized or ventilator dependent children are much more reactionary to treatment than adult tracheostomized or ventilator dependent patients. With children, even slight changes in treatment (even treatment previously assessed and found to have a positive impact) may initially cause instant compromise. The understanding that children can "crash quickly" allows less response time than there is when in working with an adult. This means that when putting a speaking valve on a child, careful assessment of medical stability, upper airway patency, patient history, behavioral issues, motivation, and patient preparation is extremely important. The valve can be utilized with children who have complex medical problems if the therapist is properly prepared and has prepared the patient and caregivers (Figures 7-18 and 7-19).

Ideally, the speaking valve is applied within a few days of the tracheostomy so the child considers it part of the tracheostomy.

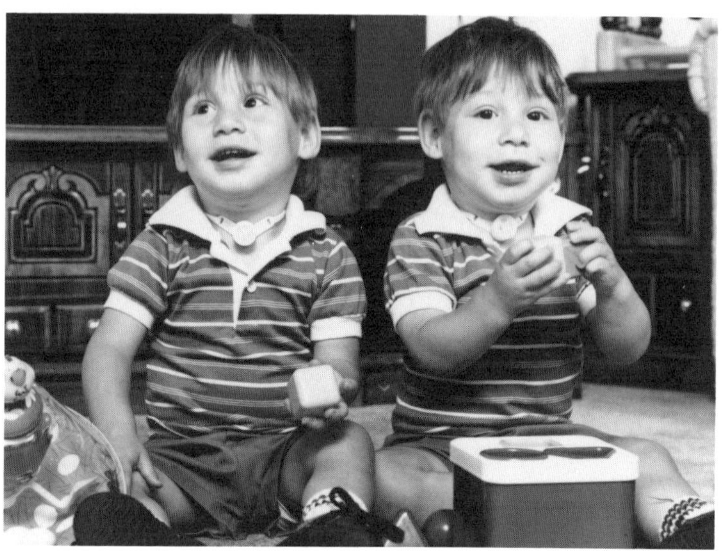

Figure 7-17 22-month-old male twins with central hypoventilation syndrome wearing speaking valves. (Courtesy of Passy-Muir, Inc., Irvine, CA.)

Children who have been tracheostomized and who did not have the speaking valve applied initially are usually very anxious and protective of their airway. Consequently, they may resist attempts made to use the speaking valve. Careful assessment prior to placing the valve is important to ensure a positive initial experience. Children, like adults may need time to become accustomed to the feeling of air flow in the upper airway.

UPPER AIRWAY OBSTRUCTION ASSESSMENT

With children, there is a higher incidence of upper airway stenosis than with adults, so it is important to first assess for upper airway patency. Many physicians will perform a bronchoscopy to evaluate upper airway patency; however, if this is not available, observing that the child can exhale and make sounds with finger occlusion of the tracheostomy tube is an alternative. Techniques for training children to exhale include blowing bubbles, using a kazoo, blowing a whistle, or even blowing a feather. Frequently, the tracheostomy tube will be too large and will need to be sized down one size to allow for improved exhalation. Children undergo bronchoscopy more often than adults and more often have tissue edema; therefore, it may be necessary to wait a few days to allow this edema to subside before using the speaking valve. If upper airway obstruction is not an issue and pulmonary compliance is sufficient, then working with the child to eliminate anxiety and overcome behavioral problems is important and may take some time. Successful transitioning techniques include play therapy and distraction methods.

Inasmuch as very young children cannot communicate discomfort, observing them while using the valve to ensure they are exhaling completely with the valve in place and not air-trapping is important. If a child is fussing or crying, one should immediately assess for the possibility of upper airway obstruction before assuming this is merely a behavioral reaction.

DEVELOPMENTAL ISSUES

Normal speech and language development is enhanced when a child can vocalize and repeat words. Many tracheostomized children who are taught sign language for communication fall behind in sound

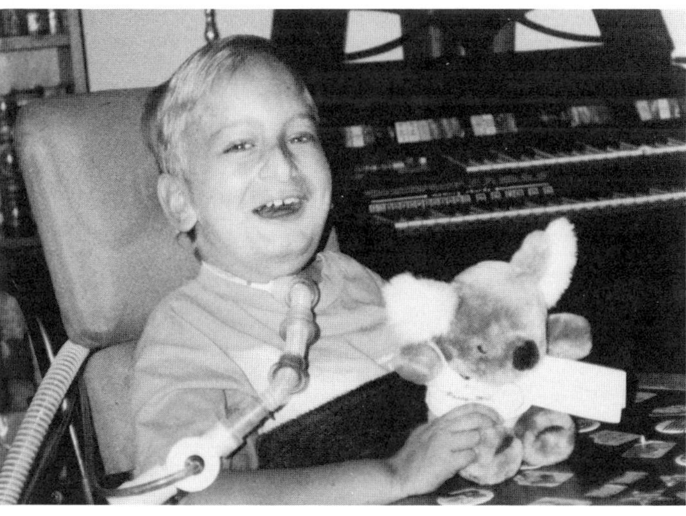

Figure 7-18 Seven-year-old child (spinal cord injury) with a Passy-Muir ventilator speaking valve in-line. (Courtesy of Passy-Muir Inc., Irvine, CA.)

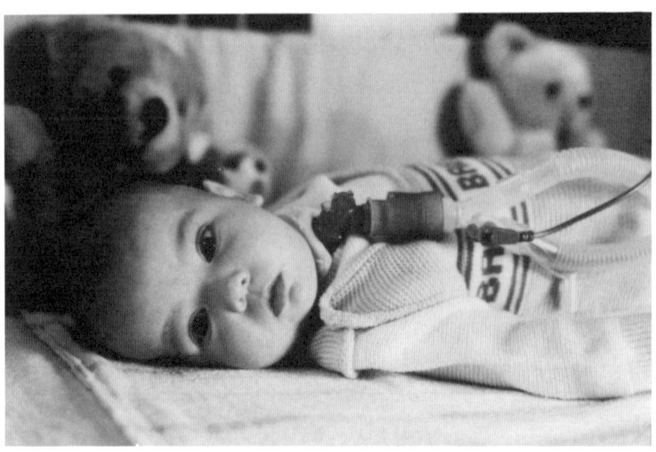

Figure 7-19 Four-month-old ventilator dependent child with central hypoventilation syndrome. Speaking valve in line. (Courtesy of Passy-Muir, Inc., Irvine, CA.)

development and in their development of expressive language. This is a devastating start for a child, especially if the tracheostomy placement is temporary. With use of the speaking valve, a child's speech and language can progress normally.

When transitioning to usage of the speaking valve, a child will often need retraining to overcome habitual chin dropping and to learn exhalation and nose blowing for the first time. Some children will develop behavioral tactics, such as coughing off the valve or taking it off, until they learn the benefits of communication.

Parents are thankful to hear their child's first cry, sound, and laughter. The speaking valve should be worn as early as tolerated to encourage the baby to babble, coo, laugh, cry, etc. As with adults, the speaking valve can facilitate a strong pressured swallow and increased pharyngeal sensation in children. In addition, children's secretions are reduced, as the airflow is evaporated naturally in the oral and nasal chambers. Tracheostomized children are susceptible to bacterial infections. The speaking valve assists in filtering and protecting the tracheal airway from particulants.

As children develop and learn to verbalize, they feel more comfortable and secure with themselves and others. With communication through use of the speaking valve, the tracheostomized child will likewise feel more comfortable interacting, playing, and integrating with other children his or her age. The child won't feel as "different" with his or her tracheostomy tube as the speaking valve provides him or her with the ability to verbalize. Using a speaking valve, tracheostomized and ventilator dependent children can be mainstreamed in school and can participate more normally with speech and singing activities while requiring less frequent suctioning.[21] Consequently, their overall self-esteem improves.

COMMUNICATION

Children begin to communicate from the moment of birth. Communication develops in five areas: pragmatics, semantics, syntax, morphology, and phonology. There are no longer "prerequisites" to communication performance. Life is communication. Communication is an innate component of every human being who interacts with his or her environment. It is also evident, from the communication research of the 1970s and 1980s, that speech and language development is interactive with and interdependent on cognitive and motoric development. When one major area of development is affected, it directly affects development in the other areas.

Several components of communication (eye gaze, social communication) are fully developed and in place by the time a child is 18 to 24 months old. The interactions that take place between caregivers and children to facilitate these processes begin at birth and some are complete by three months of age. Thus, it becomes extremely important to address communication needs via use of speaking valves or via other modes of communication (e.g., augmentative communication systems) as early as possible to avoid or decrease speech, language, and social developmental delays that may have a detrimental impact on later academic and social development.

CONCLUSION

Several vocal options for tracheostomized and ventilator dependent patients have been discussed in this chapter. Whether these patients are children or adults it is vital that their potential for achieving vocal communication (no matter how limited) be thoroughly addressed via assessment and treatment procedures. The ultimate challenge with each of these patients lies not in just establishing a functional means of communication but rather an optimal means of communication, which hopefully will be voicing.

REFERENCES

1. Bergbom-Engberg, I., and Haljamae, H., "Assessment of patients' experience of discomforts during respirator therapy." *Critical Care Medicine*, 1989; 17:1069-1072.

2. Levine, S.P., Kiester, D.J., and Ket, R.L., "Independent activated talking tracheostomy for quadriplegic patients." *Arch Phys Med Rehabil*, 1987; 68: 571-573.

3. Sparker, A.W, Robbins, K.T., Nevlud, G.N., Watkins, C.N., and Jahrsdoefer, R.A., "A prospective evaluation of speaking tracheostomy tubes for ventilator dependent patients." *Laryngoscope*, 1987; 97:89-92.

4. Siddharth, P., and Mazzarella, L., "Granuloma associated with fenestrated tracheostomy tubes." *Am J Surg*, 1985; 150:279-280.

5. Bach, John R., and Alba, A.S., "Tracheostomy ventilation: A study of efficacy with deflated cuffs and cuffless tubes." *Chest*, 1990; 97:679-683.

6. Leder, S.B., and Astrachan, D.I., "Stomal complications and airflow line problems of the Communitrach I cuffed talking tracheostomy tube." *Laryngoscope*, 1989; 99:194-196.

7. Meyers, E.N., and Stool, S.E., *Tracheostomy*, New York: Churchill Livingstone, 1985: 1-12.

8. Eggleston, G., Stanek, G.A., et al., "Utilization of Passy-Muir Tracheostomy Speaking Valve with acute CHI Patients." ASHA Annual Convention, Seattle, WA, November 16-19,1990.

9. Manzano, J.L., Lubillo, S., et al., "Verbal communication of ventilator-dependent patients." *Crit Care Med*, 1993; 21(4).

10. Mason, M., "Communication approaches for tracheostomized and ventilator dependent patients." St. Louis: ASHA, Convention Program, Scientific Exhibits, Oct. 1989; p. 203.

11. Mason, M., et al., "Protocol for use of the Passy-Muir tracheostomy speaking valves." *The European Respiratory Journal*, 1992; 5:148s.

12. Mason, M., et al., "Communication for the tracheostomized and ventilator patient utilizing the Passy-Muir valve," Presented at the California State University, Northridge, CA, March 12-14, 1992, Respiratory Nursing Society, 1992: 335.

13. Albamonte, S., and Berry, B., "Application of Passy-Muir valve with tracheostomized pediatric populations." Presented at the American Speech-Language-Hearing Association Annual Convention, Boston: November, 1988; 30(10):178.

14. Nodell, R.E., Singletary, T., et al, "Procedures for the Passy-Muir tracheostomy speaking valve." Presented at the 3rd International Conference, Respiratory Care and Speech Pathology, University of Tennessee Medical Center, 1990.

15. Frey, J.A., and Wood, S., "Weaning from mechanical ventilation augmented by the Passy-Muir speaking valve." International Conference, American Lung Association/American Thoracic Society, May 12-15, 1991.

16. Tucker, E.Z., Rogers, B., et al., "Tracheostomy speaking valve for pediatric ventilator-assisted patients." 37th Annual Convention and Exhibition, American Association for Respiratory Care, Dec. 7-10, 1991.

17. Coppola, L., and Milleori, P., "Case studies with Passy-Muir tracheostomy speaking valve." New York: Columbia-Presbyterian Medical Center, 1989.

18. Zirlen, D.M., and Haddad, L.N., "Using Passy-Muir tracheostomy speaking valves with brain injured adults." National Head Injury Foundation 8th Annual Symposium, Chicago, December 1989: 6th Annual National Traumatic Brain Injury Symposium, Maryland Institute for Emergency Medical Services Systems, 1989.

19. Scott, M., "Modified barium swallow videofluoroscopy study," 1991.

20. Light, R.W., Aten, J.L., et al., "Decannulation procedures for patients with chronic tracheostomies." Boston: Paper presented at the American College of Chest Physicians XVI World Congress on Diseases of the Chest, 1989; 96 (Suppl 2): 257.

21. Wallace, M., "60 Minutes." Wallace and Melinda Lawrence (Muscular dystrophy patient), January, 1990.

BIBLIOGRAPHY

Black, R.J., Baldwin, D.L., and Johns, A.N., "Tracheostomy, decannulation panic in children: Fact or fiction?" *The Journal of Laryngology and Otology*, 1984; 98:297-304.

Gordan, V., "Effectiveness of speaking-cuffed tracheostomy tube in patients with neuromuscular diseases." *Crit Care Medi,* 1984: 615-616.

Gordan, W.L., Dahlberg, M.A., and Montague, J.L., "Tetraplegis: Speech pathologist's role in the treatment of ventilator dependent patients." Poster Presentation at American Speech Congress and Hearing Association and American Academy and Congress of Physical Medicine, 1979.

Kluin, K.J., Maynard, F., and Bogdasarian, R.S., "The patient requiring mechanical ventilatory support: Use of the cuffed tracheostomy talk tube to establish phonation." *Otolaryngology-Head Neck Surgery,* 1984; 625-627.

Leder, S.B., "Importance of verbal communication for the ventilator dependent patient." *Chest,* 1990; 98:792-793.

Leder, S.B., "Verbal communication for the ventilator dependent patient: Voice intensity with the portex Talk Tracheostomy Tube." *Laryngoscope,* 1990; 100:1116-1120.

Leder, S.B., and Traquina, D.N., "Voice intensity of patients using a Communi-Trach I cuffed speaking tracheostomy tube." *Laryngoscope,* 1989; 99:744-746.

Lim, R.A., Salem, M.R., and Davis, G., "Airway obstruction with a fenestrated tracheostomy tube." *Anesthesiology,* 1979; 50:72-73.

Maisel, R., and Szachowicz II, E., "The Communitrach 1: Use in the vocal and non-vocal patient." Presented at the Fifth Asia-Oceania Congress of Otorhinolaryngological Societies, Seoul, Korea, October 9-14, 1983.

McReynolds, L., and Kearns K., *Single-Subject Experimental Designs in Communicative Disorders,* Baltimore: University Park Press, 1983.

Parker H., "Communication breakdown: Personal experience of being on ventilation." *News Mirror*, 1984; 158:37-39.

Szachowicz II, E., Walsh, J., and Maisel, R., "A modified tracheostomy tube which allows normal laryngeal speech while patient is on a ventilator." *American College of Surgeons 1983 Surgical Forum Vol. XXXIV.*

Wnek-Schiavoni, M., "Vocalization development using the Passy-Muir Speaking Valve." Paper presented at Language-Hearing Association, 1990.

CHAPTER VIII

PEDIATRICS

Stefanie Albamonte, *M.S., C.C.C.-SLP*
Clinical Coordinator of Speech and Hearing
Children's Specialized Hospital
Mountainside, New Jersey

Angela M. Jerome, *R.N., M.S.N.*
Pediatric Pulmonary Nurse Specialist
Children's Home Health
Pediatric Clinical Nurse Specialist
Adjunct Clinical Instructor
Old Dominion University
Norfolk, Virginia

Edited by:

Varada Diwadkar, *M.D.*
Private Practice
Pediatric Pulmonology
Scottish Rite Children's Medical Center
Kennestone Hospital
Atlanta, Georgia

Allan B. Seid, *M.D., F.A.C.S., F.A.A.P.*
Attending Pediatric Otolaryngologist
Children's Hospital and Health Center
Associate Clinical Professor
Otolaryngology, Head and Neck Surgery
University of California, San Diego
San Diego, California

INTRODUCTION

The past decade has dramatically improved the survival rate of infants and young children who suffer from prematurity, congenital anomalies, respiratory disease, and trauma. With this high survival rate, more children are requiring tracheostomies and/or mechanical ventilation. This has long-term effects on both the family and the developmental outcome of the child. The most devastating side effect of a tracheostomy is the limited ability to develop verbal communication.

ANATOMICAL DIFFERENCES BETWEEN CHILDREN AND ADULTS

Children are often thought of as small adults. This is unfortunate because it is not true. Although anatomically the structures are all the same, the positioning and the size of the structures in children are completely different from those in adults. To the untrained eye, the differences do not seem obvious. However, when reviewing a child's anatomy, the small size is a challenge to professionals working in pediatrics. With the respiratory tract, one must take into consideration the size and underdeveloped system of the small infant. Not only is the size of the child smaller, but the angles at which the structures are situated are different. The child's hyoid and cricoid cartilages larynx are higher and more anterior than the adult's. The child's larynx is one-third the size of an adult's larynx, with the adult larynx being 2 cm in breadth. With growth, the infant's larynx will descend. The hyoid bone in the infant is also higher and closer to the larynx, which creates a close approximation of the tongue and the larynx.

INDICATIONS FOR TRACHEOSTOMY

The reasons for a tracheostomy can be divided into six areas: (1) to relieve obstruction at or above the level of the tracheostomy, (2) to support mechanical ventilation for an extended period of time, (3) to decrease the potential for tracheal damage due to intubation in older

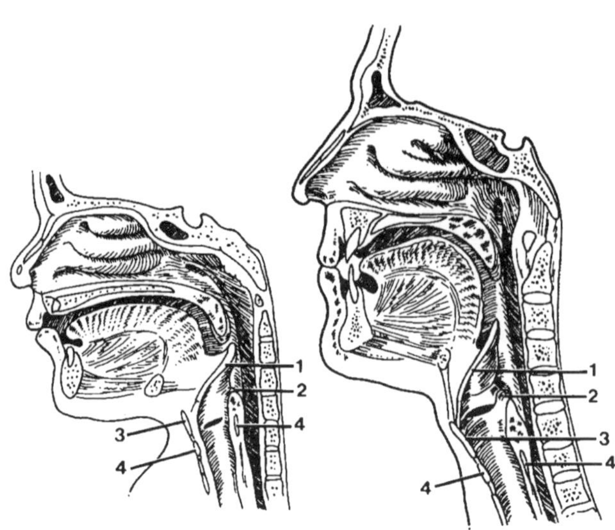

Figure 8-1 Anatomy of the larynx in an infant and an adult. Specific landmarks: ***1****, epiglottis;* ***2****, arytenoid cartilages;* ***3****, thyroid cartilage;* ***4****, cricoid cartilage. The infant larynx is situated relatively high in the cervical region. Additionally, the base of the infant's tongue is close to the larynx, and the epiglottis is located near the palate. These anatomic differences partially explain the obligate nose breathing of the young infant, as well as the relative ease with which infants develop upper airway obstructions. (From Chernick, M.D., and Kendig, E.L., Jr.,* Disorders of the Respiratory Tract in Children, *Philadelphia: W.B. Saunders Co., 5th Ed.,1990; Fig. 16-1 p. 337.)*

children, (4) to remove secretions directly when the cough mechanism is impaired, (5) to provide an airway when direct trauma of the trachea has occurred, and (6) to provide an airway during and after extensive craniofacial surgery. Approximately 85% of children requiring a tracheostomy are less than 1 year of age.

Many disorders that require a tracheostomy and/or mechanical ventilation (See Table 8-1). The length of time the tracheostomy is needed is based upon progress, if any, in the child's underlying medical condition. The amount of air that flows around the tracheostomy past functional vocal cords ("leak"), along with the child's cognitive abilities and oral-motor skills, predicts the potential for vocalization.

This affects the normal function of the airway. With the close approximation of the larynx and the epiglottis, the infant is an obligate

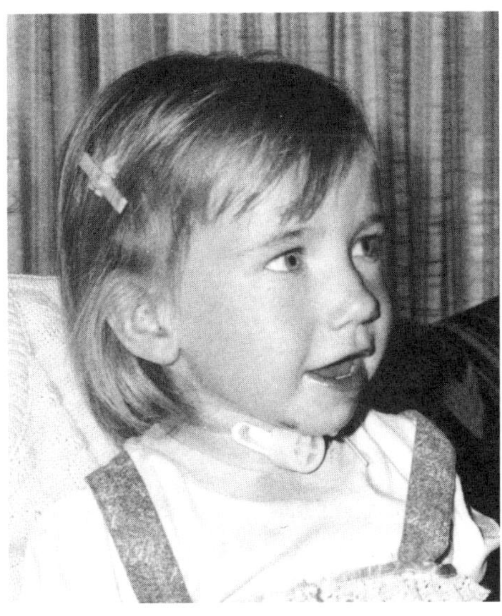

Figure 8-2 Two-year-old girl with central hypoventilaton syndrome.

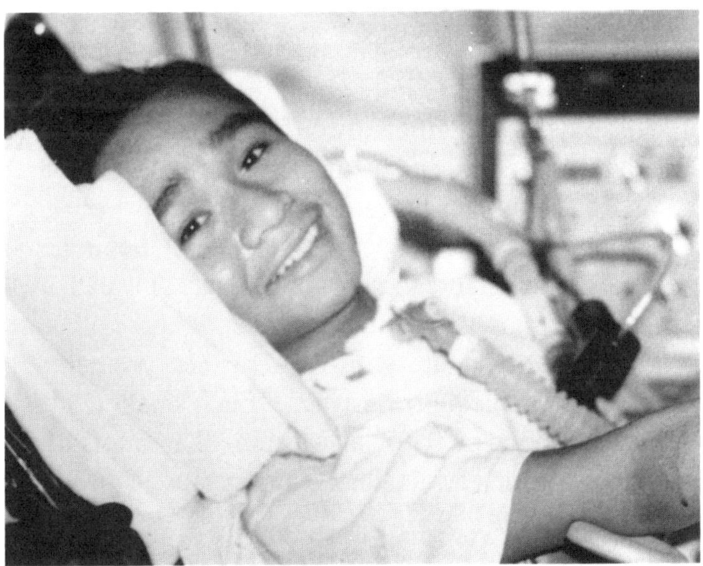

Figure 8-3 16-year-old male quadriplegic with traumatic spinal cord injury.

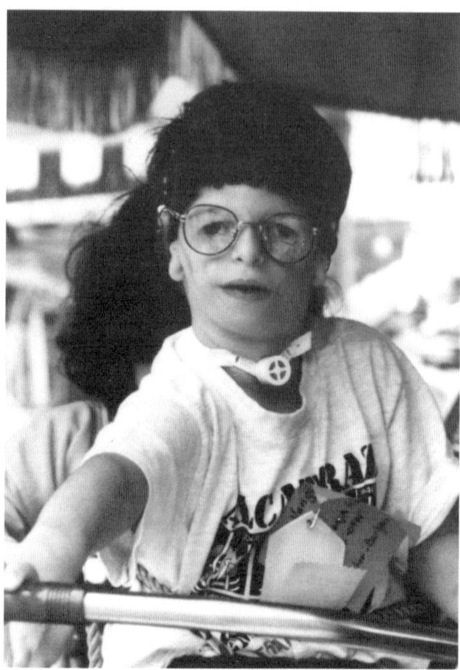

Figure 8-4 Five-year-old boy with Treacher Collins syndrome.

nose breather for the first several months of life. The closeness of the anatomical structures makes intubation difficult.

Lung tissue is also significantly different in the premature infant. Surfactant, a substance created by the body during gestation, is often lacking. Without this substance, the lung tissue does not easily expand. The lungs themselves may be pliable, but the tissues such as the alveoli stick together, creating a rubbing effect instead of expanding. This causes poor oxygenation and poor air exchange, thus causing some of the respiratory distress episodes premature infants often experience. The pediatric airway is much smaller compared to the adult airway. In the pediatric airway, small amounts of swelling largely decrease the airway diameter and can cause significant respiratory distress.

Another important aspect of pediatric anatomy is that not all bone tissue is fully calcified. The bones and cartilages are soft and pliable. With the closeness of the ribs and shoulder girdle, infants have a tendency to hold their shoulders in elevation in order to hold the weight of their head upright. Continual holding of the shoulders in an elevated position will cause tightening of the shoulder girdle musculature, creating hyperextension of the neck and head. This positioning in turn causes abnormal muscle tone and movement patterns. Due to respiratory distress, infants and children have a tendency to hyperextend the head and neck in order to enhance breathing. Since the pediatric rib cage is also cartilaginous, this may actually work against getting air into the lungs during respiratory distress. The energy needed in respiratory distress is so high so that pediatric patients fatigue easily.

IMPACT OF A TRACHEOSTOMY ON NORMAL DEVELOPMENT

Many people do not realize that a tracheostomy not only inhibits the ability to speak, but also affects the overall well-being of a child. Making the decision whether a child needs a tracheostomy is not easy for the parents. At the time the decision is made, the full side effects are not always understood no matter what the age of the infant, child, or adolescent. It is only afterward that reality sets in and the scope of changes becomes apparent.

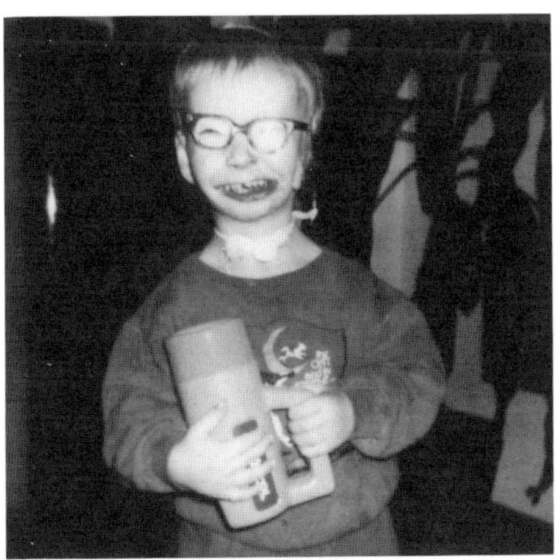

Figure 8-5 Four-year-old boy with Goldenhar syndrome.

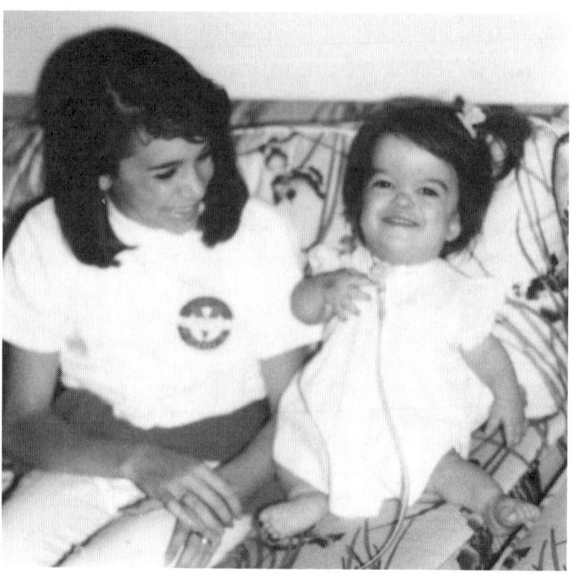

Figure 8-6 Two-year-old girl with achondroplasia dwarfism.

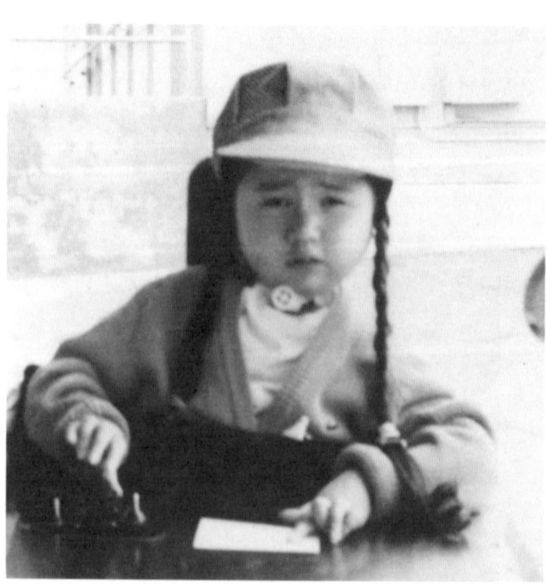

Figure 8-7 Five-year-old girl with spinal muscular atrophy (Werdnig Hoffman disease.)

Table 8-1 Pulmonary Related Disorders

DISORDER	ETIOLOGY	ILLNESS / DEVELOPMENTAL TRAJECTORY
Tracheal stenosis	Congenital or acquired fixed stricture of the trachea associated with long-term intubation, longer than 2 months in neonates and greater than 3 weeks in children.	Stenosis prevents airflow past the vocal cords. Vocalization is poor. Cognition is intact. When appropriate, laryngotracheoplasty can be performed. This surgery involves splitting the cricoid cartilage surgically and stenting open the area with a bone graft. The diameter of the trachea is increased with the goal of decannulation.
Granulation tissue	Excess tissue growth that causes narrowing of the trachea related to intubation infection and irritation to the trachea.	Granulation tissue prevents airflow past the vocal cords. Vocalization can be poor. Granulation tissue can be removed by surgery or by laser. When the airway is "clean", decannulation is possible.
Tracheomalacia	Congenital or acquired floppiness or weakening of the trachea. During exhalation, the trachea collapses instead of staying open.	A tracheostomy tube is required to stent open the weakened area. Continuous Positive Airway Pressure (CPAP) may be used to stent open the area with air pressure. As the child grows, the cartilage in tracheal rings stiffens and airway size increases, allowing for decannulation. Speaking valve may also stent airway pressures.

Table 8-1 Pulmonary Related Disorders - Continued

DISORDER	ETIOLOGY	ILLNESS / DEVELOPMENTAL TRAJECTORY
Bilateral vocal cord paralysis (adducted)	Associated with central nervous system damage and/or nerve dysfunction.	Airway obstruction prevents airflow through the vocal cords. Vocal cord functions may improve over time. Can cause airflow obstruction, making tracheostomy necessary or extended.
Pierre-Robin Apert's syndrome, Crouzon's syndrome, Treacher-Collins syndrome	Congenital syndromes associated with small mandibles and airway obstruction.	Small oral cavity prevents airflow around vocal cords; If an adequate oral/nasal airway can be created either via growth or if appropriate surgeries can be performed to mandible and other structures, decannulation is possible.
Subglottic hemangioma	Congenital ballooning and weakening of blood vessels in the subglottic area. The child has stridor and variable airway obstruction.	Vocalization varies based upon the size of the hemangioma. When appropriate, laser surgery can be performed to "scar" the area. When surgeries are complete, decannulation is possible.

DISORDER	ETIOLOGY	ILLNESS / DEVELOPMENTAL TRAJECTORY
Bronchopulmonary dysplasia	Chronic lung disease frequently associated with prematurity. Lung tissue is damaged due to required mechanical ventilation necessary to maintain adequate amounts of oxygen and carbon dioxide in the blood.	Vocalization is dependent upon the amount of tracheostomy "leak". In sicker children requiring higher ventilator pressures, it may be necessary to use a large, "tight" tracheostomy tube. Cognitive skills vary based upon history of intracranial bleeds, hypoxia, and duration of hospitalization. As the child grows, new lung tissue will replace damaged tissue. The child may then wean off the ventilator and be decannulated.
Werdnig-Hoffmann disease	Degenerative genetic neuromuscular disease. Muscles are unable to support breathing.	Vocalization depends on the status of oral-motor muscles. Deterioration of most muscle function occurs within 1 year. Mechanical ventilation and tracheostomy, if chosen, are permanent. Cognitive ability is felt to remain intact. Lifespan, if ventilated, may exceed 5 years.
Congenital central hypoventiation syndrome	Congenital dysfunction of the central nervous system's (CNS) mechanism to stimulate breathing during sleep. Requires ventilation during sleep because spontaneous breathing does not occur.	Vocalization can be good. Cognitive functions are intact. The need for mechanical ventilation is lifelong, although necessary only during sleep.

Table 8-1 Pulmonary Related Disorders - Continued

DISORDER	ETIOLOGY	ILLNESS / DEVELOPMENTAL TRAJECTORY
Bronchomalacia	Congenital or acquired floppiness or weakening of the bronchi.	Vocalization is possible if tracheostomy "leak" is present. Cognitive abilities may be intact. Episodes of respiratory distress and fatigue may occur with therapies. As the child grows, bronchomalacia may become less significant. Weaning from the ventilator is especially slow. When completed, decannulation is possible.
Arnold Chiari II Malformation (along with Spina Bifida)	Congenital malformation of the medulla which can affect nearby cranial nerves. Breathing is disorganized. Tracheostomy and/or ventilation may be required.	Vocalization is possible if vocal cords are functional and tracheostomy "leak" is present. Cognitive delays may or may not be present, but are consistent with spina bifida. Decannulation may be possible as child grows older.
Myotubular myopathy	Genetic muscle disease affecting muscle metabolism. Muscles may not support independent breathing.	Vocalization is fair to poor as oral-motor skills are poor. The child may make some sound, especially at the end of inspiration on the ventilator breath. Ventilation and tracheostomy are permanent. The lifespan is unknown, but seems to be less than 5 years. Overall body movements are slow and weak. Cognitive function intact.

DISORDER	ETIOLOGY	ILLNESS / DEVELOPMENTAL TRAJECTORY
Myasthenia gravis	Congenital disorder affecting the neurotransmitters between nerves and muscles. Severe muscle weakness is seen which is unable to support independent breathing.	Vocal cord function may be affected. Oral-motor weakness is present. Tracheostomy and ventilation may be lifelong. Cognitive function may be intact unless a hypoxic episode has occurred.
Diaphragmatic hernia	Congenital hole in the diaphragm requiring surgery at birth to correct. Lung disease may be present after surgery is complete.	Vocalization is possible if a tracheostomy "leak" is present. As the child grows, new lung tissue replaces damaged lung tissue so that the child may wean off the ventilator. Decannulation is possible.
Cervical level spinal cord injury	Injury severing spinal cord. Can affect respiratory status requires use of ventilator.	Quality of vocalization varies. Can be poor if respiratory muscles are weak. If on ventilator, quality of vocalization can be good.

Table 8-1 Pulmonary Related Disorders - Continued

DISORDER	ETIOLOGY	ILLNESS / DEVELOPMENTAL TRAJECTORY
Duchenne's muscular dystrophy	Genetic disorder characterized by progressive muscle weakness. A poor cough may lead to mechanical ventilation.	Vocalization is possible but the voice may be weak. Tracheostomy may be permanent in order to suction secretions from airway.
Head injury	Trauma to CNS "protective" centers causes impairment. A tracheostomy may be needed to remove secretions if the cough and swallow are impaired.	Vocalization is structurally possible but may not occur due to oral-motor and/or cognitive deficits. Tracheostomy may or may not be permanent, depending on how intact the cough and swallow mechanisms are.
Cerebral palsy	Perinatal damage to the CNS motor/cognitive centers. Cough/ swallow may be disorganized.	Vocalization is structurally possible but may not occur due to oral-motor and/or cognitive deficits. Tracheostomy may or may not be permanent, depending on how intact the cough and swallow mechanisms are.

DISORDER	ETIOLOGY	ILLNESS / DEVELOPMENTAL TRAJECTORY
Various craniofacial reconstructive surgeries in the post-op period	Congenital or acquired. A tracheostomy may be required after major facial bone and tissue reconstruction.	After healing of final major craniofacial surgery, the child may be decannulated; Vocalization is possible when swelling in oral structures has decreased.
Direct trauma to trachea or oral structures or oral structures preventing oral/nasal intubation	Accidental injury to trachea (example: child riding bike into wire line; dog bite, motor vehicle accident)	After injuries have healed and if airway is open (per laryngoscopy or bronchoscopy), decannulation is possible. Vocalization is based on the stage of healing, swelling, scar tissue, and/or structural damage.

DEVELOPMENTAL DELAYS

Critical Period

When an infant is tracheostomized, the audible cry is no longer available as a form of communication. The caregiver must rely solely on facial expression, body language, and knowledge of the infant's needs. The critical period for developing language is between birth and 5 years of age. Up to about 12 months of age, infants explore their voice and, at the same time, develop and refine oral movements that will emerge into intelligible speech. Without this early exploration, language development is delayed. These children often develop a unique gesture system even before they are formally taught sign language. For most families, this is heartbreaking. Their child may be several years old before they even hear a cry or laugh. During the first 2 years of life, children develop a core vocabulary using one-and two-word sentences to express themselves. Without this experience or ability, children must rely on the patience and attentiveness of the caregiver in discerning their needs and desires. This can become frustrating and may often make a child feel defeated in his or her limited ability to communicate. As a result, the child may become withdrawn or difficult to handle behaviorally. These children are able to learn receptive language from their environment; however, their expressive impact is limited. This hinders the emergence of cause and effect relationships.

Environment

Medical stability in the young infant and toddler also plays a large roll in developmental outcome. A child who has spent the first several months of life, or even a year, in a hospital setting has started off in a limited environment. Stimulation from caregivers can be noxious (needles, tracheostomy tube changes, suctioning, etc.). These experiences, although necessary, do not promote healthy communication. Instead, children may develop avoidance and mistrust. This type of environment does not promote the normal cognitive development that is a major precursor to expressive and receptive language development. Not having typical infant toys to play with and normal parent/child interactions also hinders development.

Motor Development

The advanced life support systems to which these children are attached do not allow them to move about freely. Therefore they do not fully develop age-appropriate gross motor skills. With the limited movement patterns of these children, they do not develop independent play skills or explore the environment like healthy infants. Children with respiratory compromise often do not lay prone (on their stomach) as it puts more pressure on the chest and does not allow for full expansion with breathing. It also increases the potential of accidental decannulation of the tracheostomy tube. The prone position is very important for the development of the balance between the extensor and flexor muscles of the trunk and neck and of the accessory muscles needed for breathing. Without the proper development of these muscle groups, gross motor skills will be significantly compromised, hindering higher level motor activities such as sitting independently, standing, and walking. The development of fine motor skills will also be hindered without the appropriate gross motor background upon which to build. The medically compromised infant is usually placed supine with the head turned either to the right or left and possibly hyperextended. This position feeds into the child's natural instinct to hyperextend the neck in order to compensate for respiratory difficulty. With this position, an elevated shoulder girdle and tightened sternocleidomastoid, clavicular, trapezoid, and pectoral muscles, the upper extremities do not have a solid base of support from which to move. This creates tightness in the shoulders and poor bilateral hand movement. Also, with the limited amount of time these children spend in the prone position, the weight bearing on the hands that a child needs to develop the arches within the palm of the hand is significantly lacking. Without this, grasp patterns and the ability to hold and release an object will be limited and awkward.

One may initially feel a tracheostomy to have an impact only on speech and language skills; however, all developmental skills rely on each other. Due to the size and position of the pediatric anatomy, a tracheostomy tube can be uncomfortable during movement of the larynx, oral structures, and accessory neck muscles. With any form of intubation or tracheostomy, neck and head movement is restricted, thereby limiting the child's development of full range of motion in the neck. The ability to develop a chin tuck or flex the neck is limited. Normal infants will randomly move their arms and legs as well as reach toward objects within their sight. Medically unstable children may not do this due to their overall weakness, underdeveloped central nervous system, and perhaps their inability to move freely due to the equipment necessary to assist with their breathing, intravenous lines, monitor cables, pulse oximetry, and feeding tubes. Abnormal positioning and movement patterns also limit exploration. The area in which these children can move is very limited.

Prelinguistic Development

Taking a closer look at the early stages of development, prelinguistic skills are the most critical aspect of language development. These skills begin developing at birth. It is during the first few months of life that a child uses voice to get attention in his or her environment and exercises the coordination of the oral structures for speech. An infant who has a tracheostomy and was nasally or orally intubated has suffered setbacks. These children are found to do less oral exploration such as tongue clicks, raspberries, lip smacking, and overall oral movements. Another area in which these children often show delay is in the development of cognitive skills. Medically fragile preterm infants do not have the ability to explore their environment. Sensory stimulation from caregivers is also limited and often noxious. Tactile stimulation during the early months of life is very critical to the total development of sensory integration. Infants who do not learn to process tactile information become defensive to textured, soft, wet, or mixed surfaces. These idiosyncrasies have a large impact on later development of feeding as well as further exploration of play experiences from which language and cognition evolve. Typically, early forms of play center around children putting toys in their mouth. However, tactile defensiveness, especially around the face, causes children to be hypersensitive and fearful of this kind of play exploration.

Feeding Skills

Oral defensiveness has significant impact on the development of feeding skills. The largest hurdle for children to overcome is that of allowing something near their face and inside their mouth. Transitioning a child who has been tube fed for an extended period of time to oral feeding is often challenging for the therapist as well as for the child. In many instances these children must learn how to coordinate a suck-swallow breath pattern..

Several methods of therapeutic techniques can be utilized to enhance sensory processing. For the infant, one method used is that of deep massage with lotion or a towel. The deep pressure into proximal muscle groups slowly working toward the face with a more gentle yet deep massage increases the sensory receptors of the skin and muscles. Another method of breaking down sensory defensiveness is through a brushing program. This program, however, is best used with children ages 2 years and older and should be supervised by an occupational therapist trained in sensory integration. There are several other techniques that can be used effectively. Once this is achieved, other feeding skills can be addressed. Many children do not make the transition to taking solid foods at a normal age and often take longer to tolerate regular table food. The mucosal tissues of the mouth are very sensitive on a normal child and it takes longer to break through the defensiveness of a child who has an underdeveloped central nervous system. Tactile and oral defensiveness not only affects feeding skills but also the overall environmental exploration of a child. Without touching and placing objects in the mouth, children do not explore their features and feel different textures. These experiences are important for the integration of sensory information. If a child does not touch toys or explore the texture of the rug or stuffed animal, a continued interest to play and interact with these objects will be limited. When there is a decreased interest in interaction, interest in labeling the object not played with is also limited. This in turn hinders vocabulary and communication.

Verbal Language Development

Infant to Toddler

The most obvious effect a tracheostomy has on an infant and toddler is to cause the inability to develop normal verbal language. While the normal child is cooing and babbling by several months of age, the child with a tracheostomy may still only communicate with facial expressions. As mentioned earlier, environmental exploration is also limited, whether due to medical instability, limited free movement and space, or environmental deprivation. Without these experiences, the cognitive basis for language cannot develop adequately. Receptive language skills will be directly affected by the child's cognitive skills. Unfortunately, expressive output is also directly dependent on the physical ability to coordinate oral movements and voice production. A child with a tracheostomy may be unable to vocalize. Expressive output, regardless of how intelligent a child is, will be delayed. Between 12 months and 2 years of age, children develop critical words in order to communicate effectively. Having a tracheostomy eliminates the ability to explore sound production and word approximations that will emerge into true words. Those children who are tracheostomized and have grown enough for air to flow freely upward around the tracheostomy tube cannula may develop limited verbal language. Producing speech around a tracheostomy tube is limited to one or two breathy sounding syllables. Phrases developed by a normal toddler will consist of basically one or two short words that will most easily make their verbal intent effective. A child with a tracheostomy may possibly be able to use only parts of words which in turn would make up a two-syllable utterance. When verbal communication is significantly limited, children automatically rely on gestures. Very often it is their own form of sign language. This is limiting to a child. The only people who may easily understand the child are immediate family or caregivers. The inability to be understood is frustrating for the child, as well, as the family. Parents long to hear the voice of their child. When that voice is significantly distorted and often difficult to understand or completely absent, it can be emotionally devastating for parents. Effective communication and intact cognitive skills are a key factor in overall development and well-being.

Two to Six Years of Age

A child who has had a tracheostomy since birth and is between 2 and 6 years of age is at risk to have severe expressive language delay. Children tracheostomized at the age of 2 years have already started to develop the use of morphological markers and a variety of syntactic forms. The basis for adult grammar is at a critical point in development. Once a child is tracheostomized, vocalization is compromised. Although cognitively and receptively the child may be normal, expressive language is affected until the child is decannulated or a one-way speaking valve is utilized therapeutically for vocal restoration. If for medical or psychological reasons this is not possible, the continued development of syntax and morphology may be arrested at its present state until the voice can be restored. This in itself will cause a language disorder. Once the voice is restored, intensive therapy will be needed to enhance language development. Expressive language without adequate phonation will be dependent upon gestures, an augmentative communication system, or sign language. Those children who are unable to use a one-way valve but have the ability to voice minimally around their tracheostomy tube will develop language that consists of only one or two words. Syntax will develop normally, as far as agent and action, and object and action structure. Expansion of syntactic forms is limited. If a one-way speaking valve is able to be used to provide exhalation support for voicing, then language will develop normally. This, however, is dependent upon the age at which the child is able to tolerate using a speaking valve. The more delayed language is, the more expressively delayed the child will be.

Development of phonology is not as dependent on the early exploration of the oral structures and sound play. Studies indicate that no distinctive patterns of phonological processes dominate the speech pattern. Also noted is that articulation pattern is within 6 months of the normal control group. Kamen and Watson[1] report that the most frequently noted substitutions are stops and fricatives, with velar sounds, and stops substituted for fricatives and affricates. Research in the area of the effects of tracheostomies on the development of articulation is limited. Clinical experience has demonstrated that once children are decannulated or able to use a speaking valve, the development of articulation progresses quickly if neuromotor components are not hindering the process. Children have a tendency to progress quickly from babbling to true words within 1 to 2 months, balancing their expressive language with their receptive and cognitive skills.

Social Development

These are also critical years for social development. Children who are unable to communicate are less likely to make friends. Also these children are less frequently around other children due to medical complications or general precautions to avoid getting many of the childhood illnesses. Here, too, environmental exposure is very important to the total well-being of a person. As children get older, they begin to realize that they are different, that they have fewer friends, and that they are unable to do all the things other children their age do. This is especially true for the children who are tracheostomized after the age of critical language development. They had the full ability to speak and suddenly, possibly following an accident or as a result of an illness, are tracheostomized and no longer able to communicate easily. The biggest side effect at this stage concerns the psychological aspect of the child. Children often become withdrawn and begin to hate what life has done to them. The control they once had on their environment is no longer possible. They now rely on others to anticipate their needs and desires. In case the child is an adolescent going through the growth period of independence, much of what he or she dreamed of is taken away. Fortunately, all structures of language have developed by the age of 10 and the only growth is in vocabulary. When the child is decannulated, language skills should be assessed to determine if continued therapy is warranted. If the child is still in the early years of development (2 to 9 years), therapy following decannulation may still be warranted, depending on the length of cannulation.

MECHANICAL VENTILATION

Endotracheal Intubation

There are two types of endotracheal intubation, nasal and oral. One of these two methods will be used for immediate opening of the airway in the event of an emergency situation that causes respiratory difficulty. The method of intubation depends on the physician and/or respiratory therapist performing the intubation. The most common method in infants is oral intubation, due to the ease of intubation and the need for prolonged ventilator dependency. Nasal intubation may be limited because of tube sizes and the anatomical size of the neonate. The use of nasal intubation for premature infants is usually up to the discretion of the attending neonatologist. It is, however, most likely that a premature infant will be nasally intubated after a period of time due to the ease of accidental decannulation with oral tubes. As infants try to move, they pull on the tube, which is easily dislodged. This can cause added trauma to the laryngeal area as well as anoxic episodes if the child is unable to breathe on his or her own.[2] Both nasal and oral tubes are difficult to secure and the child's head position must be kept very steady in order to avoid dislodging the tube or causing anatomical damage to the tracheal and laryngeal area.

An infant who is intubated, regardless of which method is used, may be too weak to move about and may have too many tubes, wires, and equipment attached to permit exploration of his or her environment. Many intubated infants were born prematurely and have not developed the physiological flexion of a full-term infant. With the lack of initial flexion and the extensive amount of supine positioning, gross motor skills become significantly delayed.

Oral Stimulation of the Intubated Child

Oral feeding in a child who is nasally intubated is unlikely to occur because of medical instability. The positive aspect of nasal intubation is that oral stimulation can take place during tube feeding by having the child suck on a pacifier or providing other forms of oral stimulation. Oral intubation does not allow for those experiences. In either case, a majority of these children develop oral defensiveness. Their suck pattern becomes weak and often poorly coordinated due to lack of experience.

For most adults eating is an enjoyable and effortless task. This is not so for the medically unstable child. In fact, eating often uses up more calories than the child receives in one meal. This is due to the fact that such compromised children are expending an extreme amount of energy coordinating breathing, swallowing, and coordinating movement of the oral structures. These children are often diagnosed with failure to thrive because their growth patterns are below normal. Alternative modes of nutrition are used to provide these children with an adequate caloric intake while using the least amount of energy. The most common methods are hyperalimentation, and nasogastric tube and gastrostomy tube feeding. Although these patients are not on oral feedings, it is important that they have the proper oral stimulation needed during feedings to enhance the sucking pattern and coordination of swallowing and respiratory control.

Looking at the oral structures and sucking patterns of children who were intubated for prolonged periods of time reveals interesting variations. The palate is high and narrow and the tongue is often flat. The cupping the tongue makes around a nipple is no longer adequate to form the negative pressure needed to draw liquid from a nipple. There is also inadequate lip closure around a nipple. Poor lip closure combined with poor lingual cupping causes feeding to be difficult and often ineffective for nutritional purposes. Feeding is less stressful for those who are able to coordinate breathing and eating. The most concerning side effect of a tracheostomy is the loss of internal pressure that is built up above and below a bolus of food when swallowing. Due to the open airway created by the tracheostomy, all air leaks through the tracheostomy, eliminating any positive internal pressure. Without this normal pressure, the risk of aspiration is higher. This is true whether a child is on mechanical ventilation or not. A positive aspect of a tracheostomy is the ability to easily suction immediately following feeding (sucking and swallowing) attempts.[3]

For the young infant who has never been fed by mouth, therapy will focus on establishing an adequate suck, cupping of the tongue, and building up tolerance for bolus oral feedings. A magical method for facilitating oral feedings with the medically fragile child has not yet been discovered. The placement of a tracheostomy inhibits the laryngeal muscles upon swallowing. A variety of oral stimulation programs may be applied. Working through the oral defensiveness a child may have is one of the most important factors to be addressed initially. The existence of a neuromotor disorder (apraxia) can be another equally limiting factor to overcome. Apraxia hinders overall coordination of the oral structures and is most commonly noted in the pediatric head trauma patient and the very premature infant who has suffered from interventricular hemorrhage or has an underdeveloped central nervous system. For some patients, this problem may be easily worked through with therapy and reinforcement provided from the nursing staff and family. The less neurologically impaired head trauma patients and the less impaired premature infants have the least amount of difficulty in transitioning from alternative methods of feeding to oral feeding.

Physical Barriers

Seeing their child with tubes protruding from his or her nose or mouth is a frightening experience for a family. Many parents are afraid to touch their child for fear of disconnecting the tubes that are keeping their child alive. When a child is intubated, the head and neck must be kept in a neutral position, which also makes parent interaction difficult. With the premature infant, many parents avoid getting emotionally involved fearing that their child may not live and that the emotional pain of death may be too great for them. This limited involvement has poor effects on even the smallest of infants. A child intubated either nasally or orally will not be free to move about the environment, nor will he or she be able to vocalize. Verbal language development is arrested until extubation occurs. Mechanical ventilation via either of these two modes is used in the most critical period of an illness. Speech and language development, although at a critical point in development, is not the most important aspect of the child's physical well-being. Speech therapy during intubation at this critical period need not focus on communication but rather on environmental awareness and sensory processing, which is equally as important for future development. With warmth, nurturing, and love, even a child of the smallest size will be given the internal drive to survive.

Complications of Intubation

At the time of intubation, the immediate need for the survival of the child is to maintain an adequate airway. In addition to the psychological effects intubation has on a family and on a child who understands what is happening, the possible side effects can be far-reaching. During emergency intubation, some amount of vocal cord damage can occur. This damage is not always noted until after extubation. The most obvious sign of vocal cord damage is a hoarse voice. Most patients who are intubated will experience a hoarse vocal quality until the laryngeal area completely heals. In some cases long-term intubation may cause laryngomalacia which may result in a long-term tracheostomy. When damage has occurred, the vocal quality may remain poor. In some instances, vocal cord paralysis results, which can be more damaging than vocal nodules or vocal polyps. The latter two vocal lesions are more easily treated with medical procedures and speech therapy. The focus of therapy will be on proper use of the voice and ways to avoid further vocal strain. Methods of communication should also be addressed. These side effects are uncommon and can be avoided with careful intubation procedures. Prolonged intubation can often cause laryngeal stenosis, tracheomalacia, and a buildup of granulation tissue. Granulation tissue can be surgically removed by laser. There are instances when the scar tissue grows back. Very often, the scarring will prevent the use of a speaking valve due to the limited space for airflow around the tracheostomy tube. Laryngeal stenosis, although often a reason for intubation, can be caused by the constant irritation of the tracheostomy tube in the laryngeal area and related swelling. Tracheomalacia, a softening of the tracheal wall, cannot be surgically repaired. It can be improved with the use of a speaking valves due to the added pressure of air flowing up the tracheal area, forcing the collapsed area to open. The success the valve will have in opening and strengthening the trachea will depend on the severity of the malacia.

Referral to the Speech-Language Pathologist

When a speech-language pathologist should be called in to treat patients who are intubated or recently extubated is often questioned. An important fact to remember is that any child who has been intubated for any reason may be having difficulty swallowing and/or vocalizing. Those children who are critically ill need not receive intensive therapy, as they may be too medically unstable to warrant the added stress. However, therapy to facilitate the processing of environmental stimulation and to enhance normal physical and mental development should not be discounted. Following extubation, many patients are expected to start oral feedings in order to prepare for discharge from the hospital. With the premature infant, this is not always an easy task. The child now needs to coordinate breathing, environmental exploration, sucking, and swallowing. As mentioned earlier, these children often need to learn how to adequately suck and swallow. The length of time it takes to acquire these skills and master them to a functional level for nutritional purposes is dependent on each individual child's response to therapy.

Tracheostomy Placement

A long-term tracheostomy tube is placed when intubation is required for an extended period of time, usually over 1 to 2 months. Many children remain intubated orally or nasally even longer because of medical instability and the possibility of extubation. Once medical parameters, such as cardiac and respiratory status and body temperature, are stable, a permanent tracheostomy tube will be surgically inserted.[2] In many cases of long-term tracheostomy and mechanical ventilation, weaning will not be attempted until the patient is medically stable and able to adequately maintain adequate oxygenation saturation, hemoglobin, and cardiac output. In many instances long-term ventilation is several months in duration. Once a tracheostomy is placed and the child is medically stable, therapeutic intervention may begin. It is often the speech-language pathologist who is responsible for restoring feeding skills and language skills and for enhancing cognitive skills.

Developmental Complications Secondary to Mechanical Ventilation

Prolonged mechanical ventilation has significant negative side effects on motor development. Not only is the child restricted in movement within his or her surroundings, but the quality of motor movement is also greatly affected. With constant mechanical expansion of the chest, and limited development of the intercostals, shoulder girdle, and accessory neck and respiratory muscles, the rib cage does not descend as it would in normal physical development. This results in a high barrel-chest appearance. With this type of physical stature, a child has limited trunk rotation and mobility. This affects the foundation for gross motor movement. The weakness in the muscles of the upper body also effect the muscles that support the movement of the shoulders. Upper extremity movement may be limited, in range of motion, ability, and significantly in strength. This, in turn, affects fine motor movements of the hands. Pronation and supination of the hands may be awkward or lacking. Without these movements, hand to mouth coordination for self-feeding, writing skills, and bilateral movement is limited. Intensive occupational and physical therapy is needed to facilitate normal movement patterns.

MODES OF MECHANICAL VENTILATION

In pediatrics, ventilators and ventilation modes vary based upon the child's respiratory needs. In very young children with disease processes where the lungs are severely damaged, consistently high pressures or "pushes" may be required to get air into the lungs. This type of ventilation is known as *pressure ventilation.* The child on pressure ventilation is typically less medically stable than those on other modes of ventilation. Common pediatric pressure ventilators used include the Infant Star, Bear Cub, BP 200, Sechrist, and Baby Bird.

In older children with disease processes where the lungs are relatively undamaged but breathing effort is weak and/or inconsistent, volume ventilation may be used. Breaths can be consistently provided through the ventilator using lower pressures. Pediatric volume ventilators are typically more mobile and easier to use in home care.

Continuous positive airway pressure (CPAP) involves consistent pressures of air provided through a ventilator or other device. In other modes of ventilation, "breaths" are given. With CPAP, however, a lower consistent pressure is usually given to stent open an area of tracheomalacia. The child is mobile but must always be connected to an air source such as a wall outlet, oxygen tank, or air compressor.

There are several safety issues to be aware of when providing therapy services to children on ventilators. Before picking up a child, remove excess water that has accumulated in the ventilator circuit that is connected to the tracheostomy tube. This water can inadvertently spill into the lungs via the tracheostomy tube. It is important to allow "slack" in the ventilator tubing so that it does not pull on the tracheostomy tube and cause accidental decannulation. Disconnection of ventilator tubing can occur during treatment, which will sound a low pressure alarm; this can be corrected by properly reconnecting the ventilator tubing. If the child requires suctioning, the child's chest may "rattle" and secretions may be noted in the tracheostomy tube. In this case, a high pressure alarm may sound, which can be corrected by having authorized personnel suction the child. Some children will be able to be weaned from the ventilator. Weaning will occur over several weeks or months by slowly decreasing the pressure, volume, or rate of the child's ventilator breaths. It is important to notice changes in therapy performance as this may indicate subtle signs that the child is not tolerating the weaning process. The positive side of mechanical ventilation is that the child need not breathe solely on his or her own. With mechanical support, growth and healing can occur.

CLINICAL INTERVENTION STRATEGIES OF THE SPEECH-LANGUAGE PATHOLOGIST

Role of the Speech-Language Pathologist

What is the exact role of the speech-language pathologist working with patients who have limited ability to speak due to a tracheostomy and/or mechanical ventilation? The speech-language pathologist's role has many facets, including feeding, communication, and cognition.

Most people, including those in the medical profession, think of a speech-language pathologist as a clinician whose focus is to teach children to pronounce words correctly. Unfortunately, this is a great misconception. With the medically involved child, whether an infant or adolescent, the ability to communicate and maintain nutritional status is very important. Where does one begin to treat this type of patient?

Speech for the child who is tracheostomized and/or mechanically ventilated is either totally void or absent (due to limited space available for air leakage around the tracheostomy tube up through the vocal folds) or very strained and breathy. It s the role of the speech-language pathologist to help the child reestablish or initially develop speech. Speech in a healthy child is taken for granted and the difficulty of the learning process is overlooked or forgotten. When that ability is no longer possible, the complex process of communication becomes obvious. It must be broken down not only into the formulation of words, but also the coordination of breathing and controlled exhalation. Communication now becomes a full process on the conscious level.

Language issues or communication can be separated into two areas: those children who have tracheostomies and are either mechanically ventilated or not mechanically ventilated. Both of these categories can then focus on the different age ranges and some specific diagnoses that are most likely to require tracheostomies and possibly mechanical ventilation. For the premature infant, initial mechanical ventilation may be inevitable due to lung immaturity. Once the child is stable, the speech-language pathologist may be called to evaluate feeding and nutritional needs. It was mentioned earlier in this chapter that a child who is orally or nasally intubated may not be able to eat by mouth. What is often forgotten is how communication develops. The adult may be relearning to speak, but the child is just beginning to learn. The child's learning is fully dependent on the environment and the cognitive ability he or she has to understand that environment. It is unfortunate that many people do not see communication, whether it be receptive or expressive, as important early in a child's development. A common response is that the child is only a baby and that he or she does not talk anyway. This response is upsetting for the speech-language pathologist who knows that communication starts with the first cry at birth. It is up to the speech-language pathologist to enhance the child's environment in order to facilitate cognitive and language development. Given how closely supervised that environment is, the need to communicate is limited. The nursing staff anticipates many of the child's needs before they are obvious to the lay person. This does not allow the child to develop an intent to communicate. Instead, many needs are taken care of without the child's request or the family becoming frustrated with the child's inability to express himself or herself.

Assessment

An initial assessment of the premature infant focuses on environmental awareness and the ability to react to stimuli, whether by auditory or visual means. The next aspect to be explored is that of the response to the stimuli. Does the child swipe at an object within its reach, or does he or she smile at a caregiver's face? There are many standardized tests to assess a child's early communication skills. The following is a brief list of common infant assessment tools:

St. Christopher Scale
Receptive Expressive Emergent Language Scale (REEL)
Early Intervention Developmental Profile (EIDP)
Hawaii Early Learning Profile (HELP)
Learning Assessment Profile (LAP)

What must be carefully noted when evaluating these children is the mode of communication these children currently use. Most use physiological signals. It may be as simple as looking away during an interaction, which may clearly mean, "I have had too much stimulation and I need a break from this activity." Other children become diaphoretic or have an increase in heart rate or respiratory rate. It cannot be stressed enough that the overall medical stability of a child must be prioritized when planning therapeutic intervention. Since a speech-language pathologist is geared to "make children talk," the child's ability to vocalize around the tracheostomy tube must be carefully assessed. If the child can vocalize around the tracheostomy tube, how clear and how long are the vocalizations? The child's oral motor skills should also be assessed. Is the child able to freely move his or her tongue and is he or she able to imitate oral movements? Skills that are precursors to speech need to be carefully investigated. Problems with oral motor coordination may be indicative of a neuromotor speech disorder, or more specifically, apraxia or dysarthria. Once these skills are assessed, the most appropriate mode of communication may be selected. The literature states that children who are unable to vocalize around their tracheostomy tube are taught sign language, the use of esophageal speech, or the use of an electrolarynx. For most children, learning esophageal speech is very difficult.[4] The same holds true for the use of an electro-larynx. The two most efficient modes of communication are sign language and a one-way speaking valve. In order to use a speaking valve, the speech-language pathologist will need to obtain a physician's written order and have a clear understanding of the patient's medical condition. Research also reveals that although an important precursor, a child need not actively go through the early cooing and babbling stages of development prior to learning to speak.[4] Literature continues to show that children who were tracheostomized early in life and decannulated prior to the critical period of development develop skills commensurate to those of their peers. On the other hand, those who were tracheostomized at 2 to 5 years of age and remained cannulated for an extended period of time without intervention suffered significant setbacks in language development. Intensive therapy for these patients is needed before or upon decannulation.[4]

Feeding Assessment

Another very important aspect to keep in mind is the child's ability to feed orally. Areas of concern are the ability to suck from a bottle, lip closure around the nipple, and rhythmic tongue movement. The coordination of feeding and breathing is also important to note. As mentioned earlier many children who are intubated or who have tracheostomies are at increased risk for aspiration. A blue dye test can be done to rule out aspiration. If this test is not fully conclusive or the therapist needs more information as to the area of breakdown in the swallowing process, a videofluoroscopy can be completed. Therapeutic techniques will focus on the appropriate positioning of the child to ensure total body organization in order to facilitate oral motor coordination. Other areas addressed are those of oral stimulation to enhance sucking and decrease oral and facial sensitivity. It is important to work closely with the nursing staff and other caregivers to teach them these techniques for carryover purposes. It is of utmost importance that although these children may be receiving their nutrition presently by nasogastric tube or gastrostomy tube, they receive oral stimulation during feeding times. By doing this, they associate the feeling of becoming satisfied nutritionally with the appropriate motor skills of sucking. It is very important also to encourage non-nutritive sucking. Feeding therapy should not be done during scheduled feeding times. Instead, it should be done at another time, for if the child is unable to eat adequately, he or she may associate feeding as a noxious stimulus and become adversive to it. The child's ability to handle bulk bolus feedings is important prior to encouraging total oral feedings.

Vocal Assessment

Language development is affected not only by the restricted environment but also by the tracheostomy, which inhibits vocalization. Many pediatric tracheostomy tubes do not have cuffs. Therefore, if the child has air leakage around the tracheostomy tube, a small amount of vocalization may be achieved. This, however, is not enough to allow for adequate language development or mature communication for the older child. A full assessment of the child's respiratory status should be made to determine if the child is a candidate for the use of a one-way speaking valve. The valve should be used according to the manufacturer's instructions described in Chapter 7. The most important aspect of treatment for the tracheostomized patient is to restore the ability to communicate. We may not realize how we interact with people who cannot communicate with us.

If we look at the interactions, we notice that they are very limited. Psychologically this has a big effect on a child and any patient in this situation. You can only imagine how difficult it is to make friends when you cannot speak and no one speaks to you. This can be as equally devastating as having a tracheostomy.

Assessment Considerations

Evaluation tools for the older child with a tracheostomy are quite extensive. Due to the child's limited ability to speak, most tests can be administered to determine receptive skills. However, expressive skills will need to be tested via clinical observation. If the child is old enough and has the physical ability to write, he or she can write all of the answers in the expressive portion of the test. This, however, will not count as a valid test score, due to altered testing methods. There is an extensive list of tests that may be used to evaluate the older tracheostomized child. The most important aspect of evaluating the older child is the child's ability to speak around the tracheostomy tube. Is the child able to vocalize at all? For some, it may be a matter of using a one-way speaking valve to enhance speech. For others, it may mean having scar tissue removed first in order to have enough airflow space for voicing to occur with a speaking valve. There also may be children who cannot use a speaking valve at all. In any case, if a child is able to speak using a one-way valve, the child's syntax needs to be carefully assessed. It is important to know the length of time the child has been tracheostomized and the age at which he or she was tracheostomized before deciding if the child has a language disorder.

Establishing Therapeutic Goals

Establishing therapy goals will be dependent upon the child's age, length of cannulation, cognitive level, and overall ability to communicate. Looking at the young infant, therapy will focus on motor development, feeding skills, and cognitive development. Trained staff who are familiar with the medically fragile infant and a transdisciplinary approach to treatment are best qualified to work with these children. The connection between motor skills and the ability to develop cognition is important to note when planning treatment goals. Precursors to language must be reinforced before one can expect receptive language to develop. The cause/effect relationship with the environment needs to be developed, as well as the ability to self-regulate and organize during times when the environment is overstimulating. The child's internal organization is a primary concern for the nursing staff. If these children are unable to self-calm each time they are suctioned or have a diaper changed, how are they going to learn from their surroundings? Facilitating exploration of simple rattles or spin toys may be the goal of therapy. Basic skills are needed to form a foundation from which language can be built. Once these skills are developed, more complex skills can be introduced and language can grow. Further referral for specialized services through early intervention programs is also suggested in order to facilitate age-appropriate development. Careful follow-up for the necessary special education is also important for these children.

Feeding Goals

Feeding skills for the infant should also need to be addressed. Once the child is able to tolerate bolus feedings without reflux or regurgitation, oral feedings can be introduced. Prior to this time, oral stimulation can be used to facilitate the lingual cupping and lip closure needed for adequate feeding skills. The child must be paced appropriately in order not to stress cardiac output or respiratory status. Very often, tactile defensiveness is also addressed at this time. Once these goals are achieved, feeding skills can be addressed as they would be for a less fragile infant.

Expressive Language Goals

Expressive language is the primary goal for most children, and the therapeutic options are few. The use of an electro-larynx is not practical for the young child. Teaching them how to use the device is difficult. Mastery is not always achieved by adults, let alone children. The speech produced is mechanical, monotone, and very difficult for many people to understand. Sign language is easier for small children to learn, as many have already developed their own method of gestures. However, sign language is not practical because only those similarly trained are able to understand the child.

Vocal Goals

Vocal speech is the ultimate goal. How can this be achieved? For the child who has severe stenosis and respiratory compromise, communication may be restricted to nonverbal methods. This can mean augmentative systems, sign language, or even an electro-larynx, each restricting the full development of language. For those children who are able to vocalize around their tracheostomy tube and can tolerate a speaking valve, the voice will be the primary mode of communication. Children who are the best candidates for the use of a speaking valve are those who are able to vocalize around their tracheostomy tube and have minimal stenosis. Encouraging the use of a speaking valve at as early an age as possible will enhance communication skills and, in many cases, facilitate normal language development. Children who start using a speaking valve by the age of 15 to18 months are more likely to develop normal language skills. Initial placement of the valve with the young population is challenging. Children, like adults, do not like people touching their tracheostomy tubes; therefore, it may be helpful to introduce a one-way speaking valve by using a stuffed animal or doll. It is much easier for a child to relate to a toy than to an adult. The first trials should be done in play-like settings. To encourage exhalation, activities such as singing and/or blowing bubbles, horns, and whistles are useful. Many pediatric tracheostomy tubes are not cuffed; therefore, cuff deflation does not have to be addressed prior to using a one-way valve. Further information on one-way speaking valves can be found in Chapter 7.

For the older child who has developed language skills but for medical reasons is tracheostomized, therapy will take a different perspective. The necessity for the tracheostomy needs to be investigated, as does the reason for a hospital admission. The skills focused on with the head trauma patient are much different from those of a child who has not yet developed language. With the head trauma patient, therapy will focus on cognitive skills and the functional aspects of language. Syntactic structures are usually complete and need not be a goal of therapy.

Post-Decannulation Therapy

Once a child is decannulated, speech therapy may be needed on a minimal basis, depending on the patient. If the patient is a young child who has not yet developed age-appropriate language skills, therapy will focus on overall language development. If the child has age-appropriate language skills, vocal quality should be carefully assessed and appropriate intervention used. Breath support following decannulation is very important. Many young children who were tracheostomized from birth have limited breath support to facilitate appropriate volume. These skills can be addresses with a physical therapist and a speech-language pathologist trained in the neurodevelopmental treatment approach to therapy.

CONCLUSION

As this chapter has indicated, the total development of a child who has a tracheostomy and was, or is, ventilator dependent has incurred significant setbacks. The speech-language pathologist cannot facilitate development in all areas. It is important that these children be followed by physical and occupational therapy. With the appropriate intervention, both muscle strength and physical coordination of the upper and lower body can be facilitated. Programs for young infants and toddlers, such as early intervention programs, are encouraged in order to enhance a transdisciplinary approach to development and therapy. For the older child, special education and preschool handicap programs are beneficial, giving the child a well-rounded therapy model.

Children are not small adults, but rather individuals who need special consideration in treatment in order to meet their important developmental milestones.

REFERENCES

1. Kamen, R., and Watson, B., "Effects of long-term tracheostomy on spectral characteristics of vowel production." *Journal of Speech and Hearing Research,* 1991; 34:1057-1065.

2. Koff, P., Eitzman, D., M.D., and New, J., M.D. *Neonatal and Pediatric Respiratory Care,* St. Louis: The C.V. Mosby Company, 1988.

3. Passy-Muir, *Passy-Muir One Way Speaking Valve Training Manual,* Passy-Muir, Inc., 1992.

4. Simon, B., et al., "Communication development in young children with long term tracheostomies: Preliminary report." *International Journal of Pediatric Otorhinolaryngology,* 1983; 6:35-50.

5. Tucker, E.Z., Rogers, B., Jerome, A., et. al., "Tracheostomy speaking valve in pediatric ventilator-assisted patients." Paper presented at the 37th Annual Convention and Exhibition, Dec. 7-10, 1991, Atlanta, American Association for Respiratory Care, 1991.

6. Albamonte, S., and Berry, B., "Application of Passy-Muir Valve with tracheostomized pediatric populations." American Speech-Language-Hearing Association Annual Convention, Oct., 1988; 30(10):178, Presentation SU10-PS6. Poster No. 21.

BIBLIOGRAPHY

Aloan, C. (Ed.), "Respiratory Care of the Newborn." *A Clinical Manual,* Philadelphia: J.B. Lippincott Co., 1987.

Aradine, C. R., "Young children with long-term tracheostomies: Health and development." *Western Journal of Nursing Research,* 1983.

Fujimoto, P., Madison, C., and Larrigan, L., "The effects of a tracheostomy valve on the intelligibility and quality of tracheo-esophageal speech." *Journal of Speech and Hearing Research,* 1991; 34:33-36.

Hall, S., and Weatherly, K., "Using sign language with tracheostomized infants and children." *Pediatric Nursing,* 1989; 15(4):362-367.

Hill, B., and Singer, L., "Speech and language development after infant tracheostomy." *Journal of Speech and Hearing Disorders,* 1990; 55:15-20.

Kaslon, K., and Stein, R., "Chronic pediatric tracheostomy: Assessment and implications for habilitation of voice, speech and language in young children."*International Journal of Pediatric Otorhinolaryngology,* 1985; 9:165-171.

Ross, G., "Language functioning and speech development in six children receiving tracheotomy in infancy." *Journal of Communication Disorders,* 1982; 15:95-111.

Simon, B., and Handler, S., "The speech pathologist and management of children with tracheostomies." *Journal of Otolaryngology,* 1981, 10(6):440-448.

Simon, B., and McGowan, J., "Tracheostomy in young children: Implications for assessment and treatment of communication and feeding disorders." *Infants and Young Children,* 1989; 1:1-9.

Singer, L., et al., "Developmental sequelae of long term infant tracheostomy." *Developmental Medicine and Child Neurology,* 1989; 31:224-230.

Singer, L., et al., "Developmental follow up of long term infant tracheostomy: A preliminary report." *Developmental and Behavioral Pediatrics,* 1985; 6(3):132-136.

Sweeny, J. (Ed.), *The High-Risk Neonate: Developmental Therapy Perspectives,* New York: The Haworth Press, 1986.

CHAPTER IX

PSYCHOSOCIAL

To touch another with a remembered kindness.

To impart love that continues to weave through others' lives.

To affect a change, no matter how small, that leaves others better.

To do and care for others when no one is watching.

To offer a gentle hand, a loving smile, a quiet moment of careful listening.

These are life's everyday challenges.

The greatest sadness in life is not the misfortune of illness and disabilities, but rather the missed opportunities to participate, to nurture, to heal, to make even the smallest contribution to enhance another's life.

To embrace the challenges, to look beyond the obstacles, to always sprint toward the goal, to do this with kindness and compassion, is to succeed in making a difference by changing one life for one moment in a positive way.

Anonymous

INTRODUCTION

To want to help. To offer even a small touch of healing. To make a positive difference in a patient's medical experience. These were my goals when I began my clinical practice and are still my goals today. Sometimes, however, as I travel the clinical path from patient to patient and institution to institution, it is easy to be distracted from my commitment by the technology, regulations, and conflicts of the business of medicine. First and foremost, health care delivery should be concerned with the healing of patients. Unfortunately, however, over the years, this objective has become obscured and compromised by the business of the system. I am challenged daily in my practice to deliver my therapy with respect and caring for my patients.

I remind myself always to say "Hello" to my patient before I check the ventilator settings, to ask how he or she is doing and listen intently before I review the chart, to acknowledge the person before I begin treatment of his or her physical needs. It is important to enhance the art of healing by delivering our health care with compassion and respect for the whole person.

Compassion is our ability to understand and feel the experience, situation, and emotions of another person. In order to be able to offer support and therapeutic intervention, it is necessary to have an accurate knowledge and awareness of the patient's daily challenges. If we are to provide optimum therapeutic intervention, we must be able to address the issues that are the patient's everyday reality. Awareness of the pain, frustrations, hopes, and needs of our patients will enable us to be compassionate and holistic in our rehabilitative efforts with these very compromised individuals.

It is with this philosophy that I have included the essays of several tracheostomized and ventilator dependent patients and caregivers in this chapter. I have chosen to limit the editing of these essays to avoid any alteration of their authors' histories or feelings. In so doing, I hope to give the reader the opportunity to step into these individuals' lives through their own words.

While reading these essays I challenge the reader to personally consider the vital issues of patient rights, quality of life, patient advocacy, continuity of patient care across all settings (medical and home), the dilemma of reimbursement and rising health care costs, and the role of the speech-language pathologist in treatment of critically ill patients.

It is truly the duty of each speech-language pathologist not only to incorporate these issues into his or her practice but also to constantly expand his or her professional knowledge base and then to assertively market this expertise and its application with various patient populations (e.g., tracheostomized or ventilator dependent patients) to physicians and other health professionals. It is only through ongoing individual as well as collective marketing and educational efforts that speech-language pathologists will facilitate a more accurate and in-depth understanding of our services in the health care arena and subsequently be able to better serve the needs of all communicatively compromised patients.

Mary F. Mason

Essays

Psychosocial Issues in the Care of Ventilator—Dependent Patients: A Patient's Perspective

by Jeffrey L. Santee, Ph.D.

Jeffrey L. Santee, Ph.D., is a licensed clinical psychologist specializing in behavioral medicine and treatment for ventilator dependent, cardiac, and chronic pain patients.

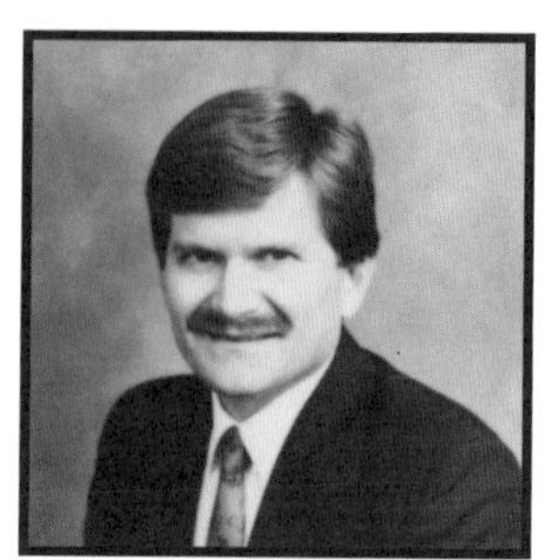

I have served as the consulting psychologist to the Ventilator Support Center (VSC)[1] for approximately five years. During that time, I have had the pleasure and challenge of working with hundreds of ventilator dependent patients and their families. I have observed many patients and families deal with the unique challenges of being ventilator dependent in a gracious and dignified manner. However, most patients and families need help in coping with numerous psychosocial issues and adjustments that come with being ventilator dependent in the hospital for long periods of time.

In this section, I will introduce the reader to some common psychosocial issues facing ventilator dependent patients and their families. I will begin by introducing you to the inner struggles of a typical ventilator dependent patient so that you may gain an inside view of the needs and feelings of this patient population. I will then follow with a discussion of the basic psychosocial needs of all people, and how being hospitalized and ventilator dependent can threaten or violate those needs. This discussion will include how such violations of psychosocial needs can lead to many negative emotional and behavioral reactions. Finally, I will offer some ideas about how the basic needs of ventilator dependent patients and families can be nurtured while in the hospital.

There are four basic human needs that are referred to in this article that are adapted from the original work of Harris Clemes and

Reynold Bean in their book entitled *Self-Esteem.*[2] The basic needs include maintaining a sense of (1) *connectedness* to important people, places, and things; (2) *uniqueness* that defines who we are as individuals and how we feel about ourselves and our personal characteristics; (3) *power* or self-control that enables us to maintain some personal control and to effect changes in our lives; (4) *models* that enable us to make sense of our experiences based on our values and beliefs. The fulfillment of these needs is important in maintaining a sense of self-esteem in adults, particularly in highly stressful situations that are chronically life-threatening.

These basic needs are inherently threatened by virtue of a person being hospitalized for long periods of time and remaining ventilator dependent. Some patients are hospitalized at the VSC for 3 months or longer. The psychological stress of hospitalization and ventilator dependency can be intensified even further by preexisting psychopathology and family dysfunction as well as direct violations of the patient's basic needs by either the caregiver or the care-giving environment. Extremely negative (dysfunctional) emotional and behavioral reactions tend to emerge under these circumstances. That is when I am often called upon to provide a psychosocial assessment of the situation and, if needed, to intervene with individual and family therapy in addition to consultation with the professional staff on how to best handle the circumstances.

A Patient's Perspective

As we look at a patient's perspective in some detail it will help to remain mindful of the four basic needs noted earlier. I would like for you to imagine yourself in the shoes of Mary Lou,[3] a 67-year-old mother of four children who has spent the last three months in the hospital. Mary Lou is an ex-smoker with a long history of emphysema. She also has high blood pressure, a weak heart, and osteoporosis, caused, in part, by the high doses of prednisone prescribed over the last five years to help her breathe. Just prior to her arrival at the VSC, Mary Lou has spent the last two weeks in the intensive care unit to stabilize her heart. During this time she has become very weak and often is in a confused and disoriented mental state. Her family tells her that while in the intensive care unit she often did not recognize them and was mumbling things that did not make any sense. It occurs to Mary Lou that she may be losing her mind.

Mary Lou is now out of the intensive care unit, and it is her first day at the VSC. She feels very frightened, unsure of herself, and unsure of what will happen next. "Why am I here? Someone told me, but I don't remember anymore. Where is my family? Maybe they are never coming! What if I stop breathing? I can't yell out to get anyone's attention. In fact, I can't tell anyone what my needs are since I can't talk to them. Will someone come in time if I need them?" As these and other frightening thoughts race through Mary Lou's mind, she begins to gasp for air and cough uncontrollably. The ventilator is going wild with the sounds of all kinds of alarms, none of which make any sense or give her the air she so desperately needs. "I can't breathe! I can't live without air! I am dying!" These thoughts scream out in her mind, and for that moment she believes them with all her heart and soul. What actually may have been only a few passing moments seemed to be her *last* moments. At long last, a therapist comes to help her. Mary Lou's frightened eyes and the expression on her face speak of her terror, but she longs to be able to speak directly to the therapist, to tell of what she feels and what she needs. Finally, after some adjustments are made to the ventilator, Mary Lou calms down and her therapist leaves the room.

She wonders, "Can I trust this machine? What if it stops working? What if no one comes to help me in time?" She then begins to think about all the things she can no longer do for herself. She feels so out of control and lost. Just a few short weeks ago she could at least do some simple things, the kind of things you and I take for granted, like being able to breathe and enjoy the fresh air, like eating real food instead of liquid food through a tube, and like talking. There are so many thoughts and feelings bottled up inside. It feels like she is about to explode. "What kind of life will I be able to have? I want my old life back!" She silently screams to herself.

And with these thoughts, Mary Lou feels her anxiety beginning to resurface. "STOP!" she shouts in her mind. "I can't count on anyone but myself. I have to take care of myself. I better not do anything too strenuous, and I better stop thinking about these things that upset me so much so I can breathe easier." But Mary Lou can't help but think about something, and so her mind drifts off to thoughts about her family. Suddenly she is hit with a profound sense of loneliness and isolation. She longs to be with her family right now and to be involved in their lives again. If she could only pick up the telephone and call them. Her husband comes to visit nearly every day and passes on little tidbits of news, but it is not the same as being home with everyone. And her friends? Well, Mary Lou lost contact with most of them years ago when she was forced to retire and then later became housebound. Besides, many of them have died already.

Mary Lou finally drifts off to sleep. It is so hard to rest with all the noises and the commotion on the unit, and so when sleep comes it is a welcomed respite. But she is suddenly awakened by loud voices in the hall and a light in her face. "What is happening? What are they doing? I'm so scared!" She thinks to herself. It is startling enough to be awakened so abruptly, but even more frightening to think that she is completely helpless and unable to defend herself.

It is another new day now, but Mary Lou feels imprisoned by the same old routine. She longs for her own privacy and space. It seems that nothing is sacred, especially her privacy and occasionally her self-respect and dignity. Each new day is a struggle for Mary Lou to keep from cashing in her old hopes for a new found sense of pessimism and despair. It is so hard to keep up her strength, to wean, to exercise, and to be probed, lifted, and poked all in the same day. The staff is friendly and helpful, but they are almost always in a hurry. Rarely do they stop long enough to get to know Mary Lou, not as a patient who needs this drug or that treatment, but as a person. She sometimes wonders, "Am I worth knowing anymore? What do I have to offer anyone?" Some days she is glad to be alive, like a real human being again; while on other days, she feels more like an object, like a block of wood that others administer to. The staff is encouraging most of the time and tells her that she is doing really well, but why doesn't she feel the same way?

The journey toward recovery seems as endless and treacherous as climbing a mountain completely blind. Mary Lou has never traveled this road before. She has never been this sick before, nor has she ever been in the hospital and away from her family for so long. She asks for directions along her difficult journey. "Am I going to die from this setback? Will I ever get off the ventilator? How much longer before I can go home?" But it seems that the doctors and staff are either as blind as she is, or they are trying to spare her the despair of knowing the truth. Mary Lou thinks, "If only I could speak to someone who has made this journey before me. Does it really have an end? Will I make it? Will it be worth the struggle? Everyone else seems to think so, but I'm not so sure."

These and other related thoughts and feelings remain with Mary Lou, day in and day out, as she makes her way toward recovery, one step at a time. For the staff who takes care of Mary Lou, she is an enigma. At times she is quiet and cooperative. Her eyes and facial expressions seem to tell a tale of sadness, if not depression. She seems nice enough, but rarely does she try to talk or communicate her needs directly. On other occasions, she is grumpy and irritable, and the staff is never quite sure what has set her off. When upset, she seems to be on the call light constantly, and she seems awfully needy, if not manipulative. The staff wavers between feeling sorry for Mary Lou and feeling angry with her at times. It is difficult for them to gain a perspective on how to satisfy her. It is difficult to develop a caring professional attitude with her that on one hand doesn't encourage her dependency and on the other hand doesn't feel too cold or uncaring and blame or shame her.

Mary Lou's issues and struggles sometimes get entangled with the staff's own issues about how to deal with a patient's dependency, demands, anger, and indifference. Sometimes, it is hard to separate her issues from their own reactions. There is never enough time, it seems, to reflect on these problems because there are more patients to see, medications to administer, blood gases to draw, and reports to fill out.

The Basic Human Needs

What reactions did you have as you placed yourself in the shoes of this patient? Can you envision why the basic needs noted earlier are so important to ventilator dependent patients? In what ways are the basic needs threatened by virtue of being ventilator dependent and hospitalized, and how does this affect patients? In the remaining portion of this chapter, I will address these important questions since they reflect on many of the psychosocial issues of ventilator dependent patients.

Maintaining a sense of *connectedness* is especially important while in the hospital. Threats to one's sense of connectedness include being away from familiar people and surroundings or in an environment where people fail to listen or respond to us as people. Other threats include multiple losses of health, the loss of important roles in the family, and having a sense of not being needed. Missing important family events and the customary ways of interacting with the family can leave a person feeling very disconnected from important relationships.

Varied reactions to these threats to connectedness include feelings of loneliness, isolation, sadness, and loss; emotional and social withdrawal; and excessive dependence on others for feelings of motivation. Caregivers who are aware of these negative reactions may nurture a healthier way of meeting the need to remain connected. These nurturing efforts might include things such as getting to know the patient on a personal level, taking time to help the patient to personalize the hospital room, and working with the patient to maintain a familiar and acceptable daily routine. Of course, frequent visits and socializing with family and friends is something families can do to help patients remain and feel more connected.

Another basic need of all patients involves a sense of *uniqueness*, which reflects how people feel about themselves and their personal characteristics. It involves what most people normally think of as self-esteem. Receiving support and approval from others as we are, even in a sickly or disabled state, helps to enhance self-esteem. Things that can threaten this basic need include losses of health and important roles and responsibilities, and the loss of self-control. Failure to reach important goals such as weaning from the ventilator also threatens a patient's sense of self-worth. Another important threat is being treated like a number or a thing rather than a person who has some unique tastes or preferences of their own.

When a sense of uniqueness is threatened it may result in the following types of negative reactions: feelings of inadequacy and worthlessness; destructive self-criticism or pessimism about one's self; and unrealistic anxiety and fears about medical procedures and setbacks. Professionals who care about more than just the patient's physical state can help by providing encouragement as well as praise and approval for what has been accomplished. Ventilator dependent patients often lose sight of the progress they are making. Encouragement from professional staff for the patient's trying, getting started, and doing parts of tasks can be very helpful and increases the patient's sense of self-worth. Helping a patient prepare for a new task or something he or she has never undertaken can be very supportive as well. Finally, a sense of uniqueness can be nurtured by allowing for the patient's own individuality, rather than forcing each and every patient to conform to one way of doing things.

Another basic need of every person is to have a sense of *power* (self-efficacy), which reflects the person's feelings about self-control and the use of skills or resources to make changes and adapt to situations. Some environments are flexible enough to adapt to the needs of others, whereas other environments such as the hospital often do not allow for much opportunity for patients to effect many changes. Some common threats to a sense of power might include things like the losses of health, finances, and decision-making control over these particular areas. Having to follow a daily routine that is somewhat unpredictable and under the control of everyone else can also contribute to a decreased sense of personal power. Unreasonable or inconsistent expectations of the staff can contribute to problems in this particular area as well. Being shamed or ridiculed for having complaints or multiple questions about the situation can result in a patient's decreased sense of power. Simply the situation of having very little knowledge about what is expected from the illness or the recovery process can leave a patient feeling powerless and victimized.

Varied negative reactions to these threats to a sense of personal power and control include feelings of helplessness or powerlessness and a tendency to blame or find fault with others, particularly the professional staff or institution in which the patient is staying. Angry, demanding, aggressive behaviors toward others also reflect a lack of inner confidence or power. Inappropriate attempts to control or test the staff may also be an indication of a low sense of power. Sometimes patients do not exercise control over things that they truly can control, but they try to exercise control in inappropriate areas. For some patients the feelings of helplessness, dependency, and a lack of control over their lives can result in tremendous internal conflicts.

Patients may be nurtured in developing a greater sense of power while in the hospital and suffering from severe medical conditions by helping them set realistic goals. Specific, realistic goals convey to the patient that the staff believes that he or she is capable of improving and reaching a higher ground. Information about what to expect as well as explaining what and why things happen, can be extremely valuable. Although the information may not help the patient control the situation, it does make it less stressful by making it more predictable. Whenever possible, giving patients choices about the timing and the way in which things are done can be helpful in increasing their sense of control. Finally, explaining the staff's expectations and appropriate ways of challenging them or raising questions and issues can help patients feel more empowered.

All people need to have a sense of *models*, which reflects how we can make sense of our experiences based on our own values and beliefs, including a sense of spirituality or transcendence. Having a model of what to expect can help guide our decisions and behavior. Most patients, like Mary Lou, need help in establishing an appropriate framework to understand what they are going through and what is normal. This is sometimes referred to as *normalization,* or providing information that helps patients to realize and deal with the reality of their experiences. One significant threat to a sense of models can be the loss of health or the threat of death. Having inadequate role models while in the hospital can be threatening since role models provide a structure of how to make sense of what is happening. Early childhood neglect or abuse can make a person feel out of control and overwhelmed in almost any stressful situation, let alone, a hospitalization.

Negative reactions to a lack of models include feelings of confusion, indecisiveness, and emptiness. They may also include an inability to set and follow any clear goals or direction. Avoidance of important issues while maintaining chronic complaints about minor problems may also reflect a lack of understanding about what is really important. Patients who seem kind of lost or who are unable to define what their direction is, may also suffer from a poor sense of models that would enable them to transcend what they are experiencing.

Patients may be nurtured in this particular area by helping them make sense of what they are experiencing. For example, it is quite common for ventilator dependent patients to make progress in their weaning from the ventilator, only to suffer a setback. When this happens it is often experienced as quite a demoralizing event for patients. Providing information that helps normalize their experiences can be helpful. It may also be helpful for hospitalized patients to maintain a comfortable routine, which gives them something of an anchor in the stress of being hospitalized. Helping the patients set realistic goals and sorting out options can be particularly helpful for them in clarifying their own values and priorities with respect to discharge options and the maintenance or withdrawal of life support.

Summary

Many of the psychosocial issues related to the care of ventilator dependent patients can be understood with respect to four basic human needs involving the fulfillment of connectedness, uniqueness, power, and models. There are many threats to the fulfillment of these needs by virtue of being ventilator dependent and hospitalized. Many of the threats to these needs are identified along with the ensuing negative reactions of patients. Ways of nurturing the needs of ventilator dependent patients are also considered. Caregivers and the hospital environment play a major role in the emotional status and rehabilitation of ventilator dependent patients, even when other psychosocial interventions are required.

It's About Attitude

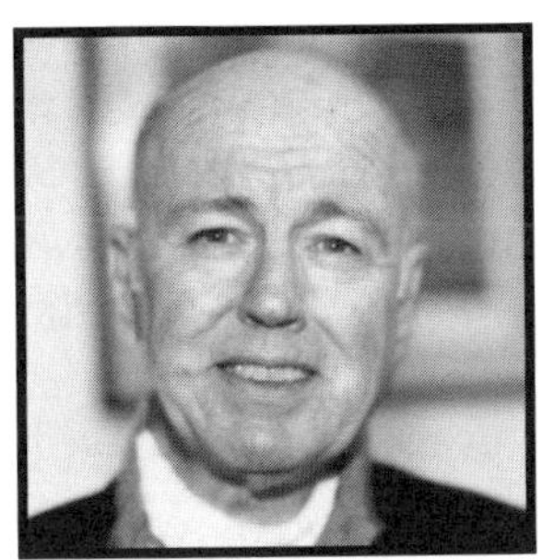

by John Connors, D.M.D.

John Connors, D.M.D., is an oral surgeon and dentist in private practice.

At sixteen years old, I developed bulbar polio. I went into a coma and the doctors told my parents I was going to die. This was in 1948 when they had very few respirators, and I was too far gone to be given one. I remember they threw a blanket over me and said, "He's gone" and then someone else said, "He's not gone yet." I could hear this but I couldn't move a muscle, which is very interesting. I did survive but I was weak, could hardly walk, and had little use of my upper limbs. They didn't have physical therapy in those days, so my father took me out in the yard, in the woods behind our house. He got me a Daisy Baby bee bee gun because I knew how to pump it and shoot it. He also bought me a bunch of balloons and said, "Now, blow up the balloon, that's good for your lungs; tie a knot in the balloon, that's good for your hands; and then let the wind blow it away. Then you pump the Daisy gun, shoot the balloon, but only with your right hand because it's paralyzed, not your left, and I'll pick you up at lunch." I was out in the yard from about 8:00 a.m. to 5:00 p.m. for seven days a week. Even when it was snowing I was out there, and my mother was inside crying, fighting with my father. "You've got to bring him in," she begged. "NO! He stays out," said my Dad. That's the way I was brought up, so I figured I better do the best I could because it was pretty cold outside, which forced me to keep moving and working all the time. The only funny side to this story was eight months later when I was really starting to come around. No one could believe it, even the doctor couldn't believe it. I was talking and walking again! I was out in the back yard shooting at squirrels, which was okay, but my father said I still had to blow up the balloons for my lungs. He was about 50 feet from where I was sitting and he was walking away from me, so

I turned around and shot him in the backside with my Daisy bee bee gun. He turned around and said, "I guess you're getting better."

I completed college, dental school, and an internship and residency in oral surgery and began my practice in New York. I began to get colds and pneumonia and would be in bed for six to eight weeks out of each year. The last two or three years I began experiencing extreme shortness of breath and I couldn't exert myself. In 1992, I was hospitalized. My vocal cords were almost totally closed when two procedures were recommended: laser surgery to remove a section of one of the vocal cords to give me more air to breathe or a tracheostomy. Because of the problems with my epiglottis and swallowing and aspiration, I decided to have the tracheostomy. Now, I can breathe easily. It was like having someone sitting on my chest for 30 years and all of a sudden they got off. I never realized the pressure I was under just to breathe. I can also communicate a little better with the tracheostomy and with the speaking valve,[4] which I received about two weeks after my tracheostomy. The speaking valve has given me a totally new perspective because without it I would be really incapacitated. With the valve I'm able to talk to you more normally. I can push air through the cords to get the vibrations for the sound because of the positive pressure. Without the valve, in order for me to talk with my patients, I would have to take off one of my rubber gloves, close my opening and talk to them; then put the rubber glove back on and go back into their mouth.

I used to be very careful when I ate and I would even choke on saliva. Now, with the valve, I can basically eat just about whatever I want. The valve also protects the trachea from dust and wind. I play a lot of golf, and out on a golf course it's windy. It literally makes you gasp because it is usually cold and you feel it. With the valve, even if you do get a sharp wind in your face, it cuts down dramatically on the amount of force of the wind entering into your bronchi and bronchial system.

After a tracheostomy you have to be very positive and have an almost arrogant attitude. I've had a lot of problems in my life, but I'm married and have six kids. Some of my roommates from college are dead and I'm still here, so I can't complain. The whole family has to be supportive of you because you can't hide this; it's out in the open and people will see it. You don't want to offend people, but at the same time you can't be ashamed of yourself. If they don't like it, you know, they don't have to look. I met a fellow the other day in the golf pro shop. He just looked at my neck and he turned around and walked out. I don't care. I'm not personally offended. I look at the tracheostomy as an inconvenience. It takes me longer to get ready to go to work in the morning and I need more maintenance as I change my inner cannula every three to four hours rather than wait until I start to cough. Sometimes I can go through a whole day if I have to, but I don't because I don't want to start coughing in front of my patients. We wear long gowns that cover the neck so my patients don't even realize I have a tracheostomy. My grandchildren just call it a boo boo and don't really react to it.

My wife loves me, I have good kids, and I have a lot of things I want to do. I dwell on the good things that have happened to me. I see people every day that are a lot worse off than me. From the way I look at it, this is just an inconvenience. I still have my voice box, and a lot of people don't even have their voice box. I'm sure that is more difficult than what I'm putting up with. When you have a tracheostomy, it's like everything else in life; you have to do for yourself, you make up your own mind and you do it. Don't get me wrong, I've been discouraged at times when I look into the mirror and see all the apparatus hanging around my neck, and I say a lot of things to myself, things that I would never verbalize to other people. You do have down days and down times. I have problems with granulation tissue that keeps coming back. It's not all roses, but I keep going and stay busy with work and with my family. I am a survivor. I have too many things to live for, and I enjoy life.

Alexa's Story

by Karen Bither

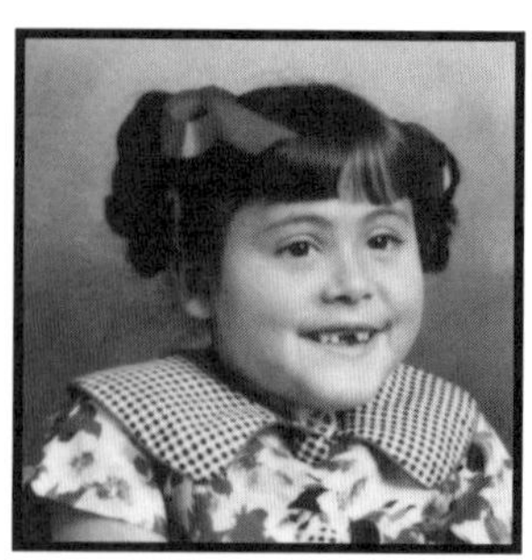

Karen Bither is the mother of Alexa who has spina bifida. Karen and her husband Harry have raised six of their own children and have adopted five more children with disabilities.

Alexa was born on June 27, 1986, in Southern California. At birth, it was discovered that she had spina bifida and was hydrocephalic. The doctors felt her lesion was low and were able to offer her parents hope that her disabilities would not be too severe. Perhaps braces to help her walk would be needed. Surgery was done immediately to repair her spine, and a few days later a ventricular-peritoneal shunt was placed to reduce the hydrocephalus. Her parents soon took her home with the expectation that with their love and medical intervention, they would be able to care for Alexa and her 18-month-old sister.

A short time later the family moved to San Francisco. At two months of age Alexa was admitted to UCSF Medical Center with a severe bladder infection. Bladder infections continued to be a problem in the following months, as other delays also began to appear. Finally, at seven months of age, after an MRI scan, Alexa's parents (Jane and Andy) were told to expect severe learning disabilities and that there were questions about her hearing. Every visit to the doctor brought new concerns. It was felt her problems were now much more severe than had first been thought.

Soon, her parents began to question how they would be able to meet Alexa's needs, their other child's needs, their own needs, and their professional responsibilities. They began looking at their options from help with Alexa at home to help outside the home. They wanted Alexa to have the best life possible in a family that could meet her needs and were very concerned with the fact that most places they looked at were nothing more than small institutions. Their decision was to place her for adoption.

At the same time we were wanting to adopt another child. We had six children who were almost all grown and a younger adopted son, Jason, who had been born with spina bifida. In our search for another opportunity to adopt a special needs child, we instead found there was a need for foster parents and had become a state-licensed small family home. In that capacity, we had cared for three other children with spina bifida and also used UCSF Medical Center for our children. Eventually, our path and Alexa's parents' crossed.

When they first contacted us about caring for Alexa, they asked us to adopt her. We suggested they take their time and place her with us first, as a foster placement while they sorted out their feelings. They had her at home for 10 months and loved her very much and we knew it would be a great loss when she was gone. They agreed to that, and on Alexa's first birthday, we brought her home.

In the following months, Alexa continued to suffer recurrent and severe bladder infections, which resulted in multiple hospitalizations. Tests revealed that she had a blocked left urethra and she underwent three surgeries to try to correct this problem. Finally, a vesecostomy was performed, which allowed her urine to drain all of the time through a little stoma. This helped her considerably and the infections stopped.

During that time, I stayed with Alexa at the hospital. At that point, Alexa was a very fearful baby who had just changed families, was constantly being hurt by painful procedures, and was terrified of all of the strangers in her life. Staying in the hospital in San Francisco was what was necessary to bond with this terrified baby and her family. Having the backing of my husband and family made it possible as that left six children to be cared for at home by Harry. By the time she was able to come home, Alexa had become very bonded to us, although she was also still very bonded to her mother. I always knew when her mother would leave us after a visit that if Alexa had a choice, she would cling to her mother.

By her third birthday, Alexa's health and temperament were much improved. She had been with us for almost two years and I felt she was beginning to accept us as her parents and her mother as a wonderful friend we saw when we were in San Francisco, which was pretty often. Jane and I had developed a close friendship in our shared concern for Alexa. It was always heartbreaking to me to watch Jane say good-bye and walk away. However, Jane had said from the beginning that she knew to make this work she could not interfere in our decisions or our family's and Alexa's relationship. Sometimes it was hard not to lean too much on Jane when I was in San Francisco and Alexa was very sick. I had to respect where she was coming from and allow her to let go.

Later that year Alexa underwent surgery in San Francisco for a tethered spinal cord and placement of a wick to drain fluid buildups that were present along her spine. After surgery, this fluid buildup continued to increase and one month later an Arnold Chiari decompression surgery was performed and another wick was placed. This latter surgery was very serious and hard on Alexa. By then she was old enough to let me know that she was very angry with me for allowing the doctors to hurt her again. For a while after surgery her beautiful little face looked as if she had had a stroke for it dropped on one side when she smiled or cried. It hurt so much to watch her go through so much. She could not turn her head and each day when the physical therapist arrived she would scream throughout the visit and be very hard to console for hours after. We held her, talked to her, and loved her for hours.

We tried to find as many fun things to do with Alexa and the other children as possible. It was important not to neglect the other children or our relationship while being so wrapped up in Alexa's needs.

Sometimes it was just a trip to the park, but it seemed so important to have a life outside the doctors' offices. We firmly believe that if you are going to save these little lives, you have to give them a life. Besides Alexa we also had three of our first seven children at home. Tim was 21 years of age and getting ready to go out on his own. Ted was graduating from high school and Jason was 15 years of age. A teenage foster child who had been with us a few months and also had spina bifida was having a hard time adjusting. Rachelle was five years of age but she was and will always be our baby as she was born with a large encephalocele. When it was repaired, much of her little brain had to be removed which left her blind and profoundly impaired.

Another teenage foster child who had been with us for some time had developmental disabilities.

By summer and Alexa's third birthday, she was very much improved and we took our annual camping trip to Hat Creek. This camp was close enough that Harry could still get to work each day. We had a wonderful time and it gave everyone a chance to relax. Also that summer we had plans to remodel the kitchen. To make it easier for Harry to accomplish this task, our oldest daughter Cindy, her two boys who were two and four years of age, myself, and our five youngest children (Robbie, Jason, Bill, Rachelle, and Alexa) went on a trip to Iowa. Of course, everyone thought we were crazy but it worked out fine and we had a wonderful time. We were gone three weeks, went 6,000 miles and stopped to see whatever we wanted. We visited Yellowstone and the Lake of the Ozarks. The kids were great and most important, everyone stayed healthy. Alexa was in the best health she had ever been in. We went with a tent trailer and just had fun. Also that summer, we asked Alexa's parents if we could take guardianship of her. They agreed to that and the process was initiated.

Later that fall, I began to notice Alexa having spells that seemed like breath holding but they happened any time and I was concerned about small seizures. I contacted her pediatrician at UCSF and a sleep study was arranged. When the results of the sleep study turned out to be negative, it was decided that Alexa's spells were a behavior problem stemming from the guardianship issue. This didn't make sense to me or to Jane because we held the same friendship and I didn't believe that at age three, Alexa knew what was happening. We continued to just watch her.

ALEXA'S TRACHEOSTOMY AND EVENTUAL USE OF THE VENTILATOR

A month later, Alexa started having very loud stridorous breathing at night but only when she was asleep. In order for our family doctor to hear her, I tape recorded her in the middle of the night, because on his examination she sounded fine.

In early November, we went to San Francisco where an MRI showed that Alexa had another fluid buildup at the base of the brain.

A laminectomy was scheduled with the hope that this surgery would correct the problem and stop the now frequent "blue spells" and stridorous breathing. Following surgery, however, these symptoms got progressively worse. Alexa had never recovered very well in the hospital and I was so scared. I remember I just kept thinking, "If I just get her out of here she will be okay." There was also a disagreement between the doctors as to how to help her and whether she should remain hospitalized. A new pulmonary doctor had been called in and we were at odds from the beginning. I finally had to ask that the doctor not come back. In the end the neurologist felt it would be okay to try taking her home but sent us for an EEG first. When I returned to Alexa's room to pack, I met the pediatrician who said I could go home but Alexa would not be leaving the hospital. I know now (and probably did then) that she was right, but it was the first time I had ever felt I did not have a choice in Alexa's care. Losing that control was a very frightening experience. I wanted to take Alexa and run because I felt there were worse things still to come and no one really knew what to do for her.

By Thanksgiving, Alexa was still in the hospital and the stridor and "blue spells" were worse. On Thanksgiving Day I took her to a special dinner for families, and it was the first time I had been able to really get her up so we followed dinner with a walk. Upon reentering her room, I began speaking with the nurse. While I was talking, Alexa started into another "blue spell" as I held her. A Code Blue was called and she was taken from me and CPR was started.

When they had finally stabilized Alexa she was moved to ICU. Once she was on continuous oxygen the spells improved but without the oxygen they returned. During this hospitalization we had received our guardianship papers. They had been rushed through, giving me the right to make medical decisions for Alexa. The following morning I overheard Alexa's mom talking to the neurosurgeon, telling him not to do anything to try to save Alexa if she became worse. It was the only time I ever felt threatened by Alexa's mother.

During the week Alexa was in ICU, there were many consultations and different ideas were thrown out as to how to help her. I'm sure from the beginning it was thought a tracheostomy would be needed. From the first mention of a tracheostomy, however, there were conflicting views expressed especially from nurses, respiratory therapists, and others. We were told she would never be able to make any more sounds, so I called Harry to rush down with a tape recorder and record her. He was also having a hard time dealing with all of this from home and not being able to see her. She never talked very much and only really said *dada*, *mama,* and *dog*, but she had a wonderful laugh and made little sounds that let you know exactly what she wanted. From the minute he sat the tape recorder down, she would not make any sounds, we tried everything to get her to talk to us. Finally, Harry had to go home and Alexa and I waited for the day of surgery.

On the morning of the surgery, Alexa's I.V. had to be taken out and a new one started. It is so hard to start an I.V. in Alexa that I asked them to wait till she was in surgery. Later, a resident came and said they had decided to go ahead with the I.V. and again I explained how difficult it was to start an I.V. and asked the resident if I could refuse to let her try till Alexa was in surgery. I was promptly told to leave ICU. As I stood in the hall listening to Alexa scream, I wanted to go in and slap the resident. Finally, after four tries the resident decided she couldn't do it and called her boss in. He assured me he had a special technique. After three more tries they waited until they could do it in surgery. The anger, frustration, and feelings of loss of control concerning our child's care were overwhelming.

After the surgery, Alexa was returned to the Pediatric floor and I was trained how to take care of her. Leaving her at the hospital was never an option we considered but we did have so many questions and fears. We were thankful we were now her guardians because as her state-licensed caregivers, they would not have let us bring her home. She would have remained in the hospital indefinitely, probability for the rest of her life.

As we brought her home shortly before Christmas, we had really mixed feelings. We were so thankful just to have her and to have her out of the hospital; however, we were very concerned about what her quality of life would be. Five days after she had come home from the hospital, Alexa had another "blue spell." After suctioning and getting her color back, I called our family doctor and asked if I should bring her in or change the tracheostomy tube. He said, "Karen, they taught you how to care for her. This is way out of my field." In the end we took her to the emergency room with oxygen. After checking her they sent us home with an antibiotic prescription and told us to fill it if we thought we needed it. That night we had to decide if we could do this by ourselves or were we going to take her back to live at the hospital. We decided God had spared her life, she was our child, and one way or another we would make it work and give her a quality life.

Alexa continued to have "blue spells." On Christmas as we opened presents, she had a spell. We had just found a new pediatrician in Redding to help us and our family doctor. I had had to beg him until he said he would see her because the alternative was to return to San Francisco.

Two days after Christmas, we took Alexa to this pediatrician and he sent us over to the hospital emergency room to get a blood test and sputum culture. While we were there, Alexa had another "spell." I tried to tell the nurses that we couldn't suction her fast enough and to change the tracheostomy tube. Instead, as she lay there blue, they hooked up heart monitors. Luckily, the doctor happened over and was surprised to see us still there. When I suggested to him she needed the trach changed, he asked if I could do it. I told him yes. "Then do it!" he said. With that the nurses threw their hands up and walked away.

A few days later, during a visit to the pediatrician's office Alexa started throwing up and food was coming out the tracheostomy tube as well. She then had a full arrest and as I suctioned in between, the doctor did CPR until his 911 call was answered. She was then admitted to our local hospital with pneumonia.

In the months that followed, Alexa began having many "blue spells" every day and was hospitalized with pneumonia every two months. Slowly, we collected the portable equipment we needed to resuscitate her when we would take her out of the house. This included a portable suction, oxygen, a mist machine, a small suitcase filled with supplies, ambu bags, and a car phone. With Alexa and equipment in tow, we began to venture out. We'd have to resuscitate her at the grocery store and on a street corner but as long as we were equipped it worked the same as if we had kept her home and not allowed her to have a life and join the family.

One day, after we had been home a few months, we found the one-way speaking valve[4] they had sent with us from the hospital. I took it out and remembered someone had said to give it to the speech-language pathologist when we got one. That was still weeks away so I read the enclosed information. A nurse was there and we were pretty good at taking care of a "blue" child by then so we tried it on. Alexa immediately started to make sounds. We were so beside ourselves we called everyone. The first call after Dad went to Jane. We would have called a national press conference if we had known how! Today, Alexa's speech is wonderful and she talks constantly. She even sings! All that might have been lost if it were not for the speaking valve.

That summer we were able to take our annual camping trip because the forest ranger at the camp allowed us to dig a trench in which Harry buried an extension cord from our trailer to the bathroom closet. This way we could use a generator at night to run Alexa's mist machine. We also got a membership to the hospital's helicopter service in case we needed to get her to the hospital. We had a few problems and it was scary but they were handled like they would have been at home and everything went fine. We were a family enjoying all of our children.

Later, after several trips to San Francisco and several tests, it was decided Alexa needed a fundoplication and a feeding tube to stop the reflux which the doctors thought was adding to her problems. I was hesitant but the medical professionals kept asking, "How many times are you going to allow her to get pneumonia before you let us do surgery?" Finally, I gave in because she was getting worse and I didn't know what else to do. During the surgery Alexa had a spell that shook the doctors up quite a bit. We were finally able to take her home again, because this time nursing care would be provided three nights a week via the Far Northern Regional Center. With that in place and because I had demonstrated I could care for her they let us take her home again.

In July of 1991, Alexa's parents agreed to let us adopt Alexa. We began to receive AAP (Aid to Adoptive Parents), which helped. We were having a very difficult time keeping up financially.

The next year was a repeat of the first with Alexa's medical condition remaining pretty much the same. Alexa was now five years old, and the school that had helped us with our other children agreed to let her into regular kindergarten three days a week accompanied by an EMT (emergency medical technician). The EMT was hired by the school to transport and stay with Alexa. She loved school so much and everyone was her friend. They did have to call 911 a few times and once they transported her to the emergency room, but she did fine. We live pretty close to the school and I could get there fast. I also acquired a pager.

Our family doctor, who had helped me through so much, retired in early 1992. His medical group refused to take his Medi-Cal patients and we had an extremely difficult time finding another doctor. This was because the doctors I found either saw only adults or did not take Medi-Cal patients. Even the residency program would not see our children.

By March, Alexa's spells were so bad that when you used the ambu bag it was hard to get a response. We were having great difficulty bringing her back. We seemed to have run out of doctors and ideas on how to help her. Finally, I picked a pulmonary doctor out of the Chico phone book, 60 miles away, and called. I found a new pediatric pulmonary doctor was coming from San Francisco and would also go to Redding. I got an appointment.

This doctor had us take Alexa to San Francisco for tests. Our overnight stay turned into 26 days. It was decided that Alexa needed to be on a ventilator at night. Again I felt I was getting mixed messages. I received the most help from a lady who stopped by to see another patient. She also had a tracheostomy tube and had used a ventilator at night for a number of years. She was so reassuring.

Finally, after many days in which California Children's Services (CCS) and Medi-Cal fought over which ventilator and humidification system they could afford for Alexa, we were able to bring Alexa home. The ventilator they sent us home with had a small cup to collect the water that builds up in the tubing. If you fell asleep and didn't empty it fast enough there was nothing to keep it from shooting water right up into Alexa's lungs. After a few sleepless nights when we didn't have a nurse, I thought of away to drill a tiny hole in the cup and attach a mist machine bag to collect the water. This worked beautifully and did not change any of the settings, but it wasn't anything I dared share with anyone. It is still working fine.

Again I had learned a lot about the fear of not getting her out of the hospital. Now, I would do anything to avoid having her admitted, because of the fear that once they are admitted you may not get them out. Far Northern also allowed us one more night of nursing. That gave us four nights of nursing coverage.

Now that Alexa was on a ventilator, summer and camping held even more challenges. We ended up buying a bigger trailer and placing the ventilator on a table inside. The ventilator improved Alexa's health more than we ever thought possible. The blue spells stopped and we were off for a great summer. The company Harry worked for was sold and he was off work, so we visited everyone from Southern California to northern Oregon. Instead of burying the extension cord at the campground as we had done before, Harry put in an electric line and the Forest Service hooked it up. Now there is electricity at the handicapped spot for anyone who needs it for medical equipment.

In January, our Medi-Cal waiver finally went into effect, three years after the trach. I had anxiety attacks every day before we went on it. It is another program that instead of asking, "How can we help," says, "Do it our way or your child could be removed for her health and safety." Where were they for three difficult years?

Through it all, we have found that the stress we experience is not with the children but with all of the agencies we deal with. Our lives are not our own and the only way to sit back and enjoy our children is to leave home. We appreciate very much all the kindness and help we are shown and the chance to have Alexa and all the children in our lives.

WHAT IS A TRACHEOSTOMY'S IMPACT ON LIFE?

FEARS: After having just seen Alexa have a Code Blue in my arms, nothing else could have been more terrifying. As we began to talk with the doctors about a trach, it was an overwhelming thought and her quality of life was certainly a concern. She was in the pediatric intensive care unit (PICU) for a week, on oxygen, before the surgery was done. During that time, we talked with a lot of professionals including doctors, nurses, respiratory therapists, etc. We got so many conflicting views and comments. Most of them were very negative. "Oh, how sad she will never talk," or "She is so beautiful, don't let them do that." Alexa has beautiful features and somehow the message we got was that because she was beautiful, she couldn't be sick. It made it so hard to go through with the trach. We felt maybe there was something else since there was so much disagreement. Of course, there wasn't, and we had to close out the comments and trust our doctors.

EQUIPMENT: When the subject of equipment was explained, we imagined from the description that it was so large we would have to build an equipment area outside of Alexa's room, then run the oxygen and mist tubes through the wall to her. Pictures would have helped a lot. When the equipment did arrive, we were so relieved to see it all fit very easily. The comments nurses made who stopped by the house to see Alexa were, "We hardly even noticed the equipment because her room, her cute room, is what you notice when you walk in."

We were also able to get everything we needed, oxygen, a nebulizer, etc., in portable equipment. The nebulizer for mist plugged into the van's cigarette lighter. I got a small case for supplies and we got a car phone so I could get help if needed. An ambu bag was always close by.

MEDICAL HELP: It was very difficult to find local doctors willing to help. We had a wonderful family doctor who was willing to work with the doctors in San Francisco but readily admitted he didn't feel he had the expertise to handle all of Alexa's needs. We luckily had a lot of experience with sick children but we were not doctors and nurses. We did feel we were pretty much on our own and needed to take control ourselves if we were going to keep Alexa at home. Finally we knew we couldn't leave her in the hospital in San Francisco and I couldn't stay with her, so we would have to learn to deal with her problems.

Having nurses come to the house was a difficult experience for me to get used to. When I get a nurse I can really talk to and enjoy having, I really appreciate it. I am pretty particular about my house being clean and staying organized. With our gang, it is just what works best. So, often I was picking up after the nurses or rushing to get ready for one to stop by. It seemed when Alexa needed help, the nurse was taking care of her and I was cleaning and taking care of the other children. I really wanted to sit down, hold Alexa, and care for her.

EXPERIENCES: There were therapy and appointments we had to take her to and trips back to San Francisco, so with the portable equipment, we started going out. If she had a "blue spell" we took care of her and waited for her to feel better with some oxygen on, then you finished what you were doing. Now that she is better, it is hard to believe we made it through two years of that. Several times, I called 911, but when I was the one who best knew what she needed, they usually had me take care of her. It was the backup I needed when the stress was too much. Sometimes when we called 911, she had been having spells repeatedly that day and would end up being admitted to the hospital with pneumonia.

COMMUNICATION: The one-way valve[4] was a real turning point. It not only helped her have speech, which was a miracle, it helped her breathing and swallowing. With the valve on she can swallow her food and it no longer comes out her trach as fast as it went into her mouth. She also seemed to breath easier and needed less suctioning. She panics if it comes off for a minute. That is hard during hospitalizations. Nurses and therapists don't understand what it is or how much Alexa needs it. They didn't think she could get air through it. I don't know how they thought she breathed with it. After I would explain it, I would come back and find it had been off for hours. This was very hard on Alexa.

Watching her start to talk was such a lift to us. The valve allows her to talk and use her hands at the same time. The public hardly notices Alexa has a trach because her speech is so good.

RECREATION: Camping became our release valve. It has helped us hang on to some form of normal life. We have a Golden Access Passport from the U.S. Forest Service. It cuts the cost of staying in federal campgrounds and national parks in half. With a trailer, we can carry all the supplies and have a kitchen, bathroom, etc.

With so many people in and out of the house, appointments,

meetings, it is really hard to just listen to and enjoy the kids. Leaving home saves my sanity and the kids get to enjoy life and have a break from all they go through. We can sleep in a little, take our time getting dressed, go fishing, play games, take walks, and visit. I always enjoy riding in the car listening to them talk to one another. I marvel at their imaginations. There are no interruptions.

At night we sleep right across from Alexa and I can open my eyes and see how she is doing. With the ventilator alarm and the apnea monitor, I feel she is safe. We have invented a better cup to collect the water that builds up in the vent tubing and now we don't have to worry about her drowning if the small cup fills too quickly.

SCHOOL: Alexa attends a regular public school kindergarten class. Before the Medi-Cal waiver took effect, the school district hired an EMT to go with her. It worked real well because EMTs are into emergencies and act quickly without a lot of supervision. It was also much less expensive than a nurse costing the district about $7.00 per hour.

When the waiver started, Medi-Cal insisted the great EMT we had be replaced with an LVN. Alexa was very attached to her aide and it was really hard on her. The cost more than tripled. We were able to get a wonderful LVN and that has helped a lot, but I have found many of the nurses we have had are used to working in a hospital setting with a lot of backup and aren't as comfortable in an emergency. I feel Medi-Cal would save a lot of money and maybe provide better care with a well-trained EMTs for trach-ventilator dependent patients.

HOW IS ONE TREATED WITH A TRACHEOSTOMY OR VENTILATOR DEPENDENCY?

LEGAL: Alexa was first placed with us as a foster child. We were a state- licensed small family home. This license did not allow catheterization, tube feedings, or any other medical procedures. We had gotten around this in the past because our children with spina bifida were older and we were just "supervising." By the time Alexa came, there was a little leeway because of our experience.

When Alexa began developing more serious problems, her

parents gave us guardianship which allowed us to care for her. Without the guardianship, we would not have been able to bring her home from the hospital after the tracheostomy. Luckily, we had already started the guardianship procedure before her hospitalization and it was rushed through and a copy was faxed to me in San Francisco.

I see little children who spend months in hospitals because of these regulations. Alexa would have had to wait for an opening in an intermediate care facility-developmental disability nursing (ICF-DDN) facility. With her "blue spells," I doubt she would have ever left the hospital.

HOSPITALS: Now that Alexa has a ventilator, she has to go to intensive care if she is admitted to our local hospital for anything. This is the same ventilator that goes in the trailer camping.

HOME: It was very hard when Alexa first came home. It consumed every minute of every day and night. Now, it almost seems like we are back to a pretty normal life.

When she first came home the medical center worried if we would have enough help and they talked about a Medi-Cal waiver. Far Northern Regional Center finally agreed to give some help while we waited for the waiver, so we were able to get Alexa home. We had three nights of nursing and 68 hours a trimester of respite so we were pretty much on our own. The first Medi-Cal worker who came by almost a year after we were home was very difficult to deal with. She was way overdressed and very intimidating.

When we brought the ventilator home, the Regional Center gave us one more night of nursing so we had a nurse four nights a week. In January of 1993, the Medi-Cal finally went through. It has language which seems very threatening and I had many anxiety attacks the week before Alexa went on it. I really did not want to go through with it, but the other agencies who were paying for services threatened to withdraw their services if I didn't take the waiver.

SCHOOL: When I first tried to put Alexa in a county preschool we met a lot of opposition and it would have taken a court battle to get her in. Once she turned five, however, our school district was very supportive. There was some concern for the other children in her class if Alexa had a spell at school, and she did a couple of times when 911 had to be called but only one parent ever expressed any concern. Alexa first went to kindergarten three days a week and repeated kindergarten this year going on a regular schedule. She is doing well and is in the top reading group.

GENERAL PUBLIC: They have been wonderful to her. Our only problem is getting people to understand that we are a family and the children are ours and we are not a group home. Once in a great while someone says something or asks a question that is upsetting to the kids. It is like they think the kids can't hear or understand.

HOW DOES ONE ACCEPT THE INITIAL TRAUMA, AND HOW DOES A FAMILY COPE?

Our first concern was whether Alexa live. Then, how would she live and how would we care for the other children and care for her. We just had to take it one day at a time. I think it was our experience as older parents that helped a lot. We had raised six natural children, four of whom had medical problems. Cindy, had been burned when she was found and had third-degree burns over 60% of her body. Harry had uncontrollable grand mal seizures from six months to six years. Tim and Ted had been born with bilateral cleft lips and palates. Ted also had a cranial stenosis which had to also be repaired. Cindy is now married with two boys and works in nursing. Harry is a graduate of Cal Poly, married with two sons and working in agriculture. Tim, an auctioneer, is as good as any auctioneer and has no sign of a speech problem. Ted is married, has a son, and is also working in agriculture.

Our adopted son, Jason, had been through a lot due to complications of spina bifida and was doing well. We had also cared for four other children with spina bifida and our little Rachelle who has encephalocele and is profoundly disabled. Two of our foster children who had spina bifida went back home as young adults and two died suddenly from Arnold Chiari complications.

This experience helped us to sit back and look at things from a little different perspective than most families would have. We knew what our fears had been with the other children and how most of it turned out OK. Our marriage had also survived and was solid. Harry and I see things pretty much the same way.

We already knew how to use the system somewhat to get what our children needed, and how to look for more help if things aren't working out and hopefully not burn our bridges behind us. Our family is pretty well known and we have already dealt with most of the people we have to deal with now.

Still our greatest fear is the loss of control we sometimes feel over our lives, our family's life, and what we believe to be in Alexa's best interest.

FINANCIAL SUPPORT SYSTEM

As a foster placement, we received the Regional Center rate of $1,200.00 a month. As Alexa's guardians the rate dropped to the SSI rate of $700.00. As an adoptive placement we received AAP (aide to Adoptive Parents) and we were allowed to keep her SSI which dropped to $490.00 with the adoption. Last year's hospital bill for 26 days was $76,000.00, so it is very cost-effective for the state to have Alexa home and they help. I do expect there will be some cuts this year.

We feel very fortunate to have the help. We know many natural families don't get any help. I believe there needs to be more help to all families (natural, adoptive, and foster) so these children can be at home and as many as possible out of institutions and hospitals. We are OK now, but at one point we did almost go bankrupt trying to care for these children and not getting the financial help we needed.

Insurance is not an option for our children because they have a preexisting condition when we get them. This leaves us at the mercy of a Medi-Cal and CCS system that is very costly and difficult to get through. It is a constant battle to get the kids needs met and we must travel 400 miles to San Francisco to get most of their medical care.

When our family doctor retired, I went door to door, first with a little resume of the kids' medical needs, then with the resume with a cute picture on it, and finally with the girls along. None of the family doctors or pediatricians wanted Medi-Cal or preexisting conditions, not even the residency program at our local hospital. At last a pediatrician I knew took them when I was at my wit's end.

EQUIPMENT

The one thing I can think of that has helped me the most is a shoe bag. I used to put everything in a box. Then I used a suitcase. In an emergency, especially if I was alone, I had a hard time finding what I needed. Finally, I took a hanging shoe bag and put a Velcro fastener at the top of each section so I could close them and prevent small things from falling out. In each pocket I put different items: tubing, suction catheters, saline vials, trach ties, wipes, small baby shampoo, tissue, etc. Then I fastened two long pieces of ribbon to the outside so I could roll the bag up with an extension cord of several plugs in the middle and tie the ribbons to keep it together. When I reached the motel room, I opened my bag and hung it on the closet door. In an emergency I could find whatever I needed fast. It was also easy to check what I had used and replenish it when I got home.

The other thing we learned was to ask a lot of questions about equipment, so we got the smallest portable equipment possible. This makes it a lot easier to take Alexa out from the beginning.

ADVICE TO PARENTS

This is really hard, because you have a hard job ahead, but it is also rewarding. Try to keep a sense of humor. It is not easy, but you will find you get further and the professionals will open up to you. It seems they feel very threatened when you lose it and they close up, making it hard for you to get what you need for your child. Stay firm, though, if you think you're right or something is being overlooked. You really do know your child best and you have listened to everything that has been said.

Take someone with you to any important appointments. Talk to that person before the appointment, exchange ideas, then write them down. After the appointment you will have help remembering everything that was said and you can sit down and rehash it again.

Go to as many training sessions and workshops as you can find, even if it is only a related matter. Not only will it give you a lot of good information, but it will empower you. You will have a lot more confidence in yourself and you will feel more like an equal partner in your child's treatment. It really helps you to be more professional and that demands respect, even where there are disagreements.

I find a lot of workshops as a foster parent, but you can also find a lot through your neighborhood school, public health agencies, a college newspaper, etc. I have also met good friends that way, and you will find others that share your concerns.

Be careful not to isolate yourself or the child with the problem. It will really eat away at you if you are alone.

Have fun. Get out even if it is only to the front yard on a nice day. So much of what has to be done is not fun. Be inventive and you'll find a way to get that mist tubing to go just a little further. Sometimes it is so much work and takes so much planning it doesn't seem worth it, but if the care and stress become all there is and you can't enjoy your child, then it will really wear you down.

Camping has been a sanity saver for us. We have a travel trailer that works well for us. Once everything is arranged it just stays set up, not like going in and out of motels, relatives' homes, etc. The vent goes on the table, we load the kids in the van in their chairs, and off we go.

Take care of yourself and your spouse. It is so easy to drift apart. Find a way to be alone together, even for a little while, visit with one another, and hold on to your dreams.

Don't Give Up, Be Persistent!

by Julia Almand, R.N.

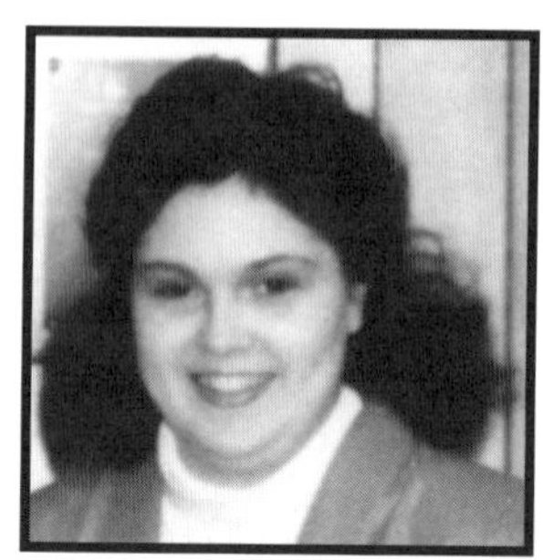

Julia Almand is a registered nurse who worked in a respiratory care unit prior to developing myasthenia gravis. She was tracheostomized and ventilator dependent and is now decannulated.

I have myasthenia gravis. Last winter they weren't able to control it and as a result I went into respiratory failure and had to be ventilated. I was hospitalized first in Arkansas where I live but due to my need for a special treatment, I was transferred to a hospital in Dallas for about five weeks. Originally, I was intubated about two weeks before they did the tracheostomy. At the time of the tracheostomy, a regular cuffed tracheostomy tube was placed. It wasn't until later that I got the talking tracheostomy tube.[5]

Having a tracheostomy is very hard on your self-esteem. I am an R.N. and I have worked in a respiratory care unit and I always said, "I'd never have a trach." I guess I can now be more sympathetic and more understanding, and I can see how the person on the other side of the bed feels. I didn't want a tracheostomy because of the cosmetic effect. I thought "My gosh, they're going to cut a hole in my neck and I'm going have this big thing in my throat. My kids are going to see it and it's going to look ugly and horrendous." That was very difficult for me.

The tracheostomy wasn't an emergency procedure but they didn't give me a choice. There was really nothing else to do because I had been intubated so long. I wasn't at the point where I could prepare because I was really sick at the time and I was kind of going with the flow of everything. When I woke up with my tracheostomy and looked into the mirror I was really upset. My nurse bought me a scarf to put around my neck so that if my kids came, they wouldn't see the trach. I was very concerned about them seeing it. They were 5 and 6 years old at the time and when they did see it they had lots of questions. I just explained that it helped me to breathe and that it would help mommy get better. They were very accepting of it and wanted to touch it and look at it. I tried to be open with them and not hide it, so they wouldn't be afraid. When I first got my tracheostomy it took me a while to accept that I had it and to deal with it. *I had to deal with it.* There wasn't anything else I could do. I could either resent it and fight it and not get better or accept it and try to get better. Because I was a nurse people thought I should accept it easier. The nurses would get frustrated with me and I with them when I was trying to communicate. I was kept in the ICU, and my husband, my children, and all my family and friends were 3 hours away. My mom was the only one with me. She could only come in during visiting hours. We had a system worked out where we could communicate, but I had a real hard time communicating with the nurses. Part of it could have been my attitude because I was resenting the trach.

Sometimes hospital staff have a difficult time interacting appropriately with a trach patient and react with, "Oh no, I've got a patient with a trach, that means I've got to do trach care," and not everybody just loves to do trach care. If it was oozing a lot or if it got infected, they would come in to clean it and would make comments like, "Ewwwe, this is really gross" or "this is really nasty," and it makes you feel awful. When I was finally transferred back to the hospital in Arkansas where I had worked, the nurses were a lot more understanding, but that could have been because they were my friends.

I had the cuffed trach for about two weeks and then I got the talking trach tube.[5] I was on a ventilator all that time. I could communicate with my mom because she bought me a Magna Doodle (writing board) which I used a lot. I also used hand motions, and later my mom was able to read my lips. She couldn't always read my lips, but I would eventually get the message across. I communicated with the nurses by trying to talk because that was the easiest thing to do, to move my lips. They would get frustrated sometimes and then wouldn't even try. Mother got to where she would just leave me the Magna Doodle and I would try to write to them. I couldn't write that well and they couldn't understand it a lot of times, and so they got to a point where they would let my mother stay in the ICU to interpret.

It was the speech-language pathologist at the Dallas hospital who told me that they wanted to put the talking trach tube[5] in and that I was a good candidate for it. She asked me if I wanted it, and I said, "Yes!" She had to push the doctors to do it. They didn't really want to do it at first. She kept asking them until they changed their minds. The doctors didn't want to put it in because they just didn't want to fool with it, that's my personal opinion. I don't know because I was in and out of it a lot. The speech-language pathologist brought the talking tracheostomy tube to me, told me how it would work and that I would be able to talk. My biggest concern was that I had been in the hospital a long time and I was away from my children. I wanted to talk to my children. I wanted them to hear Mommy. Mother would hold the phone up to my ear and tell them to talk to me, but I couldn't talk back. Before I got the talking trach tube,[5] I would cry because I was so frustrated.

At first, it was hard to learn how to use the talking tracheostomy tube.[5] I guess that is because I'd gone so long without speaking. The speech-language pathologist gave me some exercises to work on and the next day I was up and going. I could speak words, but I didn't have enough power to speak whole sentences. The first day I had the talking trach tube[5] you could understand about 50% of what I said, but the next day you could understand 100%. It wasn't my natural voice and so I just told my kids that Mommy sounded like Robo Cop or Daffy Duck, which was something that they could understand. I could talk to them on the phone and that was wonderful.

There were adjustments with the talking trach tube.[5] First, I had to remember to put my finger over the air port. By the time I got the talking trach tube[5] I was able to move my hands and my arms pretty good. At first my mom would cover the port so I could communicate with her. I would bang on the rail or something to try and get her attention so she would know to cover the air port which enabled me to talk. Another adjustment was that the trach had to stay hooked up to an air source at the wall, and it had to be hooked up to a humidifier. Consequently, it wasn't very portable. When they would get me up in a chair, they had to disconnect the air source because the tubing wasn't long enough, so then I couldn't communicate. I didn't have a portable air source with my wheelchair either. Without an air source I couldn't utilize the talking trach tube,[5] so when I was out of bed I had to use hand signals and the Magna Doodle to communicate. In general, I was just so relieved to talk that I didn't mind the air source. The biggest problem was that the nurses would sometimes forget to hook the air source back up, the respiratory therapists would forget after they had suctioned, or they would let the humidifier run dry and it wouldn't work very well. It took us a while to figure out about the humidifier. My mother and I were really frustrated because sometimes the humidifier would work and sometimes it wouldn't. When we got somebody to fill it up with water we noticed that every time it was full of water it would work and when it was empty it wouldn't.

After five weeks in Dallas, I was transferred back to the hospital in Arkansas where I had been originally. I was the first patient in that hospital to have a talking trach tube.[5] My mother was actually the one who showed the nurses how to clean it because she learned at Dallas before we left. She showed the nurses how to clean it because it is different from a regular trach. The nurses had to get used to cleaning it. The port has to be rinsed out with water and flushed. The first couple of times they did it, water would go back into my throat and I would feel like I was choking, and that really scared me because I was thinking, "Oh my gosh, they're going to drown me." It didn't scare me enough to not want to use it though. I was just so relieved to talk. I probably would have suffered through anything.

I was gradually weaned from the ventilator. I was actually taken off the vent on Mother's Day! I had been off the vent a couple of days when they changed the talking trach tube[5] to a fenestrated tracheostomy tube. They took that trach out at the very end of May.

Looking back on the experience, I'd say I have gained a whole new perspective on things. The talking trach tube,[5] compared to a regular trach, was ten times better because it enabled me to communicate. I didn't realize what a big factor that was with my patients until I had been there myself. When you can't communicate it affects a great many things because you can't communicate what you need or what you want. As for socialization, you can't talk to anybody. You can listen to somebody talk to you, but you really can't carry on a conversation. I think the hospital staff acted differently because I couldn't communicate. They would just come in and do their thing and they didn't think they had to talk to me or try to communicate with me. It's just like you are a body. It made me mad because I kept thinking, "I'm here!! Don't ignore me!" I was mad until I got the talking trach tube.[5] Once I was able to communicate with them everything was fine. A lot of my frustration went away because I could tell them what I needed or what I wanted or what was hurting. I only wish that when they had first put a trach in me, they would have put in a talking trach tube![5] The first thing I said when I was able to speak was, "When can I go home?" My neurologist in Dallas asked to speak to the speech-language pathologist on the third day that I had the talking trach tube.[5] He asked, "Why in the world did you get this? All she wants to know is when she can leave!" I was used to being really involved in talking to the doctor and finding out what's going on and how much longer or what did he think. You can't communicate with them that well when you have the trach.

One of the most difficult aspects of being in the hospital is trying to stay motivated. My mother motivated me a lot because there were times that I wasn't doing well. For instance, while in the hospital, I got pneumonia. I was resigned to just lie there and take it, when my mother said, "You've got two kids at home, you've got to get better and you've got to try and fight this." The hope of getting home to my children was motivating. Although I was still on a ventilator, the doctors in Dallas decided to transfer me back to Arkansas because they thought I would do better seeing my family and my friends.

When I got back to the hospital in Arkansas (it was actually the one in which I had worked as a nurse) I explained to my nurses and friends how frustrating having a trach was and how really hard it was on your self-esteem. I wanted to see my friends but I didn't want them to see me. It was the same way with my family. I wanted to see my brothers and sisters but I didn't because I didn't want them to see me lying there with the trach. I never told anybody they couldn't come and see me. I just told the nurses how frustrating it was.

I experienced depression, probably the most when I was in Dallas. It got better once I could communicate. Communication was the biggest thing. It's like you're isolated in your own little world and everything else is going on around you. The ability to communicate allows you to feel like you are a part of everything else. Being able to communicate helped alleviate some of my depression but not all of it. I think that it would have been wonderful if someone had given me concrete goals or something to strive for, but I didn't get any of that. My family coped with the whole situation probably a lot better than I did. I think it was hard on all of them, especially my husband. He got through it with support from his family. Family was extremely important in my recovery. For those patients without a family to provide support, I would encourage them not to give up even though I know this is easier said than done sometimes.

I think counseling would have been very helpful when I first got a trach. You need it for your self-esteem because you feel depressed. When you realize what you look like and that you might have it forever, it's very depressing. When I was in Dallas, they had a chaplain come and visit me, and I said, "I don't need you." Looking back now, I don't know what kind of counseling I would recommend but I think that there is a need for some. The chaplain would come by every day just to check on me. I guess the nurses could tell when I was down and they would try to spend some extra time with me. However, I was a nurse too, so I felt that I knew what was going on and thought I could handle it.

I also found that it's difficult to know how to make other people feel comfortable with a trach or ventilator. If you don't mention it and act like it's not there, it's very awkward. It was more comfortable with people acknowledging it than with everybody ignoring it and trying to pretend it wasn't there. I would rather them ask questions and talk about it. To walk in a room where someone is on a trach and hooked up to a ventilator, with I.V.'s, is really scary and intimidating. My mom showed my youngest little boy all the equipment the first time he came to see me and encouraged him to ask questions so he wouldn't be scared or intimidated by it. It really is important to encourage family and friends to talk about it, look at it and ask questions so they won't be intimidated by it all.

In closing, I would like to offer a few suggestions for hospital staff, families and tracheostomized individuals to consider. First, I want to stress to hospital staff the importance of remembering that trached or ventilator dependent patients who can't talk are "there."

They may not look like they're "there" but they are! Even if you think that they can't communicate back with you, go ahead and talk to them. Tell them what the weather's like outside or tell them what's going on. If nothing else, just tell them about your morning, especially when you are doing patient care. When giving them their bath and changing their sheets, talk to them, don't ignore them and make them feel like they're a slab of meat. Sometimes that's how I felt because the staff would come in and do their business and not ever say a word. Next, I would remind families not to be scared of the trach or the ventilator and to ask questions. The more you know, the less fear you have. Also, try to be supportive of your family member. There were times when I just needed to be by myself and there were times that I needed somebody, even if they weren't doing anything but just sitting in the room. It was good to just know that somebody else was there with you. Last of all, my advice to trach patients is to try and communicate with others. Don't give up easily. Be persistent!

Learning to Live...On Life Support

by Lori A. Hinderer

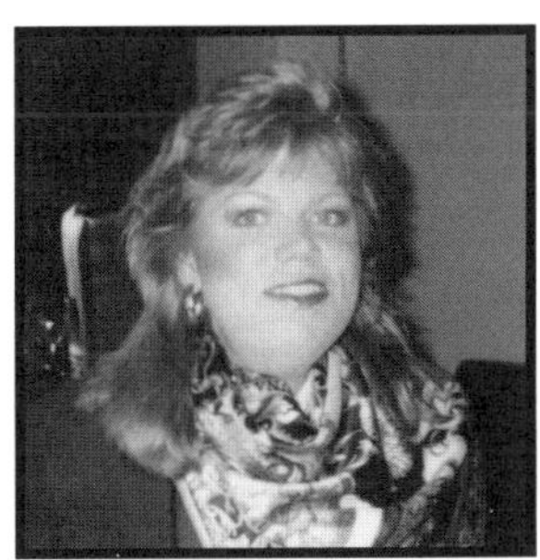

Lori A. Hinderer has muscular dystrophy and manages her own business, Ability 2000. *She lectures nationally and internationally and writes articles concerning issues for physically challenged individuals.*

It is said that nothing stays the same, and so it is true of life. Due to muscular dystrophy since birth, physical and emotional changes are a constant for me. So often, acceptance meant implementing creative alternatives to compensate for my muscle deterioration. For instance, when I could no longer walk, I turned to ceramics and drawing, or when I could no longer pick up the telephone, I used a headset. But when I could no longer breathe, my resiliency waned. I felt angry, confused, and unprepared. By age 30, people are making decisions about their career, family, or future; few must decide whether to live or die.

Yet, in June of 1990, I faced such a choice. After an emergency intubation due to pneumonia, three weeks in intensive care, and trial weaning periods, my options narrowed: either undergo a tracheotomy and use a ventilator or die. Just the thought of "life-support" conjured negative connotations. How would I speak, look, work, socialize; essentially "LIVE" again?

Despite all concerns, however, I knew for certain I loved life and somehow knew that challenges would be compensated for. And while my life literally turned upside down, I have journeyed beyond my wildest dreams. Since my tracheostomy and ventilator dependence, I have traveled extensively, spoken at numerous respiratory conferences, and met ventilator assisted individuals worldwide. It is because of my enhanced quality of life and experiences while using a ventilator that I hope to share some insight on learning to "live" with life support. I will address important issues, fears, and changes I confronted and how I integrated the ventilator into my life.

First, quality of life while using a ventilator is a common concern. When my doctor said I needed a tracheostomy and ventilator to live, I envisioned spending the rest of my life in a hospital bed at home while hooked up to a machine, never leaving the house, talking, or working again. If that really were the case, perhaps one's quality of life would be impaired. My doctor, however, felt strongly about quality of life, assuring me those fears could be overcome.

Fear of not communicating my needs, however, frightened me most. I felt like a nonperson. Nurses often talked among themselves as though I wasn't present and many were frustrated when I spelled my needs into their hand. Some respiratory therapists simply walked into the room, making vent adjustments without alerting me. Gratefully, my doctor introduced me to the one-way speaking valve.[4] Almost immediately, I was speaking as well as before, if not better, enabling me to have control over my life, resume work, and socialize again.

For me, choosing life support was the right choice even though it meant many adjustments and added responsibilities. Due to the rapid progression of my disease, I already needed full-time assistance prior to my tracheostomy. Still, I was concerned about the additional work imposed on my personal assistant who became well versed on the mechanics of the ventilator and circuit hook-ups, and was instructed on trach care, trach changes, and proper suctioning. My caregiver's knowledge is significant to maintaining independence.

In addition to learning vent and trach care, transfers had to be adapted. My assistant converted from the old "bear hug" lift, which was impossible with the trach in the way, to the "bride" technique. I, in turn, had to realize I could breathe for short periods while being lifted into bed or onto the toilet and not panic when disconnected.

Besides lifting, bathing required some changes, too. For some time, I sponge bathed and shampooed with an inflatable tray while in bed. Later I was told tub bathing was possible if the trach area was protected from water with a bib. The bib I use is just one of the products I developed and sell. With regard to dressing, I purchase high-necked shirts and cut out a slit for around the trach. Another important wardrobe addition has been scarves. This simple adaptation has afforded me more self-esteem because my hosing and trach are unnoticed.

Next, I wanted a nonhospital home environment that required little modification. A stand with two shelves was purchased and sits next to my bed. During the day, a curtain conceals the suction machine, gloves, and catheters on the shelves. At night, the top shelf is used to put the ventilator on.

Having reliable home health care is also vital. My company offers 24-hour service, many branch offices (helpful when traveling out of state), and professional respiratory therapists who take care of ventilator maintenance, supplies, and any needs.

Freedom of mobility is another factor in maintaining an active lifestyle. At first, it was hard to imagine how my 45-pound LP-6 ventilator was going to fit onto my wheelchair. Now, my ventilator is simply a part of me, and wherever I go it goes too. This ease I attribute to the medical company that restructured my electric wheelchair via the LaBac system before I left the hospital. A sliding tray holds the ventilator and batteries, allowing mobility with little inconvenience. When going out, I always carry a bag on the back of my wheelchair containing life essential items, that is, a portable suction machine, gloves, catheters, and ambu (resuscitator) bag.

Another concern was travel. Since my driver couldn't leave me to get help in the event of any van problems, a cellular car telephone was the answer, offering tremendous peace of mind. It is also the reason vacationing in Orlando, Florida, and Myrtle Beach, South Carolina, was possible. Besides the car phone, I take emergency numbers (including my home health care branch offices), an extra ventilator, and batteries. The ventilator can also be plugged into the cigarette lighter with a special adapter.

But in August of 1991, a business trip beckoned me to Las Vegas. Flying was suggested because arriving there in three hours seemed more sensible than days. With much planning, I ventured into another seemingly impossible territory: air travel with a ventilator. Six airplane trips later, including one international flight (for a medical conference on home mechanical ventilation), proved travel by plane is feasible. To help other vent users wanting to fly, I am currently compiling an airline guide and have written a couple of articles on the subject.

In conclusion, many initial fears and perceptions of ventilator dependency, like having quality of life, receiving good home health services, and changing my lifestyle, disappeared through education and experience. In fact, I have accomplished more since my tracheostomy than ever. Besides a better feeling of well-being, I attribute my success to having a positive attitude, supportive caregiver, strong family network, a marvelous doctor, and acceptance. As the Praying Hands Prayer states, it's also "having the courage to accept the things I cannot change."

When I think about visiting thc Eiffel Tower, cruising along a sandy beach, and meeting ventilator users, doctors, and respiratory therapists from around the world, it's hard to envision being on life support; that's why I like to look at my ventilator as supporting life. No one should let the ventilator stop them from enjoying life!

Desire Was the Mother of Invention

by David Muir

David Muir was the inventor of the Passy-Muir tracheostomy speaking valve. A quadriplegic with muscular dystrophy, he wrote this article, which was published prior to his death in 1990.

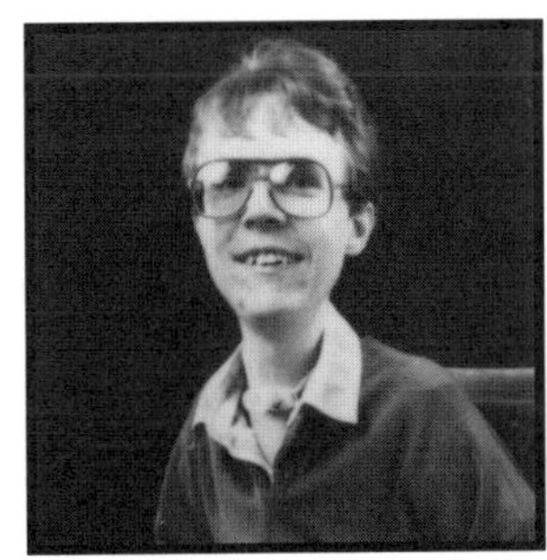

In February 1984, I suffered a respiratory arrest. I had just completed a tough semester and was starting another. This period was very difficult because it seemed as though no matter how much sleep I got at night, I was exhausted in the morning. Apparently, the arrest was coming on for a month, but I wasn't aware of how serious the sleepiness was.

One day, my mom decided to let me sleep in because I was so tired; she planned to do some shopping while my grandmother stayed with me. My mom told me later that just as she was closing the door, she had a feeling that something was not quite right with me. My mom discovered me. I was blue and barely breathing so she pushed the Medic-Alert box. The paramedics arrived about ten minutes later. They intubated me and rushed me to the hospital.

A day or two later, I woke up. The first thing I noticed was a room full of balloons and my family all around the bed. It was a strange but reassuring sight. I was wondering what was I doing here and why I couldn't talk. My mouth was incredibly dry and my nose and throat were sore from being intubated. I became painfully aware of the importance of speech when I wasn't able to communicate even the simplest of needs. I remained optimistic. After all, how long could this last?

We went through several different methods of communication. We tried charades; we tried going through every letter of the alphabet; and I tried using a list of commonly used phrases. Although these methods were adequate, they sure were maddening. I was intubated for a few days and I wasn't exchanging gases adequately enough. It was decided that a tracheostomy was necessary. It was definitely not what I wanted.

A funny thing happened on the way to surgery, at least if you don't really believe Dr. Welby. I was given a local and, after a few minutes, two doctors came up to the gurney. One of them was a short intern who needed to use a step stool just to reach me, which was bad enough, but then he started to make a horizontal incision as is done for children. Luckily, the other doctor was paying attention and stepped in and did the incision vertically and the tracheostomy was completed smoothly.

A friend, who had been trached a few months before, was kind enough to come by and offer some advice about living with a trach. I left the hospital on a hopeful note. When I got home, however, I became very depressed and angry because I wasn't able to wean myself from the ventilator. I tried to plug my trach, but I just didn't have the strength.

I've always felt that I was indestructible. Then my respiratory arrest shook me to my foundation. I felt betrayed, angry, and bitter. How could this happen? What had I done to deserve this? I had accepted that I was not able to walk, I had accepted that I had lost arm strength after an operation to correct a curvature of my spine, but I felt that I couldn't take any more. I became more and more withdrawn as it seemed my world had ended. I lost interest in everything—family, friends, even food and personal comfort. I had awful thoughts of suicide. Life became merely an existence that I had been imprisoned in.

Even though I was sinking into an abyss of despair, something in me was not ready to give up. I said to myself, "Wait a minute! You've never given up this easily before and you're not going to this time. There has to be a way around this problem." These thoughts became my theme for three agonizing months.

A couple of months went by before the idea came to me. One night, I noticed a valve in my ventilator circuit. This was a one-way valve designed to allow an extra breath to be taken between the inspiration and closed on exhalation. All I needed was to take this valve and adapt it to fit the hub of the inner cannula of my trach. My valve would allow me to breathe through the trach and then the air would be forced up through my vocal cords and nasal passages. I explained my idea to a psychologist I was seeing. She told a friend who knew Dr. Victor Passy.

I contacted Dr. Passy at UCI and told him of my idea. He was interested enough to invite me to his office to discuss my idea. When I arrived, Dr. Passy was a little surprised that I was a patient and not a doctor or an engineer. I showed him the valve and told him of my desire to help other trached patients. He seemed excited about its effectiveness.

That night Dr. Passy told his wife, Patricia, about my visit. Having had previous business experience, she was very interested in the prospects of the valve. Patricia did some investigating and later contacted me with the results. I learned that over two million trach tubes are distributed a year and that trachs were not limited to just quads like myself. So Patricia and I formed a corporation and began letting people know about my ideas for the valve.

Our prototype worked, but I found that it was difficult to use for long periods of time because the flap inside was made of rubber and was hard to move. Another problem was appearance. It protruded too much from the trach, and the red flap was unattractive. We experimented with different materials and designs until we found the right combination. One of our failures would have made a perfect duck call because it made a very loud QUACK! I discovered that I could sound like a woodcock or even a Canada goose. Finally, we came up with a valve that was smooth with a relatively short protrusion and a light, easy to move, silicone flap.

We took our valve on the road, so to speak, starting with a local meeting of otolaryngologists (ear, nose, and throat surgeons who specialize in airways and trachs). I've been to conventions before, but it feels a lot different on the other side of the table. Then we attended a national meeting in Atlanta. This was my first trip on an airliner and my first big meeting. We had some literature made up and I had appeared in an ad in many magazines. I was interviewed by a few reporters and I even received a congratulatory letter from Dr. Robert Schuller. All this was fun and flattering, but the most rewarding aspect of the valve is that it has helped many people.

I learned many things from this experience. I learned that anger, if turned toward a problem rather than toward oneself or circumstances, can be overcome and God can work wonders. Indeed, just as I thought God had turned his back on me, he, in reality, gave me an incredible opportunity to help myself and others. Another important lesson is that no matter how far you sink into despair, never shut out your loved ones because there is nothing more selfish than to cause pain to those who are there for you.

As corny and trite as it may sound, "In every rain cloud there is a silver lining." This is absolutely true. Ask me, I know firsthand.

"I'm Sorry, Your Baby Has a Congenital Birth Defect."

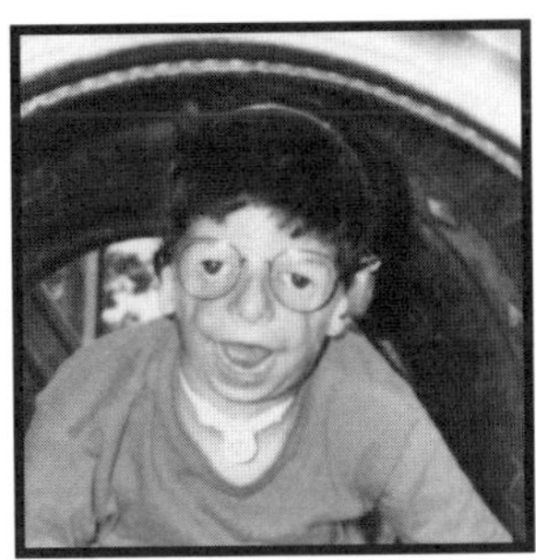

by Angela Vangalis

Angela Vangalis is the mother of three, including Alex Vangalis, who was born with Treacher Collins syndrome.

Stunned. What do you mean he's born with a congenital birth defect? Treacher Collins syndrome? What's that?

At 5 days old, the gastrostomy gave Alex the nutrition he needed to survive, and the tracheostomy allowed him to cry without turning a bluish gray color.

The physical anomalies associated with Treacher Collins syndrome in Alex's case are the absence of his outer ears and cheekbones along with underdeveloped jaw/mandibles. Neurologically, Alex is normal.

So, I had a baby who looks "different." The most difficult anomaly to accept during his infancy was his silent cry. The tracheostomy had robbed him of voice, which made him sound like a hissing cat. I remember my tears welling up when I'd hear someone's baby crying in the grocery store or a restaurant. I wanted to hear *my* baby cry. I felt cheated. There were times when we would cover his trach with a finger to listen to him "goo goo, gaa gaa" or, yes, cry frantically. We clearly had a unique advantage to hear his voice only when we wanted to.

Then we had the good fortune of acquiring a speaking valve[4] when Alex was about a year old. The valve enhanced Alex's vocalization dramatically. He became more self-confident as he became more easily understood. Now at the age of 5 years, the speaking valve is an important part of getting ready for the day.

Upon first impressions, people notice that Alex looks different before they even notice the trach. Usually, Alex will say "hi" with a smile or even extend his hand in friendship. This gives Alex the power of controlling the introduction and it helps ease the feelings of uncertainty to those who are unaware or afraid of his condition. We call his hearing aids and trach valve "helpers," so Alex can hear, breathe, and talk better.

Dealing with such a challenge has been accomplished by asking positive questions like: How can I use this situation to our advantage? How can we help others understand? What can I do to give my child the self-confidence he needs? Writing about the experiences, assisting support networks with newsletters to increase awareness, and above all, communicating with people who care are all emotional incentives to keep motivated.

Ventilator Dependent Limb Girdle Muscular Dystrophy

by Tedde Scharf, M.A.

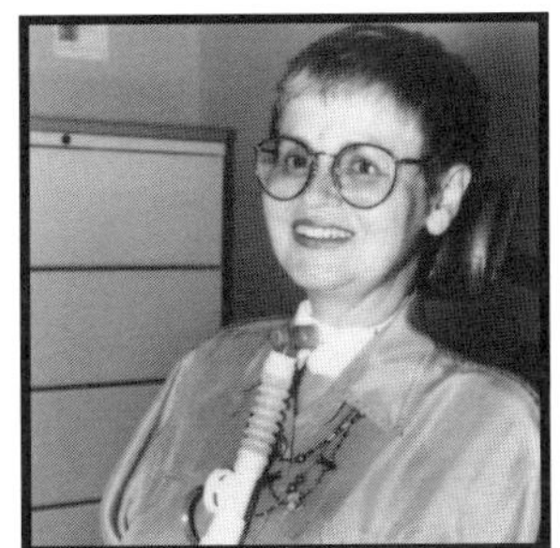

Tedde Scharf, M.A., directs the Disabled Student Resources Program at Arizona State University. She is on the National Board of Directors for the Muscular Dystrophy Association and the MDA National Task Force on Public Education, and consults on Accommodations and Americans with Disabilities Act (ADA) compliance in higher education.

I direct a large, comprehensive program for over 1300 students with disabilities at Arizona State University. My job involves supervision of 12 full-time staff and over 100 part-time employees. As a person who is ventilator dependent 24 hours a day, it is necessary for me to be mobile and to be able to communicate easily with many people individually, on the phone, and in groups. I speak clearly and without hesitation because I have a one-way speaking valve[4] located in-line in my ventilator system. The portable ventilator is conveniently placed on a tray under the back of my power wheelchair.

In 1988 before I was ventilated, my speaking volume had dropped to a whisper because of gradual respiratory failure and the resultant low volume in breathing. Other symptoms included unusual sleepiness during the day, lapses of memory, swollen and bloated body tissue, and loss of appetite. Today, with adequate ventilation, my day starts at 5 and ends at 10:30 or 11:00 each evening. I am suctioned a couple of times in the morning before work and again before bed. At the age of 51 years, I work 10 to 12 hours a day, lead an active social life, travel, speak at state and national conventions, pursue volunteer activities locally and nationally, and enjoy my hobby of portraiture and painting.

In this account, I will discuss the psychosocial aspects of disability and how they relate to persons who use ventilators. Key factors that affect the psychosocial development of individuals with any disability are self-concept, physical perceptions, emotional reactions, social behaviors and attitudes, interpersonal relationships, the rehabilitation process, persistence, and motivation. One of the most important aspects is the ability to communicate. Communication is a developmental process that starts at birth and continues through life. Senior citizens who lose their hearing and withdraw from social contacts and the world around them lose the ability to communicate. This can be very debilitating and isolating. The speaking valve[4] has provided a real breakthrough for individuals who are ventilator dependent or trached. It permits speech, which opens the door to all other aspects of the rehabilitation process. Restoring speech as early as medically possible is essential to the successful rehabilitation of patients who are ventilator dependent.

Initially, there is a great deal of fear associated with a tracheostomy, ventilation, and the introduction of a new system (e.g., the speaking valve) to the breathing mechanism. The medical procedures of suctioning, care of the trach, and knowledge of the ventilator can be overwhelming. The constant threat of infection, pulmonary plugs, choking, or aspiration are frightening. It is important that all members of the patient's family or caregiver team overcome these natural fears in order to help the patient successfully rehabilitate.

A major part of the rehabilitation process is educating the medical professionals about themselves. As ventilator dependent "patients," we develop a close relationship with medical professionals: physicians, respiratory therapists, speech therapists, nurses, and lab technicians. Many medical caregivers in the current HMO medical programs have not had exposure to ventilator dependent persons. Often the initial prognosis offered by physicians is based on disabilities, not abilities. They will advise the family not to expect their loved one to return to work or to leave the house more than a few times a year. They warn of the dangers of infection. They are not aware of the technological advances in wheelchairs that allow the ventilator to be built into the chair. Many physicians do not know how to provide what we really need. We must be able to communicate our expectations after rehabilitation: functional communication, mobility, return to home, work, and society. In other words, we must take responsibility for our own full rehabilitation process. If we are enthusiastic, willing to learn new procedures, knowledgeable about our needs, and able to communicate our goals to medical people, they will work unceasingly for us. Physicians will not give up if we don't give up on ourselves.

We need to be educated, too. It's important that we, as patients, learn everything about the concept that is keeping us alive: ventilation. What is a ventilator? How does it work? How can one avoid colds or respiratory infections? How can a ventilator dependent person live in a social environment, work, and stay healthy? It takes a great deal of special knowledge about ourselves and the medical resources that are available. Thus, resourcefulness is a major factor. We must find out all we can about the medical procedures that surround our physical well-being and the special equipment that will help us function optimally.

The patient can learn about ventilation through literature, videotapes, and role models of other persons who have been successfully ventilated. He or she needs to know about the tracheostomy tube (fenestrated and nonfenestrated), the inner cannula, the functioning of inflated and deflated cuffs, and how to avoid infections. Also, it is essential to understand how the ventilator works: the purpose of volume, breath rates, airflow, ventilator alarms, insufflation and exhalation tubes, the cascade system.

Knowledge about vocal communication options will increase the patient's ability to accept them. Demonstrate how the various devices look and work. If demonstrating a one-way valve and if medically advised, teach the patient to deflate the tracheostomy cuff and practice speaking. This is not a comfortable process. There will be some bubbling and sputtering, but the patient will feel the sensation of speech after having been unable to speak for a period of time. It is helpful to have speech therapy instruction when the communication options are first utilized and for several additional sessions, until the patient learns to use the ventilated air appropriately for breathing and speaking smoothly.

I have found that smooth, nonhesitant speech is a primary advantage of the one-way speaking valve I use.[4] Other positive aspects are a normal sounding voice because the air is directed past one's own vocal cords. The ventilator, in combination with the speaking valve,[4] increases speech volume, enabling normal speech levels and the ability to address groups or larger audiences without a microphone. There is reduced mucus buildup, which means less seepage and suctioning. The senses of taste and smell are more normal, which leads to increased appetite.

The ability to communicate our needs impacts heavily upon the development of self-concept. If one isn't allowed or able to express oneself, self-esteem is significantly lowered. The ability to communicate and express our needs to others, the socialization process, is what distinguishes humans from other animal forms. Independent living is difficult without some method for communication to be able to tell others how to assist us when we need help. Effective communication builds self-esteem and self-confidence in our individual abilities.

Management of caregiving is a major part of being severely disabled. Ventilator dependent patients require extra kinds of personal care, medical procedures, and equipment maintenance. Important keys to successful caregiving are a bright, sunny environment, arrangement of medical supplies and ventilator equipment in a well-organized manner for easy access, and a consistent daily routine that can be easily taught to new caregivers. Once routines are established and organized, we are free to lead our daily lives. A physical challenge doesn't have to excessively interrupt the living process, the work process, or social activities. An orderly caregiving procedure saves many hours for more important pursuits!

Training personal care attendants is very important. Whoever is helping us needs to know the procedure and routine well. They must understand the need for "clean" procedures when providing trach care, suctioning, cleaning cascade and ventilator tubes, or handling the trach area or pieces at any time. The ventilator dependent person must take responsibility for ensuring appropriate care. The depressed or negative person will show little interest in his or her own care and will be little motivated to develop a close vigilance of daily care.

Successful psychosocial development after trauma or onset of severe disability is relative to the levels of motivation and persistence.

The patient who remains in a prolonged depressed, negative state requires special care and may need psychiatric assistance. A good professional counselor can discover the positive and negative motivators that stimulate the patient's behavior. A doctor must be up-front and honest to gain the confidence and respect of the patient. The patient needs to express his feelings of loss, anger, resentment, and depression. Eventually, those feelings will become more positive and accepting. At that point, the patient takes control of his own rehabilitation and life. Always keep the ventilator dependent person reaching a little beyond his or her limits so that feelings of accomplishment are maintained. If this stretching stagnates for too long, the patient will feel that there is no reason to go on, and the rehabilitation process will stop, as will the ability to acclimate to his or her medical situation, home, workplace, or life. Successful rehabilitation means control of all circumstances in one's life.

Expectations that include someone else (e.g., medical professionals or family members) in control will create a further deterioration of self-esteem and sense of self. The development of self-esteem is the single most essential goal the patient needs to achieve. As caregivers and medical professionals, we must view the patient's situation from the patient's own shoes. Although we may not agree with choices the patient makes, we must accept and respect the right to choose. Internalizing the acceptance process is a bumpy road of ups and downs that each person with a disability must travel. Family and professionals can reinforce the positive, try not to reinforce the negative behaviors, and understand the process.

Sometimes it is difficult for medical experts to work with people who are disabled because it is difficult to let the patient take control. Taking control of one's life means integrating all of the aspects of the disability, the physical condition, and the qualities of persistence, motivation, self-esteem, anger, frustration, and pain until it is all part of the patient himself. For myself, the ventilator is my breathing mechanism. I can't imagine being without it, not because I'm dependent on it, but because it really gives me a chance to live my life more completely.

Since becoming ventilator dependent, I have had a lot of interesting experiences and adventures such as interviewing blind applicants for a job in the office before I had the speaking valve! The applicant couldn't see or hear me since I couldn't speak. It was a confusing situation that required a sense of humor and creative thinking!

Don't let seeming barriers keep you from doing what you want to do. I'm a great football fan of the ASU Sun Devils. When I returned to work and received my packet for season tickets, I wasn't sure how I would be able to attend games as the weather cooled off. I enthusiastically attended the first few games during the hot weather. As the night temperatures dipped down to 40 to 50 degrees, I was unable to keep the air I breathe warm and moisturized. I didn't renew my season tickets the following year. The Athletic Department Box Office continued to send me renewal notices, and the promotional ads on television kept repeating, "What will it take to have YOU renew your season tickets to the football games?" Finally, I called the Athletic Director and said, "It will take an electrical outlet for me to renew my season tickets!" I haven't missed football season since. I attend all the games with the aid of a long-range extension cord provided by the stadium management!

All people face challenges in life. Resourceful, creative, persistent thinking and actions help each person build and rebuild his or her life. Every new barrier develops increased self-esteem and self-confidence, which helps us cope with new life challenges more easily. Ventilator dependence is not the end of the world, it's another beginning.

REFERENCES

1. The Ventilator Support Center (VSC) is a 33-bed inpatient unit devoted to the rehabilitation and weaning of ventilator dependent patients. Comprehensive treatment is provided by the multidisciplinary teams consisting of services from pulmonary, psychology, nursing, respiratory therapy, speech pathology, physical and occupational therapy, dietary, and social work.

2. Clemes, H., and Bean, R., *Self-Esteem,* New York: Zebra Books, 1982.

3. Mary Lou is not an actual patient, but represents the composite experience of many ventilator dependent patients.

4. Passy-Muir Tracheostomy Speaking Valve.

5. COMMUNItrach™ I.

CHAPTER X

DYSPHAGIA

Jo Puntil, *M.S., C.C.C.*
Dysphagia Clinical Specialist
Private Practice
Seal Beach, California

Mary F. Mason, *M.S., C.C.C.-SLP*

Edited by:

Melissa Scott, *M.A., C.C.C.-SLP*
Specialist in Ventilator Dependent Patients
Private Practice
La Grange, Illinois

INTRODUCTION

Dysphagia can be found in a diverse array of clinical populations, for example, following an acute neurological event, surgery, respiratory failure, and secondary manifestations that involve muscular, neuromuscular, or structural components of the alimentary tract. The presence of a tracheostomy tube can result in the development of a dysphagic symptom/disorder.[1] Many patients have normal swallowing function and no aspiration symptoms until the placement of a tracheostomy tube.

Swallowing requires pressure both above and below the food mass to propel the food safely into the esophagus.[2-10] The presence of a tracheostomy tube alters these pressures generated by swallowing because air pressure escapes through the tracheostomy tube and, as a result, swallowing becomes abnormal and aspiration a risk. Some tracheostomized patients also develop tracheoesophageal fistulas secondary to an ill-fitted, large, or overinflated tracheostomy tube cuff.[11] These swallowing problems are directly related to tracheostomy tube placement.[12]

CLINICAL EVALUATION

With some minor alterations, a comprehensive clinical evaluation with a tracheostomized and/or ventilator dependent patient primarily involves the same type of evaluative approach that would be performed on a non-tracheostomized dysphagic patient. The tracheostomized patient is not complicated to assess at bedside due to the availability of a direct access to the lower airway via suctioning (by authorized personnel) before, during, and after the assessment of the upper airway. The tracheostomized patient's secretions in the lower or upper airways give vital information about the risk or presence of aspiration. In reality, bedside assessment of a non-tracheostomized patient is more difficult, as direct airway access for lower airway suctioning is not available.

TEAM ASSESSMENT

The most comprehensive evaluation can be achieved with a team approach. This team would include the physicians involved with the patient, that is, the internist, pulmonologist, physiatrist, otolaryngologist, pediatrician, gastroenterologist, and others; the nurse; respiratory therapist; dietician; and dysphagia clinician (Table 10-1). Responsibility of each team member is within his or her own discipline with a mutual awareness of each clinician's role and goals with the patient. Effective communication among the therapists, nurses, and physicians on the team is vital in order to set appropriate goals and rationales for a swallow evaluation. It is also important that the patient be involved in the process of goal setting and informed of the steps of the evaluation process.

The evaluation should begin with the patient's subjective complaint or problem. This is followed by a review of the relevant health and medical history. The examination of the dysphagic patient will include an assessment of swallowing function, history, pertinent clinical observations, detailed physical examination, and type of tracheostomy tube the patient currently has in place, including size

- Physicians
  - Internist
  - Pulmonologist
  - Physiatrist
  - Otolaryngologist
  - Pediatrician
  - Gastroenterologist
- Dysphagia clinician (e.g., speech-language pathologist, occupational therapist)
- Respiratory therapist
- Nurse
- Dietician
- Audiologist

Table 10-1 Team Members.

and whether the tube is cuffed or cuffless and air-filled or foam-filled. (Table 10-2). At times, modification of the evaluation procedures may be necessary due to the medical status of the patient. The dysphagia clinician should perform the clinical evaluation of a tracheostomized patient in the presence of a respiratory therapist or nurse unless the clinician is well trained and approved by the institution to suction the patient without medical supervision.

The primary objective for the dysphagia clinician is to understand what complaint or problem was identified to necessitate a dysphagia evaluation. At times, evaluation of a tracheostomized and/or ventilator dependent patient's swallowing abilities is requested to ascertain whether or not the patient tolerates his or her own secretions. Referral for evaluation also may be made to determine if the patient's swallowing function is adequate to enable safe oral intake or to facilitate weaning from the ventilator (and/or possible decannulation of the tracheostomy tube). The dysphagia evaluation is a valuable contribution to the management team and is often provided by the speech-language pathologist who assumes the role of the dysphagia clinician. It is often possible to transition a tracheostomized/ventilator dependent patient more quickly and appropriately in regard to feeding, decannulation, and weaning when the dysphagia clinician plays an advocate role in these areas. When the dysphagia clinician is a speech-language pathologist, he or she should take this opportunity to educate the other team members as to the important role speech-

---

Subjective complaint (provided by the patient)
Medical history
Swallow function history
Clinical observations
Physical examination
Tracheostomy tube
- Size
- Fenestrated/nonfenestrated
- Cuffed/cuffless

Table 10-2 Evaluation.

language pathology plays in the treatment of dysphagia.

Once it has been determined why the referral was requested, the clinician should obtain information from the medical chart and nursing personnel pertinent to the swallowing disorder. Depending on the setting, that is, whether acute care, inpatient rehabilitation, skilled nursing facility, or home, a varying amount of information can be made available to the dysphagia clinician. The clinician should obtain as much information as possible prior to the oral presentation of any type of consistency of food or fluid.

ELEMENTS OF THE CLINICAL EVALUATION

Medical Review

A thorough review of the medical chart is vital and is a crucial part of the evaluation. The dysphagia clinician needs to obtain as much information on the patient's medical status as possible prior to meeting with the patient. The most pertinent information the dysphagia clinician will need to note when reviewing the chart includes: why the patient has been admitted to the facility (acute diagnosis), what caused the patient to have respiratory problems or go into respiratory failure, how long the patient has been on a ventilator, current ventilator settings, the reason for tracheostomy tube placement, the length of time the tracheostomy tube has been placed, and the type and size of the tracheostomy tube. Understanding the dynamic process the patient is experiencing in his or her course of the hospital stay is important. The level of dependence the patient has on the ventilator as well as where the patient is in the weaning process should be noted. Patients who are dependent upon ventilators and who are beginning their process of weaning become very fatigued and have decreased endurance when they are attempting to breathe on their own. The clinician should understand what the patient is experiencing in the effort to breathe on his or her own and that beginning a feeding program may affect and possibly decrease the patient's endurance. The primary goal should be to wean a patient off the ventilator if this is medically feasible and then to maintain or institute normal oral feeding (Table 10-3).

Reason for admission
- Diagnosis
- Respiratory status
- Length of time on ventilator
- Length of tracheostomy tube usage
- Reason for tracheostomy tube placement
- Type of tracheostomy tube
    - Size, cuffed/uncuffed, air-filled/foam-filled
- Weaning attempts/schedule

Table 10-3 Medical Chart Review.

Nutritional Assessment

Nutrition plays an important role in the endurance of the respiratory compromised patient and the ability to maintain ventilatory workload. If the patient is feeding orally, it is ideal to assess a patient during the course of a meal in order to ascertain elements of fatigue. Often this is not possible due to the time constraints of the dysphagia clinician. The clinician should note the number of swallows needed to consume a meal, which (depending upon how much the patient can eat) can vary from approximately 50 to 150 to 250 swallows.[13] If the patient is being weaned from the ventilator, the dysphagia clinician should be aware of the stress (decrease in endurance) that oral feeding may produce if it is the primary means of nutrition rather than tube feeding.

Nursing notes provide detailed nursing observations as to whether the patient has been receiving trials of oral fluids and taking oral medication and any relevant observations regarding swallow that the nurses have made regarding the patient's vital signs, secretion levels, mental status, and medications administered (Table 10-4).

Respiratory Review

Respiratory care notes play a vital role in the evaluation of a dysphagic tracheostomized or ventilator dependent patient. A dysphagia clinician needs to know how often the patient is suctioned, what is the

Medications
Fluid intake
Daily observations
Secretion levels

Table 10-4 Nursing Chart Notes.

consistency of the secretions, and what contributes toward that consistency. Secretion thickness, color, and amount may provide information about the presence of infection, disease progression, or the need to assess humidification. Presence of thick secretions may hinder an optimal swallow.[1,14] Respiratory care notes also will indicate what type of bronchial hygiene regimen is in place to control secretion levels, such as humidification, medications, or chest physical therapy (Table 10-5).

The dysphagia clinician should also review the patient's chart to determine the patient's physical mobility, results of any recent radiological procedures or of gastrointestinal procedures, nutritional status, and any other pertinent information to obtain comprehensive evaluation.

It is important to thoroughly review the pulmonologist's reports, primary physician's reports, and dietician's notes as well as the patient's diagnosis, current pulmonary status, and code status. The dysphagia clinician should know the patient's code status (resuscitation orders) so that appropriate procedures will be followed in the event that a problem occurred during the evaluation.

After extensively reviewing the medical history, the dysphagia clinician should ask the nursing staff how the clinician should also inquire as to the patient's cognitive status, level of alertness, medications,

Secretion status
Secretion management
Bronchial hygiene regime
Ventilatory status

Table 10-5 Respiratory Chart Notes.

secretion levels, and presence of infection. Any information that the nurse can give the dysphagia clinician as to how the patient is doing medically and emotionally will offer the clinician a comprehensive picture of the patient's status at that particular point in time. Collaboration with nursing and respiratory care therapists enables the dysphagia clinician to proceed with a comprehensive evaluation. After the clinician has reviewed the patient's chart and spoken with the nursing and/or respiratory staff, the clinician is ready to initiate the evaluation of the patient (Table 10-6).

Oral-Motor Examination

The initial part of the clinical evaluation should include an oral-motor examination of the patient with the inclusion of a blue dye test. The dysphagia clinician should explain his or her role to the patient and the need for the procedures included in the evaluation. It is important that the patient understand all of the steps involved in the evaluation as well as the benefits of the evaluation. The oral-motor examination includes looking first at the patient's overall body position, head/neck control, and facial symmetry. Poor positioning can interfere with an effective swallow. The dysphagia clinician should then assess the patient's salivary function (presence or absence and amount of oral secretions), dentition, and mandibular function. Following this, the dysphagia clinician should assess labial range,

- Interview staff
- Mobility
- Gastrointestinal procedures
- Nutritional status
- Cognitive status
- Secretion status (infection)
  - Bronchial hygiene
  - Control regimen
- Ventilator weaning information
- Code status

Table 10-6 Respiratory Patient Assessment.

strength, and coordination; lingual range, strength, and coordination; and velopharyngeal elevation. The presence or absence of reflexes such as the gag (bilaterally) and cough should be noted as well as any type of abnormal reflex that may be present (Table 10-7).

Cognitive/Communication Assessment

The patient's cognitive and communication status is assessed to determine how efficiently the patient is communicating with his tracheostomy tube and/or ventilator dependency. This can be done using formal and informal tasks. The level of the patient's ability to answer questions verbally or nonverbally (with tracheostomy cuff deflated if present), follow directions, and attend to the entire evaluation procedure can affect the way in which the dysphagia clinician will proceed with the assessment. If possible it is important to ask the patient questions as to his or her current status regarding, for example, eating efforts, problems encountered when attempting to eat, and specifically any subjective complaints with respect to the ability to swallow and/or communicate. Often, if the patient has a cuffed tracheostomy tube and is able to tolerate cuff deflation[15] (see next section for details on this procedure), this may be the first time that the patient will be able to communicate verbally since being tracheostomized or ventilator dependent. Consequently, it is often a positive experience for the patient.

Educate patient to procedure and rationale of the evaluation

Physical exam:	
	Body position
	Head/neck control
	Facial symmetry
Oral motor exam:	
	Salivary function
	Dentition
	Mandibular function
	Labial function
	Lingual function
	Velopharyngeal function

Table 10-7 Clinical Examination.

Pharyngeal/Laryngeal Function Assessment

Cuff Deflation

In order to fully assess pharyngeal/laryngeal functions, it is recommended that if the patient has a cuffed tracheostomy tube the cuff be deflated. Approval by the referring physician is necessary to deflate the cuff. If the patient is ventilator dependent, the respiratory therapist may need to compensate for the change from a "closed system" to an "open system" by adjusting the ventilator settings,[15,16] as there will be air leakage up through the laryngeal and oral airways once the tracheostomy cuff is deflated. The clinicians and therapists that are involved with the evaluation need to reassure the patient beforehand that he or she may hear some alarms on the ventilator and that the respiratory therapist is there to ensure that the patient gets enough air and that the patient's ability to breathe will not be compromised throughout the procedure. If the ventilator does alarm, it is important to assure the patient that the respiratory therapist is there to ensure that monitoring of the patient is appropriate.

Prior to cuff deflation, the patient must be suctioned by the nurse, respiratory therapist, or other authorized professional according to the facility's protocol. Prior to any type of laryngeal status assessment, the dysphagia clinician, respiratory therapist, and/or nurse should note the tracheostomy tube size, the presence of a cuff and/or fenestration, and whether the inner cannula is disposable or nondisposable. It is important to suction the patient orally before as well as during cuff deflation to retrieve any oral secretions that may mobilize after cuff deflation. Prior to cuff deflation, the dysphagia clinician should advise the ventilator dependent patient that he will feel a rush of air into his mouth and that this is very normal, and that it is this rush of air that will enable him to vocalize. The patient may feel secretions shifting or moving in the oropharynx and trachea and may need reassurance that these can be suctioned if necessary. A patient who is ventilator dependent, should be advised that he or she may feel air traveling upward into the mouth after cuff deflation, which may contribute toward anxiety, and that this is a normal process. Throughout the evaluation, the therapists involved in the evaluation should closely watch all monitors that may be connected to the patient to assess oxygen saturation levels, heart rate, and blood pressure. These should be compared to their baseline levels. It is recommended that the minimal monitoring system acceptable is an oximeter. Using the oximeter the dysphagia clinician can constantly assess the patient's oxygen saturation levels and heart rate throughout the evaluation period (Table 10-8).

If the patient is unable to tolerate complete tracheostomy cuff deflation due to poor ventilatory status, a minimal leak procedure can be used throughout the evaluation. (Please refer to Chapter 3). There should be a minimal leak between the cuff and the tracheal wall in order for the dysphagia clinician to be able to detect the presence of aspiration. If the cuff is maximally inflated so that it is in full contact with the tracheostomy wall, the assessment cannot be accurate because the dysphagia clinician will be unable to determine if the patient is aspirating.[17] This is because food and/or liquid will pool on top of the inflated tracheostomy cuff instead of falling down into the airway, where it can be suctioned and aspiration revealed. It is recommended and beneficial to the patient to conduct the dysphagia evaluation with the cuff fully or at least minimally deflated. Besides facilitating the detection of aspiration if present, cuff deflation allows the larynx to elevate in a more timely and effective manner[18] and allows airflow into the pharynx for a more adequate swallow, as well as increased pharyngeal sensation and improved expectoration of secretions.[17]

Cuff deflation should occur slowly as secretions will begin to

---

Physician authorization
Educate patient to procedure
Respiratory therapy participation
Ventilator compensation
Monitoring and oximetry
Suctioning of secretions
Type of tracheostomy tube and cuff type

Table 10-8 Cuff Deflation Assessment.

mobilize to the airway during the procedure. Slow cuff deflation will prevent the occurrence of a large rush of air into the upper airway, which may initiate coughing.

Laryngeal Function Exam

In assessing laryngeal status, the dysphagia clinician should evaluate the patient for the presence of a dry swallow. It is important to assess the patient's ability to elevate the larynx during a dry swallow as well as to assess the integrity of the vocal folds. At this point in the bedside assessment, cuff deflation in combination with the introduction of gloved finger occlusion will enable assessment of vocal fold strength and integrity. It should be noted that a one-way valve could be used in place of finger occlusion to assist in this vocal assessment (Table 10-9). There are a number of one-way valves manufactured; however, at this time for ventilator dependent patients, the only valve that is registered with the Food and Drug Administration for in-line use is the Passy-Muir ventilator speaking valve.[16] Speaking valves are discussed in detail in Chapter 7.

If voicing with finger occlusion or a one-way valve in place is weak or faint, the dysphagia clinician should review the length of time the patient has gone without utilizing the vocal folds for phonation. The intubation history of the patient should also be reviewed again, as there is a risk of vocal fold damage associated with intubation. Vocal fold pathology should be investigated when no voicing is achieved after proper cuff deflation and occlusion of the tracheostomy tube. If vocal fold damage has been ruled out via laryngoscopic assessment (performed by a physician), vocal fold retraining may be necessary in conjunction with the use of finger occlusion or a one-way valve to achieve voice. The dysphagia clinician should assess vocal fold

Dry swallow assessment
Cuff deflation (in conjunction with gloved finger occlusion or one-way valve)
Vocalization attempt

Table 10-9 Laryngeal Function Exam.

closure and the quality of voice as these are important aspects related to swallowing function.

This assessment may be the first time in a long time that the patient has heard his or her own voice. Depending on the level of success in producing voice, the patient's reaction can be negative or positive.

Once it has been established that the patient is able to tolerate cuff deflation and the status of laryngeal function has been determined, the dysphagia clinician should listen to the patient's breath sounds to assess the patient's respiratory status. The respiratory therapist and/or nurse as well as the dysphagia clinician are responsible for listening to the patient's breath sounds to assess secretion accumulation, breathing depth, breath patterns, or dyspnea. (Further information on assessment of breath patterns and sounds is delineated in Chapter 4.)

If the patient is medically tolerating the assessment procedure, that is, oxygen saturation, heart rate, and blood pressure are stable and within the patient's normal ranges, then the next step in the assessment is to complete a blue dye test (Table 10-10).

Blue Dye Test Procedure

The blue dye test is used to ascertain whether the tracheostomized or ventilator dependent patient is aspirating. It is easier to assess a tracheostomized or ventilator dependent patient for aspiration than it is a nontracheostomized patient because there is direct access to the airway. If the patient aspirates, the patient's airway can be suctioned immediately via the tracheostomy tube. Blue food coloring is effective to use in this assessment.

The dysphagia clinician should note that a blue dye test needs to be completed over a period of time. The swallowing function of a

---

Breath rate/sounds
Oxygen saturation level
Heart rate
Blood pressure

Table 10-10 Continuous Monitoring During Evaluation.

patient cannot be accurately assessed for all consistencies of food via the blue dye test. This is due to the fact that if the blue dye test reveals that the patient has aspirated, and the patient consumed two or three different food consistencies, it will be impossible to determine which food consistency administered (liquid, pureed, or solid) was actually aspirated.

It should also be noted that the patient's oral and pharyngeal cavities will be stained blue as a result of the blue dye test procedure, thus causing oral secretions to be blue.

It is generally advisable to utilize liquid material when first assessing the patient's swallowing. If possible, this procedure should be carried out over a period of at least 24 to 72 hours.[18] The blue dye test is a dynamic process that is extremely comprehensive in assessing the patient's ability not only to tolerate liquids but also his or her own secretions throughout the day and night.[18] This procedure gives the dysphagia clinician significant information as to the patient's tolerance of secretions and liquids during periods of alertness as well as during periods of fatigue. In this case, the procedure involves adding blue food coloring to either ice chips or liquid material. The patient should be made aware that the tracheostomy tube will be suctioned to assess the color of the secretions returned. If the secretions from the tracheostomy tube are the color that is normal for that patient, then the patient is tolerating the consistency of the food well. If the secretions that are suctioned out of the tracheostomy tube are blue or blue tinged, then this is evidence of aspiration.

1. Assessing Swallowing for Ice Chips/Small Amounts of Liquid

The first step in the blue dye test is to administer a small amount of blue dye via a toothette or in various amounts of ice chips. Initially, the patient should be given a small amount, for example, 2 to 5 cc or a teaspoonful, of blue-dyed liquid or ice chips and then be observed during the oral and pharyngeal phases of the swallow.

Assessment of the oral phase involves determination as to whether the patient is able to control the bolus in the mouth without drooling and thrust it posteriorly toward the pharynx without a delay in the initiation of the swallow.[13,20,21,22,23] Assessment of the pharyngeal phase of the swallow includes observation of laryngeal elevation.[20] This is accomplished by palpating the neck to feel the superior and anterior elevation of the larynx during the swallow.[20]

During this procedure, the patient should be given one teaspoon at a time. Immediately following each teaspoon presentation and assessment of the oral and pharyngeal phases, the patient should be monitored very closely. Optimal monitoring involves mechanical means, for example, heart monitor and oximetry, as well as assessing behavioral manifestations, such as coughing, choking, or voice quality changes. It is recommended that the dysphagia clinician occlude the tracheostomy tube with a gloved finger or one-way valve to assess voice quality throughout the evaluation.

If the patient is able to tolerate a single teaspoon of the blue-dyed ice chips or liquid, the procedure should continue with successive teaspoons of material utilized as long as the patient can medically tolerate it. The dysphagia clinician should then give the patient another teaspoon, and then ask the patient to cough. This is to assess whether the patient is able to clear the airway. If the patient is able to cough and no blue secretions are expectorated from the tracheostomy tube site, then the test should continue. If the patient coughs and bright blue secretions are expectorated from the tracheostomy tube, then it is obvious that aspiration has occurred in the upper airway.

Some patients will not have the ability to cough, for example, patients with advanced neuromuscular disorders or high-level spinal cord injuries, so care should be taken to check the airway via suctioning by authorized personnel. If the patient has aspirated, then it is necessary to make a team decision as to whether the procedure should continue. The team should be aware that when some patients aspirate, they do not always aspirate with every swallow; thus the team may observe inconsistent aspiration. Every patient is individual; therefore, the patient's medical/pulmonary status as well as anxiety level should be considered when determining whether or not to continue the procedure at bedside or if continued assessment should occur under fluorography.

2. Assessing Swallowing for Increased Amounts of Liquid

If the patient is tolerating the small amounts of blue-dyed material, the dysphagia clinician should allow the patient to give himself or herself the blue-dyed liquid via cup or straw in order to assess swallowing function for larger bolus sizes. The same procedures in suctioning and observations at the tracheostomy site apply.

3. Monitoring of the Patient

If the patient is able to tolerate 50 to 100 cc of liquid material[18,19] without any evidence of aspiration, such as coughing or suctioning blue secretions from the tracheostomy tube, then a team decision should be made regarding how long the blue dye test should continue. It is advisable that the blue dye test continue over a 24 to 72 hour period in collaboration with nursing and respiratory therapy.[18,19] Nursing or respiratory therapy should apply blue dye to the patient's tongue every shift and/or give the patient water with blue dye in it for the next 24 to 72 hours. The respiratory therapist and nurse should document the color of the secretions retrieved from the tracheostomy tube when appropriate. Optimally, the cuff of the patient's tracheostomy tube should remain deflated for the entire 24 to 72 hour period so that aspiration, if present, can be detected. If this is not possible due to the patient's inability to tolerate cuff deflation for an extended period, then a minimal leak should be maintained throughout the 24 to 72 hours. It should be noted that, in some facilities, a physician's order may be required for the cuff to be deflated completely or minimally for this 24 to 72 hour period.

4. Posting a Blue Dye Test Notice

To facilitate completion of the test, the dysphagia clinician should place a sign above the patient's bed, indicating (1) that "a blue dye test" for secretion and/or oral feeding management is in progress for *X* amount of hours; (2) that blue dye should be applied to the tongue every shift; and (3) that any signs and amounts of blue secretions observed during tracheostomy tube suctioning or around the stoma should be documented.

During the 24 to 72 hour period of the blue dye test, it is recommended that the dysphagia clinician leave his or her name and telephone number at the patient's bedside in plain view. This will allow family members and/or any ancillary professionals to contact the clinician in the event that they become alarmed and do not understand why the patient has a blue tongue, blue lips, blue oral secretions, and possibly blue tracheal secretions (Table 10-11).

5. Documentation of Blue Dye Test Findings

As previously mentioned, nursing and/or respiratory therapy will be monitoring the amount of secretions suctioned or expectorated from the tracheostomy tube or observed around the tracheostomy site. The appearance of blue secretions in notable amounts calls for discontinuation of the study at that point as recommended by the physician or the dysphagia team.[18,19] Documentation of any blue dye test findings should include the amount, color, and consistency of any secretions and the clinical appearance of the patient, including position, level of alertness, low-grade fever (infection), and any signs of respiratory distress. The dysphagia clinician should assess the patient daily for continued tolerance of secretions and continuation of the blue dye test as indicated to assess for oral feeding tolerance.

The team, usually the respiratory therapist, nurse, physician, and dysphagia clinician, should collaborate after the first 24 to 72 hour period to discuss the testing process, results, and/or impressions. If results indicate that the patient is able to tolerate thin liquids without any signs of distress, then pureed foods should be assessed via the blue dye test procedure.[18,19]

Blue Dye Test Procedure
Educate staff to test in progress
Time frame: 24-72 hours monitoring
Liquid bolus - ice chips (2-5cc)
Palpatation of swallow
Suction for evidence of aspiration
Physical observations
Larger bolus introduced 50-100 cc
Monitor 24-72 hours

Table 10-11 Blue Dye Test Procedure.

6. Assessing Swallowing of Pureed Food

The blue dye test procedure can continue with pureed material (dyed blue) following the previous steps. At this point, the dysphagia clinician must remember that if the previous blue dye test indicated that the patient has difficulty tolerating his or her own secretions and/or thin liquids, a false positive sign of aspiration may occur during the blue dye test for pureed food. This is because the patient will now be ingesting pureed material that is dyed blue, and that pureed material will dye the patient's oral and pharyngeal areas as well. As the patient is eating this material, he or she is also swallowing his secretions. If the patient aspirated secretions before, he or she may aspirate again, thus giving the dysphagia clinician a false positive result, that is, observation of blue tracheal secretions, when it appears the patient is aspirating the pureed material but in reality is aspirating his secretions.

The dysphagia clinician should monitor the oral and pharyngeal phases of the swallow with pureed material, as was described for thin liquid material, assessing the ability to maintain a cohesive bolus in the oral cavity and to thrust the bolus posteriorly, the presence and extent of laryngeal elevation, vocal quality, and any signs of respiratory distress. Throughout the evaluation, the dysphagia clinician should monitor the patient's heart rate, oxygen saturation level, and blood pressure. After the patient has swallowed the first teaspoon of pureed material, he should be asked to cough. Coughing and/or suctioning should be done as needed by authorized personnel. If the secretions are clear, then the procedure should continue. The amount of pureed material that is given to a patient should correlate with the patient's medical tolerance of the procedure. If the patient is tolerating the pureed material without signs of aspiration, then increasing amounts should be given until an amount considered by the team to be functional is consumed. It is important that the dysphagia clinician assess the patient's fatigue level and cognitive status while the patient is eating and, if possible, while the patient is feeding himself or herself.

When the administration of pureed material has been completed, the team should once again determine the length of time that the blue dye test should continue, preferably over a 24 to 72 hour period. If possible, the tracheostomy tube cuff should again remain completely deflated or deflated with minimal leak during the test. Nursing, the respiratory therapist, and the dysphagia clinician need to collaborate through written documentation as well as verbal communication as to what the patient has eaten, as well as the consistency, color, and amount of secretions being suctioned or expectorated from the tracheostomy tube over the 24 to 72 hour period.

As mentioned previously, food of one consistency should be assessed at a time in order to determine how the patient is going to tolerate each consistency. The period of 24 to 72 hours will allow for positional changes, fatigue, and other environmental factors that may affect swallowing function.[18,19] After the 24 to 72 hours have been completed, the clinician may want to assess solid foods and/or recommend that a modified barium swallow study or other swallowing evaluation be performed.

7. Assessing Swallowing of Solid Food

The blue dye test procedure can continue with the presentation of solid food material following the same procedures described for the thin liquid and pureed materials. The only difference between solid food and pureed food in regard to swallow function is the presence of mastication (chewing)[13,20] that is needed to formulate a cohesive bolus and the increased amount of time spent in the oral and pharyngeal phases of the swallow.

8. Determining Goals and Recommendations for Oral Feeding

Once the blue dye test has been completed, the team should determine the goals and recommendations for oral feeding. It is important for the team to decide which consistencies of food the patient can safely tolerate. The team should remember that if the patient is being weaned from a ventilator, fatigue and endurance levels will play a major factor in aspiration risk. It is best to work on weaning the patient from the ventilator if possible prior to aggressively pursuing oral feedings. When a patient is weaning, he or she can also be maintained on non-oral feedings in conjunction with trial oral feedings or small amounts of oral feedings. This will allow a gradual transition from non-oral to primarily oral nutrition as appropriate.

DOCUMENTATION OF BEDSIDE DYSPHAGIA ASSESSMENT

Documentation of the results of the bedside dysphagia assessment and treatment recommendations is vital. Documentation should include the following (Table 10-12):

Background Information

It is extremely important to document all behavioral manifestations that have been observed throughout the evaluation, both subjective and objective. Documentation of the bedside evaluation should include the patient's diagnosis, onset, and background medical information, including the physician's history and physical examination, reasons for referral, prior oral intake, flow sheet information, nursing notes, patient report notes, physical status, cognitive status, medications, patient's level of alertness, tracheostomy tube size, type of tracheostomy tube (fenestrated, cuffed, uncuffed, inflated or deflated cuff), respiratory status, and ventilator status.

Oral-Motor Examination

Oral-motor physical examination documentation should include: (1) observation of the patient's head and trunk symmetry; (2) mandibular control; (3) sensation; (4) dentition; (5) any normal and abnormal reflexes present; (6) labial range, strength and coordination;

Background information
Oral-motor examination
Trial feedings
Impressions
Recommendations
Goals
Follow-up issues

Table 10-12 Documentation.

(7) lingual range, strength and coordination; (8) velopharyngeal elevation/retraction; (9) laryngeal elevation and excursion; (10) quality of voice; and (11) breath sounds.

Trial Feedings

Documentation in this area should include: (1) the total amount given for each consistency of food; (2) the types of consistencies that were administered; (3) observations made in the oral and pharyngeal phases; (4) oxygen saturation levels; (5) any type of behavioral manifestations observed; (6) color, type, and quantity of secretions noted from the tracheostomy tube or around the stoma site and from lower airway suctioning; (7) patient's position; (8) compensation maneuvers; and (9) coughing and noted aspiration.

Impressions

The dysphagia clinician should determine the level of severity of the patient's dysphagia.

An example of minimal dysphagia would be a patient who tolerates all consistencies of food with no signs of aspiration, but exhibits a slight disorder in the oral preparatory phase of the swallow. A patient with a minimal dysphagia may also evidence difficulty in learning recommended compensatory strategies needed to enable that patient to be an independent eater.

A mild dysphagia disorder would include the need for an altered diet such as ground or chopped meat and three meals a day with possibly some supervision needed to ensure safe swallowing.

A moderate dysphagia disorder would include non-oral treatment and possibly some limited oral feedings. Documentation should indicate the risk for aspiration, the consistency of food the patient may be aspirating, and the need for some level of supervision or alteration of diet. A severe dysphagia disorder is characterized by the patient who is unable to eat by mouth and thus requires non-oral feedings to maintain nutrition.[18,19]

Extremely severe dysphagia describes a patient who is unable to eat any consistency of food by mouth and may have extreme difficulty tolerating/managing his own secretions.[18,19]

Recommendations

The recommendations section of the documentation should summarize the team's collaborative decisions regarding continuation of the evaluation, continuation of therapy, need for a modified barium swallow study or some other swallowing evaluation procedure, type of oral diet or need for non-oral feedings, obtaining consultation from a gastroenterologist and/or otolaryngologist, the possibility of tracheostomy occlusion trials, the possibility of trials of tracheostomy plugging and decannulation, and the scope of patient and family education/training to be provided. It should be noted that this list is not all inclusive and that recommendations might consist of a combination of these factors. Those listed above are the primary recommendations that are commonly addressed when evaluating tracheostomized and ventilator dependent patients. Results, concerns, and recommendations stemming from the evaluation should be provided to and discussed with the patient and with the patient's attending physician.

Goals

The team should establish both the long-term and short-term goals. An overriding goal is to achieve adequate nutrition and hydration. The patient and family should be included in the formulation of these goals. These goals should be measurable, functional, and related to the patient's ability to successfully achieve weaning from the ventilator, decannulation, and oral feeding. For instance, an example of a long-term goal might be to have the patient manage his or her own secretions. The short-term goal to effect this outcome might be to improve his or her ability to cough.

Follow-up Issues

After the evaluation has been completed, the dysphagia clinician needs to be concerned with the therapeutic techniques that will facilitate the patient achieving the goals that have been set. There is no cookbook method to follow when evaluating and treating a patient who is tracheostomized or ventilator dependent. A team approach is vital as it will facilitate the decision-making process. Monitoring the patient closely as well as educating the patient and family throughout the evaluation will help to decrease any surprise or anxiety that may occur during the evaluation. Evaluation for these patients is ongoing and can affect treatment intervention. Furthermore, follow-up should also include continued monitoring of oral feedings to prevent recurrence of difficulties and to ensure that the patient has the endurance to consume meals orally.

MODIFIED BARIUM SWALLOW STUDY (VIDEOFLUOROSCOPIC ASSESSMENT)

A videofluoroscopic swallowing evaluation is a dynamic assessment of the swallow and may be an adjunct to the clinical evaluation.[9,10,13,21,22,23,24,25] After a clinical bedside evaluation has been performed with a tracheostomized or ventilator dependent patient, a radiographic dysphagia evaluation **may be performed** to more directly observe and assess all phases of swallowing (especially the pharyngeal and esophageal phases).[26-29] This is particularly important when failure with a particular consistency is noted during clinical assessment or if silent aspiration is suspected. It is recommended that this be done as a team process, in which the team members include the radiologist, dysphagia clinician, nurse and/or respiratory therapist, and the patient.

Use of the Passy-Muir Tracheostomy Speaking Valve to Facilitate Swallowing

Speech-language pathologists have reported that the use of the Passy-Muir tracheostomy speaking valve (Figure 10-1) during the modified barium swallow study has facilitated the patient's ability to swallow.[17] Explanation of this finding is related to the positive closure[30,31] provided by the Passy-Muir valve, which parallels normal reintroduction of airflow in the upper airway, increasing overall oral and pharyngeal sensation and normalizing pressure relationships.[17] This in turn decreases the pocketing of food in the buccal cavities, valleculae, and the pyriform sinuses where it can often become trapped.[17] With the use of the valve, the patient can sense the pocketed food bolus and encourage its movement through the oropharynx via successive swallows.[17] Using the valve also provides the patient with increased airflow in the upper airway, and subsequently pressures are equalized in the oropharynx. Thus, the patient may be able to clear food particles with functional expectoration out of the oral and pharyngeal cavities so they are not aspirated later.

It is recommended at this time that the modified barium swallow study be performed both with and without the Passy-Muir valve to clinically determine its efficacy for use during swallowing.[17] This device functions more efficiently than finger occlusion in simulating the "closed" system usually present in the swallowing process. It reduces radiation exposure to the dysphagia clinician by eliminating the need for finger occlusion and it gives the tracheostomized patient the benefit of still being able to use the tracheostomy tube for inspiration.

It should be remembered that all three phases of the swallow will be assessed via the modified barium swallow study.[28] However, even though this is a dynamic assessment of deglutition, it is a static point in a patient's life. Therefore, results from a radiographical assessment should not be considered as the final word but instcad as a tool to support clinical judgment and to assist in the determination of appropriate therapy intervention (Figure10-2).

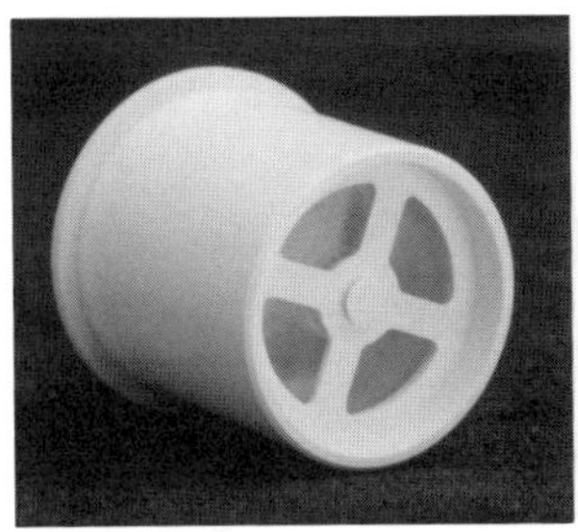

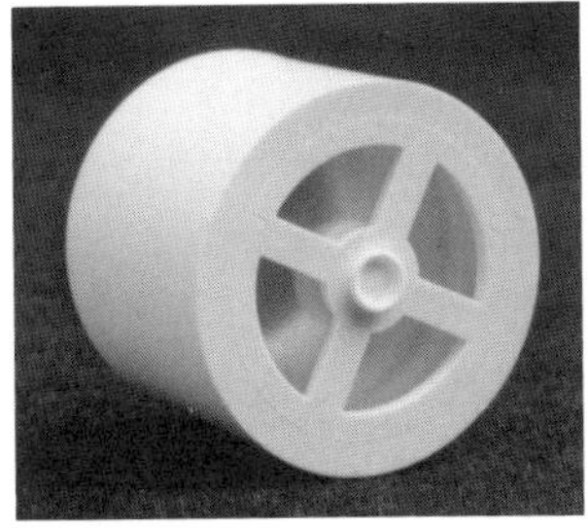

Figure 10-1 The Passy-Muir speaking valves. (Courtesy of Passy-Muir, Inc., Irvine, CA.)

Evaluation Process

Medical Review

The dysphagia clinician should carefully review the patient's history prior to examining the patient in radiology. A bedside evaluation should be completed prior to a radiographic dysphagia evaluation. Medical information should be obtained from either the patient's chart (if an inpatient) or the referring outside therapist, physician, or family member. It is imperative that the dysphagia clinician who is conducting the radiographic study have sufficient background information in order to formulate an idea of how the assessment will be executed as well as to anticipate any possible problems and/or concerns. It is necessary to have the following team members present in the radiology suite when working with a tracheostomized and/or ventilator dependent patient: radiologist, dysphagia clinician, respiratory therapist, and/or nurse.

Pertinent information should be gathered in the initial radiographic evaluation. (Please see previous section of medical review of this chapter.) If the patient is an outpatient, much of this data can be obtained from the patient, the patient's family, the treating therapist, and/or the referring physician.

Preparation of the Patient

Prior to giving the patient any amount of a bolus, the patient may need to be suctioned. This should be performed according to hospital protocol by the respiratory therapist, nurse, or dysphagia clinician (if the latter is authorized to perform this procedure). If the patient is ventilator dependent, ventilator adjustments will be necessary if the patient's tracheostomy cuff is to be deflated so that the ventilator alarms do not activate and increase the patient's anxiety. If at all possible, adjustment of the patient's tracheostomy cuff from the inflated minimal leak position to the completely deflated position should be made to allow for observation of a relatively normal swallow with a tracheostomy tube in place.

It is important for the therapist to discuss with the patient the steps of the procedure in the radiological suite prior to the patient

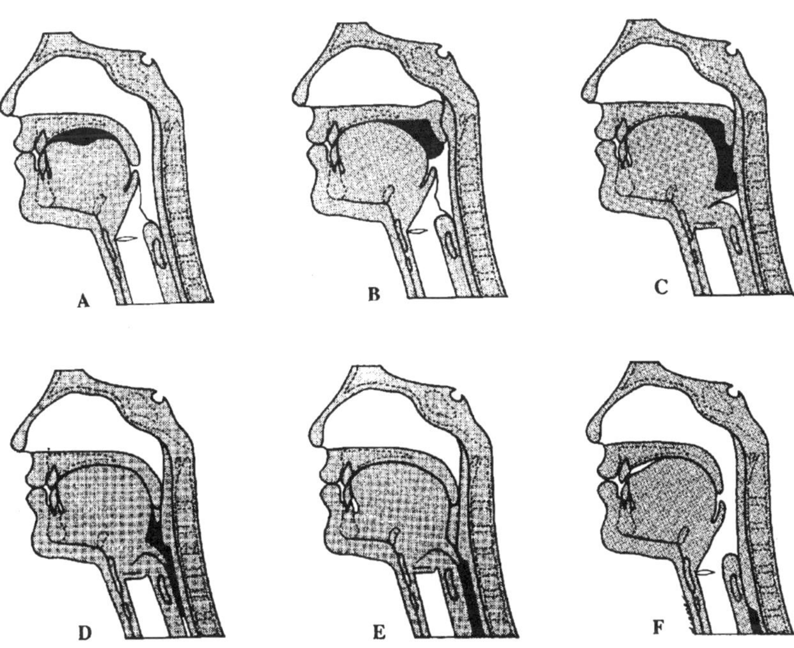

Figure 10-2 Summary schematic of the pharyngeal swallow of a large liquid bolus in an adult, as demonstrated by radiography in the lateral projection. ***A****, The bolus is retained in the oral cavity by approximation of the velum with the tongue; nasal portal respiration can be continued.* ***B****, The bolus is conveyed through the faucial isthmus and into the oropharynx by the tongue. The velum is displaced upward and backward and is approximated by a protrusion on the posterior pharyngeal wall, the beginning of the pharyngeal peristaltic wave.* ***C****, The bolus extends into the laryngopharynx. The epiglottis is tilted downward, and the hyoid and larynx are fully displaced upward and forward. The peristaltic wave is descending in the constrictor wall.* ***D****, The bolus penetrates the opened pharyngoesophageal segment. The peristaltic wave has descended further. The upper portion of the palatopharyngeal isthmus has reopened.* ***E****, The bolus has nearly traversed the pharynx. The peristaltic wave has reached the hypopharynx. The oropharynx is beginning to reopen.* ***F****, The mouth, now empty, and the pharynx have returned to reference position. (Reprinted with permission from Springer-Verlag, From Donner, M.W., Bosma, J.F., and* Robertson, *D., Anatomy and physiology of the pharynx.* Gastrointest Radiol *1985; 10:196-212.)*

being taken to the suite. The patient needs to be informed of the benefits and the results of the assessment as they relate to receiving oral nutrition and possibly weaning from the ventilator, as well as possible weaning from the tracheostomy tube. The patient should be informed that he or she will be eating a variety of consistencies of food in both the sitting up and supine positions and that he or she just needs to do the best that he or she can. The patient should be instructed to advise the dysphagia clinician if he or she becomes uncomfortable so an attempt can be made to minimize the discomfort or, if this is unsuccessful, a decision to terminate the assessment can be made.

Oral-Motor Examination

It is strongly recommended that the dysphagia clinician performs an oral-motor exam prior to the radiographic evaluation. Please see previous text on oral-motor assessment (Table 10-7).

Modified Barium Swallow Study Procedure

1. *Materials*

a. liquid barium
b. liquid (water)
c. barium paste
d. pureed food (e.g., pudding)
e. solid food (e.g., vanilla wafer cookies)
f. several plastic cups
g. several plastic spoons
h. straws
i. thickener (to thicken liquids, if needed)
j. VCR and tape (to videotape the radiographic examination)

2. *General Considerations*

Persistence and creative approaches to obtaining transportation with a patient who is on life support are imperative. This may involve internal transit or transit to another facility. Achieving transportation to conduct this study may mean achieving safe and successful swallowing. Once it is determined that the patient is going to be able to tolerate this radiographic examination, the team members need to decide how the patient will be positioned during the procedure. The best way to assess a patient is in both the sitting erect and lateral/supine positions (if the patient can tolerate these positions). The radiographic evaluation of a patient with dysphagia should assess all phases of the swallow. Thus, it must involve observation of all anatomical structures involved in the swallowing process, including the lips, tongue, soft palate, pharynx, larynx, and esophagus. These observations should be made with all consistencies of food. The best position to assess the esophageal function with all consistencies of food is both in the upright sitting position (to assess with gravity assistance) and in the horizontal or what is known as the RAO (right, anterior, oblique) position (which eliminates gravity assistance).[13,18,19]

Once positioning of the patient has been determined (ideally, in both the sitting erect and supine positions), the next team decision is whether the patient with a cuffed tracheostomy tube can tolerate the procedure with the cuff deflated. If the patient is already taking some oral nutrition, it is strongly recommended that the dysphagia clinician conducting the evaluation know if the patient is eating with the cuff inflated or deflated. Based on this information, the evaluation should proceed using the most functional means possible, that is, by trying to simulate how the patient has been eating in whatever environment he or she is in, be it hospital, nursing home, or private home.

The tailored examination involves assessment of swallowing in a variety of different positions as well as the ability to deal with the tracheostomy tube. This may include inflating or deflating the cuff.

3. Preparing Bolus Consistencies

Prior to the start of the examination, the dysphagia clinician should have prepared approximately (at minimum) 250 cc of thinned barium.[18,19] Some barium that is being utilized in a variety of hospital settings is thicker than the consistency of water. If the dysphagia clinician is being asked to assess the ability of a patient to tolerate his or her secretions and/or thin liquids, then the barium consistency needs to be comparable to that of a thin fluid. The barium can be thinned down by using a barium-to-water ratio of 1:2.[18,19] This mixture is a bit more difficult to see during the radiographic evaluation than is the high-density (undiluted) barium that is used to coat the mucosa. In addition to the 250 cc of thinned barium, a thicker consistency of barium (approximately the consistency of honey) should be prepared so an assessment of the patient's ability to tolerate thickened liquids can be completed.[18,19]

A pureed food consistency should also be prepared for administration to the patient during the radiographic assessment. This will allow evaluation of the patient's ability to tolerate pureed food. Esophatrast paste mixed with food of a pudding consistency or powdered barium mixed with any type of pudding consistency can be used quite effectively in this procedure. It is difficult to get a pureed consistėncy with applesauce or custard, because they thin down at room temperature.[18,19]

Solid food tolerance is assessed by using vanilla wafers (or a wafer type of cookie) covered with barium paste. For edentulous patients, it is possible to prepare barium brownies or to dip the solid food into a prepared barium material.

4. Preparation for the Procedure

If possible, the patient should be in the erect sitting position. This may be done with the use of positioning aids such as pillows, cushions, or special videofluoroscopic chairs. If the patient is unable to sit up, the patient should be placed in the RAO position. The radiologist needs to focus on the head and neck, so as to include a view of the lips, tongue, palate, pharynx, larynx, and the cricopharyngeal area.[18,19]

It is recommended that the consistencies of food be utilized in the same order (e.g., thin, thickened liquids, pureed, solid). This will allow the dysphagia clinician and radiologist to review each section of the procedure and know the order of material administered. Some patients may aspirate on a thin liquid. In this circumstance, some radiologists will abort the study. However, the patient may do better on subsequent swallows or materials. It is recommended that the dysphagia clinician either try to establish and follow a routine or utilize a consistency first that the patient is expected to tolerate, then proceed to the consistencies expected to be more intolerable.

5. Presentation of Thin Liquid Barium

The evaluation usually begins with the administration of liquid of thin consistency. If in the erect sitting position or lateral supine position, the patient should be given a small teaspoonful (approximately 5 cc)[18,19] in order to assess the ability to tolerate a small bolus size.[18,19] At this point, the respiratory therapist should be ready to suction the patient immediately if needed. It is advisable that if the patient can feed himself or herself, this should be allowed. This enables the dysphagia clinician to observe the cognitive aspects that control feeding and swallowing. If the patient tolerates the small bolus[18,19] of thin liquid, the patient's system should be stressed by introducing larger and larger bolus sizes. It is advisable that the patient be given a cup that contains approximately 20 cc of barium so that the patient will be required to extend the head when drinking.[18, 19] A 13- mm barium tablet may be given to assess the ability to take medication safely.[18,19] It is best to observe as much functional behavior in radiology as possible. In other words, the patient's daily routine should be simulated as closely as possible in regard to the size and type of boluses, for example, by spoon versus drinking by cup or straw, as well as the method of presentation, for example, feeding the patient versus letting the patient feed himself or herself.

The radiologist should focus on the oropharynx during the initial portion of the evaluation. Once the oral and pharyngeal phases have been assessed, it is advisable that the esophageal phase be assessed in the sitting position. Optimally, if the patient is able to tolerate it, larger amounts of liquid barium should be administered, one to two mouthfuls at a time. Observation should be made of multiple swallows from the oral cavity to the stomach.

The best way to assess esophageal function is in the RAO position. This adds stress to the process because gravity assistance is absent. This method also helps the radiologist and dysphagia clinician assess the function of the gastroesophageal junction (which allows barium to enter into the stomach) as well as how efficiently the stomach empties.

If the patient is unable to tolerate thin liquids and begins aspirating on small bolus sizes and is unable to cough the barium out of the tracheostomy tube, the patient should be suctioned. Before continuing with the evaluation, the reason for aspiration needs to be determined. If the dysphagia clinician understands why the aspiration occurred, then he or she will be able to determine whether compensatory techniques (i.e., positioning or swallowing maneuvers) should be attempted.

Depending on the amount of aspiration, the dysphagia clinician may want to consider trying to present larger bolus amounts in order to assess esophageal function in the erect position. In this case, thorough suctioning of the patient via the tracheostomy tube should be performed afterward as needed if the patient cannot cough the material out. This is obviously done only if the team feels the patient can tolerate it, as exhibited by the patient's endurance, ability to follow multiple commands, and respiratory status.

If the patient flagrantly aspirates large amounts of the thin liquid consistency, it should be determined why the patient is aspirating and when the patient is aspirating (i.e., before, during, or after the swallow) to determine whether or not more liquid barium should be administered. Once it is sufficiently determined that the patient can or cannot tolerate certain amounts of thin liquids, presentation of the pureed consistency or thick liquid may begin. The same procedures used with thin consistencies will be followed with pureed and solid food consistencies.

Determining whether the evaluation should proceed to the next consistency should be based on the severity of the dysphagia evidenced thus far by the presence and amount of aspiration and the patient's ability to continue the study. Consideration of which, if any, compensatory positioning techniques or compensatory swallowing maneuvers might facilitate a more functional and safer swallow should be constantly reviewed throughout the radiographic procedure. As described with the thin liquid consistency, if the patient has tolerated small amounts of pureed food, the swallowing system should be stressed by presenting several spoonfuls of the pureed material.

If the patient is physically able to tolerate it, he or she should be moved to the recumbent position and all three phases of the swallow should be assessed with all three consistencies of food.[18,19] This will enable the dysphagia clinician to assess the esophageal phase with all consistencies of food and fluids. The patient should be asked to consume the thin liquid via straw by taking 2 to 3 swallows. The patient should be instructed not to swallow until told. This will enable the team to visualize the material going from the mouth to the lower esophageal segment without the effects of gravity. This provides a good assessment of esophageal motility and can identify the presence of various possible esophageal disorders.

It is highly advisable that one, two, or three swallows be completed because it is necessary to fill the entire esophagus with barium in order to adequately view the primary peristaltic wave. If the patient is able to tolerate this procedure with the thin liquid barium, it should be repeated using the pureed and solid food consistencies.[18,19]

It is highly advisable to observe esophageal motility with various consistencies of food. Patients may complain of choking when eating and indicate that the food is sticking in the throat; however, the source is actually in the esophagus. In order to accurately determine what type of diet a patient should be placed on, it is important to know what consistencies of food are being cleared through the esophagus.

Study Termination

There are various reasons to terminate a study in radiology. These reasons can include severe dysphagia (inability to tolerate any consistencies of liquid or food without vast amounts of aspiration), patient noncompliance, intolerance of the procedure, or absence of swallow response. If aspiration occurs, the clinician should determine the rationale and timing in which aspiration occurred. Optimally, the information gathered from this procedure should be sufficient to determine a clinical plan of action.

During the entire process of the evaluation, the respiratory therapist, nurse or other authorized personnel involved in suctioning the patient and the dysphagia clinician and radiologist need to work together to determine step-by-step what needs to happen next. It is highly recommended to try to perform compensatory strategies during the procedure to determine if the patient can swallow without aspiration. The compensatory techniques commonly utilized with nontracheostomized patients are often effective with tracheostomized and ventilator dependent patients.

Interpretation of the Study

Once the study has been completed, the team (including the patient) should develop appropriate goals. The patient needs to be informed of the results of the radiological evaluation, including what difficulties were observed, why he or she had difficulties, and what needs to be done in order for him or her to be able to achieve the goals set by the team. The entire study should be recorded on videotape and the team should review the study immediately on its completion. This ensures that everyone has a clear understanding of the results and recommendations.

Documentation

Documentation of the procedure is mandatory. It is highly advisable that the dysphagia clinician be able to document behavioral and physiological manifestations with all consistencies of food. Documentation should be completed in whatever format has been designated by the facility where the radiographic study took place. The primary referring physician should be telephoned and notified of the results of the study. If the patient is an outpatient, a copy of the written report should also be sent to the primary/referring physician. The report should generally include the following sections:

A. General Information

1. The patient's medical background information
2. All information that was gathered during the referral for the dysphagia evaluation
3. The oral-motor evaluation results
4. Trial feedings that have taken place prior to the radiographic procedure
5. Events occurring in radiology

B. Radiographic Procedure

1. The total amount of barium given to the patient
2. Whether the barium was given in controlled bolus sizes (i.e., 5 cc or teaspoonful) or in uncontrolled and multiple swallows
3. All behavioral manifestations observed at each phase of the swallow

4. What disorder(s) is evident
5. When the disorder(s) occurred during the swallow process
6. What consistency of barium was aspirated
7. Approximately how much barium material was aspirated
8. When and why the aspiration occurred
9. What (if any) compensatory strategies were attempted and which were successful

C. Impressions

The impressions section should provide a dysphagia severity ranging from minimal to extremely severe.

D. Prognosis/Goals

Prognosis involves many aspects such as judgment of the patient's potential for safely tolerating and/or possible decannulation of the tracheostomy tube. The team (including the patient) should be sure to determine long-term and short-term goals that are measurable and functional. Communication with all ancillary professionals involved in the case also should be included in the report to facilitate a coordinated effort toward achieving these goals.

In review, the dysphagia clinician needs to understand the significance and importance of the radiographic procedure with tracheostomized and ventilator dependent patients, particularly if symptoms of a swallowing dysfunction were observed through the clinical assessment (e.g., evidence of aspiration during the blue dye test procedures). The modified barium swallow is an extremely useful tool in determining the prognosis of a dysphagic tracheostomized patient.

ADDITIONAL TYPES OF DIAGNOSTIC METHODOLOGIES

The following procedures can be utilized in coordination with bedside assessment, blue dye study, or videofluoroscopy to further identify pathology with the difficult-to-diagnose dysphagic patient: videoendoscopy, ultrasound, and scintigraphy. Most of these methods are currently being used in research studies of swallowing physiology in an effort to better understand this complex mechanism. These methods, although not commonly used as of yet, can be incorporated into diagnostic assessment in order to better quantify disorders.

Videoendoscopy

Videoendoscopy is a procedure whereby the function and appearance of the epiglottis or the larynx can be examined and recorded.[26,27,28] It can be utilized in conjunction with a modified barium swallow study (videofluoroscopy) in the management and diagnosis of dysphagia. Rationale for use of videoendoscopy stems from some limitations inherent in the modified barium swallow study. Such limitations include repeated exposure to radiation, lack of availability of equipment, scheduling difficulties, patient transport difficulties, or the requirement of a waiting period for test results to be analyzed. In addition, videoendoscopy may be more readily accessible as it is often used for other diagnostic purposes at a medical facility.

Videoendoscopy involves the use of a fiberoptic scope, which can be used to view the esophagus, pharynx, and larynx and has the ability to record that data on videotape. Videoendoscopy allows the dysphagia clinician clear viewing and assessment of the function of the oropharyngeal airways, including the tongue, palate, pharynx, and larynx. With the introduction of food materials or colored liquids, the pharyngeal and laryngeal structures and musculature can be dynamically examined for dysfunction. Types of dysfunction that can be viewed include the pooling of food materials, sensory deficit, spillage, filling or pooling of the laryngeal vestibule, visualization of weakness, and even aspiration. Slow motion viewing can be helpful in a more precise diagnosis.[26,27,28]

Videoendoscopy allows only for indirect examination of structures. Due to limited viewing of structures it does not provide a complete assessment of oral cavity function or complete bolus transit during swallow or information for esophageal disease diagnosis.

Ultrasound

An ultrasound test will not penetrate bone. It is best used to view soft tissue and muscle. It is useful for the viewing of swallowing and tongue movement as it readily displays images of muscle, tissue, and bone dynamically.[32,33,35] An advantage of ultrasound is that there is no risk of exposure to radiation.[32,33,34] Therefore, it is safe and repeatable. A limitation of this procedure is that it does not track bolus transit or confirm presence of aspiration.[32,33,34]

Scintigraphy

Scintigraphic bolus analysis is useful for the detection of occult aspiration that may not be readily apparent in fluoroscopic modified barium swallow studies. Further studies of its usage are being conducted in the hope of using scintigraphy to assist in the prevention of pneumonia and the identification of the passive leakage of oronasopharyngeal secretions. Scintigraphy is useful in quantifying the amount of bolus material retained in the pharynx after the swallow.[35,36] It is a three-dimensional assessment that provides quantitative information.

CONCLUSION

The treatment of swallowing disorders has provided therapists with a new field of science for clinical research. Each year more data are available for analysis. This acquisition of knowledge affects our selected modes of treatment for this patient population.

All team members must work together to address the needs of the dysphagic patient. It is particularly important for the dysphagia clinician and respiratory therapists to develop an effective working relationship to be able to closely monitor and address the needs of this fragile patient population.

The control of aspiration plays a vital role in the prevention of ventilator complications due to infection risk. In addition, the ability to maintain weight is crucial to maintain stamina for the work of breathing and directly affects a patient's ability to wean from the ventilator. Budget restraints mandate expeditious patient transitioning, which, for the ventilator dependent, requires the coordination of many health care specialties. Only with good team effort and patient care management will we develop the state-of-the-art care that the current competitive health care profession demands.

REFERENCES

1. Elpern, E., Jacobs, E., and Bone, R., "Incidence of aspiration in tracheally intubated adults." *Heart and Lung*, 1987; 16:527-531.

2. McConnel, F., "Analysis of pressure generation and bolus transit during pharyngeal swallowing." *Laryngoscope*, 1986; 98:71-78.

3. McConnel, F., and Mendelssohn, M., "The effects of surgery on pharyngeal deglutition." *Dysphagia*, 1987; 1:145-151.

4. McConnel, F., Cerenko, D., and Mendelssohn, M., "Manofluorographic analysis of swallowing." *Otolaryngologic Clinics of North America*, 1988; 21:625-635.

5. McConnel, F., and Cerenko, D., "Timing of major events of pharyngeal swallowing." *Archives of Otolaryngology, Head and Neck Surgery*, 1988; 114:1413-1418.

6. Miller, A., "Swallowing: Neurophysiologic control of the esophageal phase." *Dysphagia*, 1987; 2:72-82.

7. Miller, A., "Deglutition." *Physiol Rev*, 1982; 62:129-184.

8. Miller, A., "Neurophysiological basis of swallowing." *Dysphagia*, 1986; 1:91-100.

9. Jones, B., Kramer, S., and Donner, M., "Dynamic imaging of the pharynx." *Gastrointestinal Radiology*, 1985; 10:213-224.

10. Jones, B., and Donner, M., *Normal and Abnormal Swallowing Imaging in Diagnosis and Therapy*, New York: Springer-Verlag, 1991.

11. Sasaki, C.T., Gaudet, P.T., and Peerless, A., "Tracheostomy decannulation." *American Journal of Diseases of Children*, 1978; 132:266-269.

12. Stauffer, M., and Silvestri, M., "Complications of endotracheal intubation, tracheostomy, and artificial airways." *Respiratory Care,* 1982; 27, 417-433.

13. Groher, M., *Dysphagia, Diagnosis and Management.* 2nd Ed., Boston: Butterworth-Heinemann, a division of Reed Publishing, Inc., 1992.

14. Martin, B., Corlew, M., et al. "The association of swallowing dysfunction and aspiration pneumonia." Presented at Conference, *Swallowing and Swallowing Disorders: From Clinic to Laboratory*, Evanston, IL: Oct. 1991.

15. Bach, J.R., and Alba, A.S., "Tracheostomy ventilation: A study of efficacy with deflated cuffs and cuffless tubes." *Chest*, 1990; 97:679-683.

16. Manzano, J.L., Lubillo, S., et al. "Verbal Communication of Ventilator Dependent Patients." *Critical Care Medicine*, April 1993; 21(4):512-517.

17. Scott, M., Speech Care, Videofluoroscopy study, LaGrange, IL: 1991.

18. O'Sullivan, N., Puntil, J., et al. *Dysphagia Care Team Approach with acute and Long term patients*, Los Angeles: Cottage Square Press, 1990.

19. Huntington Memorial Hospital, *Dysphagia Team, Policy and Procedure for Evaluation and Blue Dye Testing*, Pasadena, CA: Huntington Memorial Hospital, 1990.

20. Logemann, J., *Manual for the Videofluorographic Study of Swallowing*, Waltham, MA: College-Hill Press, Little Brown & Co., 1986.

21. Dodds, W., "The physiology of swallowing." *Dysphagia*, 1989; 3:171-178.

22. Dodds, W., Steward, E., and Logemann, J., "Physiology and radiology of the normal oral and pharyngeal phases of swallowing." *Am J Radiol*, 1990; 154:953-963.

23. Dodds, W., Man, D., et al. "Influence of bolus volume on swallow-induced hyoid movement in normal subjects." *Am J Radiol*, 1988; 95:1307-1309.

24. Rubesin, S., Jessurun, J., et al. "Lines of the pharynx." *Radiographics*, 1987; 7:217-237.

25. Linden, P., and Siebens, A., "Dysphagia: Predicting laryngeal penetration." *Archives of Physical Medicine and Rehabilitation*, 1983; 64:281-284.

26. Bastian, R.W., "Videoendoscopic evaluation of patients with dysphagia: An adjunct to the modified barium swallow." *Otolaryngology, Head and Neck Surgery,* 104(3):339-350.

27. Bastian, R.W., "Videoendoscopic evaluation of dysphagia in an office setting." *Clinical Geriatric Otorhinolaryngology,* St. Louis: Mosby Year-Book, 1992; 13-20.

28. Bastian, R., Kaniff, T., et al., "Indirect videolaryngoscopy versus direct endoscopy for larynx and pharynx cancer staging: Toward elimination of preliminary direct laryngoscopy." *Annals of Otology, Rhinology & Laryngology,* 1989; 98(9):693-698.

29. Langmore, S., and Logemann, J.A., "After the clinical bedside swallowing examination: What next?" Second Opinion, *American Speech-Language and Hearing Journal*, Sept. 1991:13-20.

30. Mason, M., and Watkins, C., "Protocol for use of the Passy-Muir Tracheostomy Speaking Valves." *The European Respiratory Journal*, Aug. 1992; 5:148s No. p0469.

31. Mason, M., and Watkins, C., "Communication for the tracheostomized and ventilator patient utilizing the Passy-Muir Valve," Presented at the California State University, Northridge, CA: Technology and Persons with Disabilities Conference, 1992; *The Respiratory Nursing Society*, March 1992.

32. Sonies, B.C., Parent, L.J., Morrish, K., and Baum, B.J., "Durational aspects of the oral-pharyngeal phase of swallowing in normal adults. *Dysphagia*, 1988; 3:1.

33. Sonies, B.C., and Baum, B.J., "Evaluation of swallowing pathophysiology." *Otolaryngology Clinics of North America*, 1988; 21:4.

34. Sonies, B.C., "Beyond Pu, Tu, Ku." *Evaluation of the Speech and Swallowing Mechanisms* (Videoconference), Rockville, MD: American Speech-Language-Hearing Association., May 13, 1988.

35. Hamlet, S., Muz, J., et al., "Scintigraphic quantification of pharyngeal retention following deglutition." *Dysphagia,* 1992; 7:2-16.

36. Silver, K. H. and Van Nostrand, D., "Scintigraphic detection of salivary aspiration: Description of a new diagnostic technique and case reports." *Dysphagia*, 1992; 7:45-49.

BIBLIOGRAPHY

Buchholz, D.W., Bosma, J.F., et al., "Adaption, compensation, and decompensation of the pharyngeal swallow." *Gastrointestinal Radiology*, 1985; 10:235-239.

Cameron, J.L., Reynolds, J., et al.,"Aspiration of Patients with Tracheostomies." *Surgery, Gynecology & Obstetrics.* 1973; 136:68-70.

Cerenko, D., McConnel, F., Jackson, R.T., et al., "Clinical application of the manoflourogram." *Laryngoscope*, 1988; 98:705-711.

Cerenko, D., McConnel, F., et al., "Quantitative assessment of pharyngeal bolus driving forces." *Otolaryngology, Head and Neck Surgery 100*, 1989; 1:57-63.

Davidoff, G. L., Thomas, P., et al., "Closed head injury in acute traumatic spinal cord injury: Incidence and risk factors." *Archives of Physical Medicine and Rehabilitation*, 1988; 69:869-872.

Eisele, D., "Surgical approaches to aspiration." *Dysphagia*, 1991; 7:71-78.

Fornataro, L.M., and Wyse, M.A., "The tracheostomized patient: Evaluation and management of communication and swallowing." Paper Presented at the *American Speech-Language and Hearing Association,* Seattle, WA, 1990.

Gilbert, R.W., Mcllwain, J.C., et al., "Management of patients with long-term tracheotomies and aspiration." *Annals of Otology, Rhinology and Laryngology*, 1987; 96:561 564.

Horner, J., and Massey, E., "Silent aspiration following stroke." Neurology, 1988, 38:317-319.

Kahrilas, P., Logemann, J., and Gibbons, P., "Food intake by maneuver; an extreme compensation for impaired swallowing." *Dysphagia,* 1992: 7:155-159.

Levine, R., Robbins, J., and Maser, A., "Periventricular white matter changes and oropharyngeal swallowing in normal individuals." *Dysphagia*, 1992; 7:142-147.

Nash, M., "Swallowing problems in the tracheostomized patient." *Otolaryngologic Clinics of North America*, 1988; 21:701-709.

Splaingard, M.L., Hutchins, B., et al., "Aspiration in rehabilitation patients: Videofluoroscopy vs. bedside clinical assessment." *Archives of Physical Medicine and Rehabilitation,* 1988; 69:417-433.

Vinod, A., "Surgical Considerations in Trachael Stenosis." *Laryngscope* 1992; 102: 237-242.

GLOSSARY

Access method: The physical method in which the user will indicate items on the communication system; may be directly (i.e., pointing) or indirect (i.e., stopping a cursor on a desired letter)

Achalasia: Failure of a ring of muscle (as a sphincter) to relax

Acidosis: A condition characterized by the presence of excessive quantities of acids in the blood; used mostly to indicate a decrease in the alkaline reserve below normal levels

Adenocarcinoma: A malignant adenoma arising from a glandular organ

Adenoma: A neoplasm of glandular epithelium

Agenesis: Failure of an organ or part to develop or grow

Airway: The path air travels from the atmosphere to and from the alveoli; in anesthesia or resuscitation, a mechanical device used to keep the passages of the upper respiratory tract open for the passage of air

Airway obstruction: The presence of a foreign body, growth, or swelling that occludes the air passageways and interferes with normal breathing

Alkalosis: A condition in which the alkaline content (hydrogen ion concentration) content in the blood increases above normal limits; used most often to indicate an increase in alkaline reserve above normal levels

Alveoli: Microscopic air sacs located at the end of the respiratory tract. The total number of these sacs has been estimated at 300 million. (Singular: alveolus.) Grape-like clusters of sacs that allow inhaled oxygen (O_2) to enter the bloodstream. Carbon dioxide (CO_2) leaves the bloodstream and enters the sacs where it is exhaled through breathing

Anastomosis: The surgical union of parts and especially hollow tubular parts

Angiofibroma: A tumor consisting of fibrous tissue

Anoxia: Literally means *without oxygen;* used generally to indicate lack of oxygen in the blood and tissues of the body

Apnea: Complete cessation of respiration

Adult respiratory distress syndrome (ARDS): Shock lung or wet lung. A symptom secondary to initial pathology (e.g., pneumonic or trauma) that results in injury to alveolar capillary units causing acute pulmonary edema due to capillary leak from capillary membrane damage. High mortality rate, approximately 50%

Arrhythmia: Irregularity or loss of rhythm, especially of the heartbeat

Artery: A vessel through which oxygen-rich blood passes to various parts of the body

Artificial airway: Surgical airway route that bypasses the normal airway (mouth and nose)

Arytenoid: Resembling a ladle or pitcher mouth. Relating to the arytenoid cartilage, gland, ligament or muscle

Asphyxia: A condition caused by insufficient intake of oxygen in the environment

Aspiration: Inhalation of any foreign matter, such as food, saliva, or stomach contents (as after vomiting) into the airway

Asthma: A disease state characterized by difficult respiration and wheezing on expiration. Wheezes are caused as exhaled air flows past air passages narrowed by spasms of circular muscles around bronchi and bronchioles; usually complicated by secretions inside the airway that increase the difficulty of breathing. This condition may lead to infection

Atelectasis: A collapsed or airless area of the lung. May be caused by excessive secretions, obstruction by foreign bodies or compression

Atmospheric: Of or relating to air

Atresia: Congenital absence or closure of a normal body opening

Ausculation: Process of listening for sounds produced in some body cavities (i.e., chest and abdomen)

Barotrauma: Injury caused by a change in atmospheric pressure between a potentially closed space and the surrounding tissue (e.g., lungs)

Bolus: Food formed into a cohesive mass (in preparation for swallowing)

Bradycardia: A slow heart beat characterized by a pulse rate under 60 beats per minute

Bradypnea: Decreased respiratory rate

Bronchi: The air passages of the lungs, beginning with the first bifurcation at the carina, through all their branches, to the smallest tubes at the distal portions of the lungs (singular: bronchus)

Bronchiectasis: A chronic dilation of the bronchi or bronchioles marked by fetid breath and paroxysmal coughing with the expectoration of mucopurulent matter

Bronchiole: The smallest conducting airway with cartilage construction in the respiratory tract. The bronchioles connect to the atria and alveoli to complete the lung unit

Bronchiolitis: Inflammation of the bronchioles

Bronchitis: Inflammation of the bronchial tubes due to exposure to cold, to the breathing of irritant substances, and to acute general disease

Bronchodilator: Any of a number of drugs that enlarge the bronchial air passage either by shrinking the mucous membranes or by relaxing the smooth muscles that constrict the air passages

Bronchorrhea: An abnormality in which the cells in the walls of the bronchial tubes secrete an excessive amount of mucus

Bronchoscopy: A technique to view inside the trachea and main bronchial tubes by means of a tube and light that are passed through the mouth into the trachea and bronchi

Bronchopulmonary dysplasia: Abnormal development of tissue, pertaining to bronchi and lungs

Bullae: Large blebs or blisters inside the lung, as in emphysema

Cannula, inner: Removable inner tube of the tracheostomy tube that acts as a passageway for airflow and secretion removal after tracheostomy

Cannula, outer: An external tube (tracheostomy tube) that is inserted into the trachea through a surgical opening to provide an artificial passage for breathing may house a removable inner cannula

Capillary network: Group of tiny blood vessels that connect arteries to veins

Capnography: Noninvasive, in-line, infrared analysis of carbon dioxide levels. Infrared light is absorbed by carbon dioxide and water but is not by oxygen, nitrogen, argon, helium, and other atmospheric gases. An infrared frequency is selected that will not be affected by water so that carbon dioxide content will be measured

Carbon dioxide: Heavy, colorless, odorless gas that passes out of the lungs during respiration. By-product of the body's metabolism

Carbon monoxide (CO): A gas caused by incomplete combustion that, when inhaled, forms a semipermanent bond with the hemoglobin. Death from carbon monoxide poisoning is caused by low oxygen tension in the tissues

Cardiopulmonary: Relating to the heart and lungs

Cardiovascular: Pertaining to the heart and blood vessel system

Cardiovascular accident (CVA): Stroke, rupture of a blood vessel in the brain

Carina: Bifurcation of the trachea; area of the tracheobronchial tree where the first two branches leave the trachea

Choana: A funnel-shaped opening, especially one of the posterior nares, the communicating passageways between the nasal fossae and the pharynx

Chemoreceptors: Small bodies located in the brain and on the carotid and aortic arteries that are sensitive to changes in blood oxygen and carbon dioxide pressure and that help regulate the rate and depth of respiration

Chronic: Continuing over a long period, as a persistent ailment or sickness

Cilia: Minute, hairlike structures found in the respiratory tract that propel foreign matter on a thin layer of mucus toward the pharynx where the mucus is normally swallowed or expectorated

Coarctation of the aorta: Narrowing of the aorta caused by a localized malformation

Coded systems: A pattern or code of signals to indicate message elements; used by nonvocal patients

Congenital goiter: Enlargement of the thyroid gland present at birth

Connector, 15 mm: The part of the inner cannula that secures the outer cannula to the inner cannula and adapts to standard respiratory equipment, such as a ventilator

Connector, low profile: A part of the inner cannula designed to reduce tube protrusion at the neck. Not compatible with respiratory equipment

Connector, snap-lock: Part of the inner cannula that is discarded after one use. The 15 mm connector secures the inner cannula to the outer cannula. It also provides a universal attachment that adapts to standard respiratory equipment, such as a ventilator

Connector, twist-lock: A 15 mm connector that attaches the inner cannula of the tracheostomy tube to the outer cannula of the tracheostomy tube by twisting into place

Continuous positive airway pressure (CPAP): The application of positive pressure to the airways and alveoli throughout the respiratory cycle when the patient is breathing spontaneously

COPD: Chronic obstructive pulmonary disease. A general term describing disorders that result in chronic airflow obstruction of the lungs (e.g., emphysema, chronic bronchitis and asthma. COPD involves decreased expiratory flow rates with increased total lung capacity

Copious: Abundant; much; of an extraordinary amount. Usually used to describe the volume of secretions

Cor pulmonale: Failure of the right side of the heart to empty properly as a result of pulmonary hypertension

Costal breathing: Respirations produced solely by use of the intercostal muscles

Cricopharyngeal sphincter (Pharyngoesophageal junction): Muscle located between the pharynx and esophagus that opens during normal swallowing. Its function can become impaired due to swallowing disorders

Croup: Disease condition of the larynx that is characterized by harsh, raspy cough, a crowing sound, and difficult respiration

Cuff: Balloon-like component that, when inflated with air, acts as a seal to eliminate or reduce airflow through the mouth and nose. With the cuff inflated, breathing is directed through the tracheostomy tube

Cuffed tube: A tracheostomy tube that has a cuff which, when inflated with air, acts as a seal to eliminate or reduce airflow through the mouth and nose. With an inflated cuff, breathing is only through the tracheostomy tube

Cuffless tube: A tracheostomy tube without a cuff that allows airflow through the mouth, nose, and tracheostomy

Cyanosis: Blueness of the skin often due to cardiac malformation that causes insufficient oxygenation of the blood

Cyst: A closed sac or pouch, with a definite wall, that contains fluid, semifluid, or solid material. It is usually an abnormal structure resulting from developmental anomalies, obstruction of ducts, or parasitic infection

Cystic fibrosis: An inherited disease of exocrine glands affecting the pancreas, respiratory system, and apocrine glands; usually begins in infancy and is characterized by chronic respiratory infection, pancreatic insufficiency, and increased electrolytes in sweat

Cystic hygroma: A rapidly growing hygroma of lymphatic origin; usually located in the neck but may be in the thorax

Dead space, anatomic: The air that is always in the tube system of the lungs, normally 150 ml in the normal adult or approximately 1 ml per pound of body weight

Dead space, mechanical: The volume of the apparatus or tubes into and out of which thc patient may be forced to breathe and from which carbon dioxide is not effectively removed

Dead space, physiologic: Areas of the lung in which oxygen is not exchanged through the alveolar wall as a result of any interference with ventilation or diffusion of blood supply, such as atelectasis or embolism

Decannulation: Removal of the tracheostomy tube or endotracheal tube

Decannulation plug: A button that attaches to the outer cannula of a fenestrated tracheostomy tube when the inner cannula has been removed; it blocks airflow through the tracheostomy tube and directs breathing through the nose and mouth

Decompensation: Failure of the heart to circulate the blood properly or at a fast enough rate

Deflation: Collapse by removing air or gas

Dermoid: Resembling the skin

Diaphoretic: Stimulating the secretion of sweat. A medicine that increases perspiration

Diaphragm: Main muscle used in breathing. It separates the abdomen from the chest cavity. During inhalation, it flattens out downward, allowing the bottom parts of the lungs to expand. During exhalation, it elevates, allowing the lungs to restore to their natural shape

Diaphragmatic hernia: Congenital or traumatic protrusion of abdominal contents through the diaphragm

Direct laryngoscopy (fiber-optic evaluation): Examination of the larynx by direct vision with the aid of a flexible scope

Direct selection: Technique in which the message sender indicates elements of his message by directly pointing to them in some manner

Double pneumonia, bilateral: Inflammation of both lungs

Dry swallows: Swallowing without taking food or liquid into the mouth; Refers to swallowing saliva only

Dyspnea: Air hunger resulting in labored or difficult breathing, sometimes accompanied by pain. Normal when due to vigorous work or athletic activity

Edema: Accumulation of fluid in the tissues

Elasticity: Ability to stretch

Emphysema: Abnormal condition of the lungs caused by air trapped in lungs or tissue as a result of a disease process or aging

Encephalocele: Protrusion of the brain through a cranial fissure

Encrustation: Buildup of hardened mucus

Endobronchial: Within a bronchus

Endotracheal: Within the trachea, as an endotracheal tube

Epiglottis: Elastic cartilage covered by mucous membrane, diverts food from the mouth to the esophagus by closing over the trachea

Epiglottitis: Inflammation of the epiglottis; most common in young children. If left untreated, may cause death. A more appropriate term for this condition is supraglottitis

Esophagus: Tubular structure through which food and fluids are directed into the stomach

Expectorate: To expel sputum through the mouth

Expiration: Act of exhaling air from the lungs

Faucial pillars: Located in the posterior fauces (the constricted opening between the oral cavity and pharynx). The pillars line the side of the fauces. Place in rear of mouth to apply ice during thermal stimulation

Fenestration: A hole or holes in a cannula that allow air to be directed past the vocal cords and through the mouth and nose

Fetid: Having a rank or disagreeable smell

Fistula: An abnormal tube like passage from a normal cavity or tube to a free surface or to another cavity. May be due to congenitally incomplete closure of parts or may result from abscesses, injuries, or inflammatory processes

Forced expiratory volume (FEV_1): A flow rate calculation based on a forced vital capacity and normally expressed as a percent of FVC; equals forced expiratory volume in 1 second

Forced vital capacity (FVC): The amount of air that can be exhaled forcefully after a maximum inspiration

Gastrostomy tube: A feeding tube surgically inserted directly into the stomach

Glioma: A sarcoma of neuroglial origin

Glottis: Area between the vocal cords

Granulation tissue: Abnormal tissue comprised of granulations

Hemangioma: A benign tumor of dilated blood vessels

Hemolytic disease of the newborn: Disease of the newborn characterized by anemia, jaundice, enlargement of the liver and spleen, and generalized edema. Due to transplacental transmission of maternal antibody, usually evoked by maternal and fetal blood group incompatibility

Home health care provider: Clinician who provides medical support for the patient and family

Humidification: A moderate degree of wetness, especially in the atmosphere. Air the patient breathes must be humidified to keep the tracheal mucosa moist and thereby facilitate mucociliary transport of secretions and prevent crusting and eventual obstruction of the airway

Hyaline membrane disease: A respiratory disease of the newborn. Formed after initial tissue injury from alveolar epithelial cell debris. Bronchopulmonary dysplasia can result from this disorder. See *Adult Respiratory Distress Syndrome*

Hyperalimentation: Intravenous administration of total nutrient requirements

Hypercapnia: Elevated CO_2 level in the blood

Hyperoxemia: Excessive acidity of the blood

Hyperthermia: An abnormally high body temperature; fever

Hypertrophy: Increase in size of an organ or structure that does not involve tumor formation. Generally describes to an increase in size or bulk not resulting from an increase in number of cells or tissue elements, as in the hypertrophy of a muscle

Hyperventilation: Abnormally prolonged, rapid, and deep breathing; also the condition produced by overbreathing oxygen at high pressure. It is marked by confusion, dizziness, numbness, and muscular cramp brought on by such breathing. Also called O_2 poisoning

Hypoglycemia: Deficiency of sugar in the blood; a condition in which the glucose in the blood is abnormally low

Hypotension: Decrease of systolic and diastolic blood pressure to below normal

Hypoventilate: To underaerate the alveoli; to put less air into the lungs than a patient needs for adequate oxygenation as a result of a decrease in rate and/or depth of ventilation

Hypoxemia: Insufficient amount of oxygen in the blood

Hypoxia, anemic: Hypoxia caused by low hemoglobin or too few red cells

Hypoxia, demand: Increased use of oxygen by the cells, caused by high fever or thyroid dysfunction

Hypoxia, histotoxic: Inability of cells to use oxygen as a result of poisoning of the cell

Hypoxia, stagnant (ischemic): Hypoxia in the tissue cells, caused by slow circulation of the blood

Idiopathic: Occurring without known cause

I/E Ratio (Inspiratory/expiratory ratio): Amount of air that a person takes in and breathes out, which is controlled by a ventilator. Expiration is a longer process than inspiration

IMV (Intermittent mandatory ventilation): A technique that guarantees a specific amount of mechanical ventilation to a patient. At preset low respiratory rates, it may be used to wean a patient from the ventilator. At high preset respiratory rates, it may be used to control a patient's respiration

Infarct: An arterial blood clot that occludes a blood vessel, causing a triangular area of tissue being supplied by that artery to die

Inflation line: Thin plastic line connected to cuff, pilot balloon, and luer valve, which allows the cuff to be filled with air

Inspiration: Act of drawing or breathing air into the lungs

Inspiratory capacity (IC): Maximum amount of air that can be taken into the lungs on forced inspiration from resting expiration; normally 3500 ml in adults

Inspiratory reserve volume (IRV): The amount of air that can be breathed in after normal resting inspiration; normally 3100 ml in the adult

Insults: Any effort, disease, or trauma that adds to any abnormal condition that the patient may already have; for example, pneumonia insults the respiratory ability of the emphysema patient

Intercostal: Located between the ribs

Intermittent positive pressure breathing (IPPB): Pressure on inspiration, followed by a passive exhalation, which usually refers to a short-term breathing treatment; also refers to inspiratory positive pressure breathing

Intermittent positive pressure ventilation (IPPV): See *Intermittent positive pressure breathing*. Usually refers to continuous mechanical ventilation

Internal respiration: Exchange of gases (oxygen and carbon dioxide) between the tissues and bloodstream

Intrathoracic: Inside the rib cage or chest wall

Intratracheal: Inside the trachea

Intubation: The process of passing a tube through the mouth or nose into the trachea

Ischemia: A decrease in blood supply to a localized area as a result of constriction of blood vessels

Kyphoscoliosis: Humpback and curvature of the spine to the side and forward

Laminar flow: Straight line movement of fluid through a passageway. Most desirable in terms of volume moved per unit of time at a given pressure gradient

Laryngitis: Inflammation of the larynx that may obstruct ventilation

Laryngocele: A congenital air sac connected to the larynx. Its presence is normal in some animals but abnormal in man

Laryngomalacia: Softening of the tissue of the larynx

Larynx: Structure that houses the vocal cords and connects the upper and lower airway

Leak: Expired air that escapes past a tracheostomy tube, either room air or during ventilation and passes through the glottis and allows vocalization

Leukocyte: White blood cell, responsible for fighting infection

Liter (L): 1000 ml or 1.0567 quarts

Liter/minute: Measure of flow; liters per minute, L/min, or lpm

Lobe: A globular part of an organ separated by boundaries; for example, lobes of a lung

Long-term tracheostomy: Tracheostomy that extends past the seven- to ten-day acute care phase. In long-term tracheostomy, aphonia may be present part or all of the day secondary to cuff inflation. Oral-motor weakness may or may not be present; however, there is a strong likelihood of eventual extubation

Lumen: Space within a tube; for example, tracheal lumen

Lung abscess: Enclosed, pus-filled area or cavity inside the lung

Lymphangioma: Tumor comprised of lymphatic vessels

Lymphosarcoma: A malignant disease of lymphatic tissue. Clinically may be quite similar to Hodgkin's disease. Diagnosis is made by biopsy rather than by clinical examination

Macroglossia: Hypertrophied condition of the tongue; a congenital disorder

Malacia: Softening of the cartilage

Manometer: Device for measuring the pressure of a liquid or gas

Manometry: Technique to evaluate the speed and the pressure changes of a bolus as it moves from the pharynx into the esophagus. Only the passage of the bolus is noted; no anatomical information is given

Maximum ventilatory volume (MVV): Previously called maximum breathing capacity (MBC); the maximum volume of air a patient can move in 1 minute

Meconium: First feces of a newborn infant, made up of salts, liquor amnei, mucus, bile, and epitheal cells

Mendelsohn maneuver: Technique used to increase the opening of the cricopharyngeal sphincter during swallow. The patient is instructed to hold the larynx elevated during the swallow. This technique is taught and practiced by speech and occupational therapists

Metabolic: Pertaining to the sum of the cellular and tissue changes, physical and chemical, whereby the body functions and energy is produced

Metabolism: Sum total of all chemical activity in the body

Micrognathia: Abnormal smallness of jaws, especially the lower jaw

Minute volume: Volume of air breathed in a minute

mm: Abbreviation for *millimeter*. 1 millimeter = .039 inch

mm Hg: A measurement of pressure. 1 millimeter of mercury represents a pressure equal to 1.36 cm H_2O (centimeters of water)

Mucoid: Resembling mucus. Any of a group of mucus-like conjugated proteins of animal origin

Mucolysis: The breaking down or loosening up of mucous secretions by chemical means

Mucopurulent: Containing both mucus and pus

Mucosa: Mucous membrane; the tissue that lines the inside of the nose, mouth, trachea, bronchi, and bronchioles

Mucous plug: Thick, dry piece of mucus that is large enough to occlude the lumen of a bronchi or bronchiole

Mucus: Clear, viscid secretions of the mucous membranes (consisting of mucin, epithelial cells, white blood cells, and various salts suspended in water)

Myasthenia gravis: Disease of the sixth thoracic nerve that causes progressive paralysis of the muscles of breathing

Myocardial infarction (MI): A heart attack resulting from injured heart muscle

Nasogastric tube: A tube inserted through a nostril down to the stomach, used for feeding

Nebulization: The process of breaking down a fluid into fine particles and suspending them in a gas; this forms a mist called an aerosol

Nebulizer: A device for making a mist (aerosol) of small particles of a solution

Negative pressure: Pressure less than ambient

Neonatal: Pertains to the newborn infant

Neurofibroma: A tumor of connective tissue of a nerve including medullated layer of a nerve fiber; may occur in mouth, pleura, or stomach

Nosocomial: Pertaining to a hospital or an infirmary

NPO (Not per oral): Instruction not to give a patient anything by mouth, including food, drink and medications

Obstruction: Anything that blocks a structure and prevents its normal function

Oral apraxia: Difficulty initiating and sequencing movements of the lips and tongue to swallow foods or to produce oral movements on command

Orthopnea: Shortness of breath except when in an upright position

Oximetry: Measurement of the oxygen saturation of arterial blood by means of bichromate photoelectric infrared colorimetry

Papilloma: Any benign epitheal tumor

Paradoxical respiration: Expansion on expiration and contraction on inspiration of the lungs

Patent: Open, clear

Patent ductus arteriosus: Persistence of a communication between the main pulmonary artery and the aorta after birth

Penetration: Entry of material into an unprotected airway

Peristaltic motion: Wavelike muscular motion, for example, in the intestine or esophagus

Perinatal: Concerning the period beginning after the 28th week of pregnancy through 28 days following birth

Permanent tracheostomy: The placement of a tracheostomy tube for an extended period of time, often with no plan for extubation. Aphonia may be present part or all of the day secondary to cuff inflation. Oral-motor weakness may or may not be present.

Population may include neuromuscular disease (i.e., amyotrophic lateral sclerosis), end-stage pulmonary/respiratory disorders (i.e., chronic obstructive pulmonary disease)

pH: A measure of the hydrogen ion concentration of a substance

Pharyngitis: Inflammation of the pharynx

Pharynx: An area of mucous membrane behind the mouth and nose and above the esophagus and trachea

Phospholipid: A lipoid substance containing phosphorus, fatty acids, and nitrogenous base, as lecithin

Physiologic: Concerning normal body function

Pickwickian syndrome: A restrictive disease of the chest that is caused by obesity and is characterized by somnolence, hypoventilation, and erythrocytosis

Pierre Robin syndrome: Unusual smallness of the jaw combined with cleft palate, downward displacement of the tongue, and an absent gag reflex

Pigeon breast: Malformation of the front of the chest wall causing the sternum to be elevated and pushed forward into a point

Pilot balloon: Plastic sac-like component connected to the inflation line and luer valve, which acts as an indicator for the amount of air pressure within the cuff

Plasma: Fluid portion of the blood

Plethora: Congestion causing overfullness of blood vessels

Pleura: The tissue that lines the inside of the chest walls and the outside of the lungs. These two layers are side by side with only a potential space between them

Plug: A button that is used to close the tracheostomy tube, to allow for upper airway breathing. Used during the decannulation process.

Pneumoconiosis: A disease of the respiratory tract that results from inhalation of dust particles

Pneumonia: Inflammation of the lungs; fluid in the lung tissue causes consolidation

Pneumonitis: Inflammation of the lungs; often a viral pneumonia

Pneumoparesis: Progressive congestion of the lungs

Pneumothorax: Air leaking into the pleural space from the lung or through the chest wall; if uncorrected results in a collapsed lung

Pocketing: Food collected between the teeth and cheek, usually on the affected side (weaker)

Poliomyelitis: Inflammation of the gray matter of the spinal cord, sometimes causing paralysis

Polymyositis: Inflammation of many muscles; sometimes affects the chest muscles

Positive end expiratory pressure (PEEP): The application of positive pressure to the airways and alveoli during expiration when the patient is breathing with a mechanical ventilator. Maintains a small amount of air in the lungs, preventing complete emptying on exhalation to avoid airway collapse

Postural drainage: Gravitational assistance to empty the secretions from a body cavity by positioning; in respiratory therapy, specifically, the draining of mucus from any part of the lung so that it can be expectorated or removed

Pressure: Amount of air needed to inflate the lungs

Pressure-relief valve: Replaces standard luer valve. When connected to a luer syringe, it inflates or deflates the cuff. The pressure-relief valve automatically limits internal cuff pressure to approximately 25 mm Hg (34 cm H_2O)

Prognosis: An estimate of the probable outcome or course of a disease

Prolapse: The falling or sinking down of a part

Prone: Lying face downward

Protrusion: A part that bulges or extends beyond the tip (end)

Pseudomonas: A bacterium that produces a blue-green pigment and is infectious

Pulmonary: Pertaining to the lungs

Pulmonary edema: The leakage of fluid from the capillaries into the alveoli as a result of increased pressure inside the capillaries or a leaky capillary wall

Pulmonary emboli: Blood clots in the vessels of the lung; often fatal

Pulmonary flora: Organisms that normally live inside the lung, trachea, and bronchi; they cause no disease and may often prevent the implantation of other organisms that could produce disease

Pulmonary hypertension: Increased pressure within the pulmonary circulation

Purulent: Consisting of or containing pus; associated with the formation of or caused by pus

Pyriform sinus: Space on each side of the larynx, in the lower part of the pharynx. Place where food can collect when swallowing function is impaired

Rales: Bubbling sounds heard when mucus or fluid is present in the lumen of the trachea and bronchi

Rate: The number of inspiratory/expiratory cycles set on a ventilator

RDS: Respiratory distress syndrome. See ARDS: Adult Respiratory Distress Syndrome

Residual: Undigested contents remaining before a tube feeding is given. If more than 100 cc remains, the next tube feeding should be postponed

Residual volume (RV): The volume of gas remaining in the lungs after a maximum expiration

Respiration: The exchange of oxygen and carbon dioxide between the atmosphere and the cells of the body. The physical and chemical processes by which an organism supplies its cells/tissues with the oxygen needed for metabolism

Restrictive: Hindering normal motion. In a pulmonary study, any condition that hinders normal chest wall motion or normal expansion of the lungs, such as kyphoscoliosis or cystic fibrosis

Retrolental fibroplasia: A bilateral disease of the retinal vessels present in premature infants, some of whom were exposed to high postnatal oxygen concentrations

Rhinitis: Inflammation of the mucous membranes of the nose

Rhonchi: Abnormal, course sounds heard during auscultation of the chest. These sounds occur in the larger air passages and throat; they may be called dry or sibilant rales

Sarcoma: Cancer arising from connective tissue such as muscle or bone. May affect the bones, bladder, kidneys, liver, lungs, parotid glands, and spleen

Scanning: Technique in which message elements or groups of elements are presented one at a time to the message sender who signals the desired element

Sclerosis: Abnormal hardening of tissue

Secretions: Liquid drainage, either normal or disease-produced

Septum: Dividing wall made of bone or tissue as in the nose

Single use only: For onetime use only. Do not reclean, re-sterilize, or reuse

Sinusitis: Inflammation of the sinus cavities of the face; if chronic, may be a cause of some pulmonary diseases

Spirometer: Instrument that measures vital capacity or volume of inhaled and exhaled air

Spirometry: Technique to measure the breathing capacity of the lungs

Spontaneous: Happening by itself without apparent cause

Sputum: Secretions of the lungs, bronchi, trachea, and other secretions coughed or expectorated

Stenosis: Narrowing of a passageway

Stent: A mold formed from a resinous compound and used for holding a surgical graft in place

Sternal: Pertaining to the flat bone in front of the chest wall

Sternum: Breast bone; the bone to which the ribs connect in the front of the chest wall

Stretch receptors: Nerve cells inside the lung that react to deep inhalations and cause the chest to rebound to its resting position after inhalation

Stridor: Abnormal, harsh, high-pitched sounds that occur during difficult or obstructed respiration

Stroke volume: Amount of blood pumped by the ventricles at each heartbeat

Subarachnoid: Beneath arachnoid tissue in brain or spinal cord

Subglottic: Beneath the glottis

Subluxation: A partial or incomplete dislocation

Suctioning: Procedure in which a small catheter is placed into the tracheostomy tube to remove accumulated secretion from the tube and lungs

Supine: Lying with face upward

Supraglottic swallow sequence: Technique to protect the breathing tube (trachea) from food and liquid entering during the swallow. The patient is instructed to hold breath, swallow and then cough (taught and practiced with speech and occupational therapists)

Surfactant: Substance within the lungs that reduces friction and tension and prevents the alveolar walls from sticking together

Swivel neck plate: The swivel neck plate contains information on the size and product designation of a tracheostomy tube. The neck plate, with the tracheostomy ties properly attached, helps secure the tube to a patient's neck. The swivel assists the tube in positioning properly within the trachea

Syndrome: A collection of symptoms that are associated with a morbid process and that constitute a distinct clinical picture

Tachycardia: Abnormal rapidity of heart action, usually defined as a heart rate over 100 beats per minute

Tachypnea: Excessive rapidity of respiration, characterized by quick, shallow breathing

Teratoma: Congenital tumor containing one or more of the three primary embryonic germ layers

Thermal stimulation: Technique to quicken the initiation of the swallow response. An iced laryngeal mirror or long cotton swab is applied to the faucial pillars on each side in the mouth (taught and practiced with speech and occupational therapists)

Thyroglossal: Pertaining to the thyroid gland and the tongue

Tidal volume (Vt): The amount of air passing in and out of the lung during normal resting respiration

Total lung capacity (TLC): The total amount of air in a forced maximum inspiration and a forced maximum expiration, including the residual volume; normally 6000 ml in the adult

Toxic: Resembling or caused by poison

Trachea: Muscular breathing tube that is 4 to 5 inches in length and directs the passage of air into the lungs

Tracheal stoma: An opening in the neck that forms an additional path for airflow to the lungs, usually bypassing the mouth and nose

Tracheal wall: Mucosal lining of the trachea

Tracheitis: Inflammation of the trachea; may be acute or chronic and may be associated with bronchitis and laryngitis

Tracheitis sicca: Dry inflammation of the trachea

Tracheobronchitis: Inflammation of the trachea and bronchi

Tracheocutaneous fenestrations: Abnormal cavities beneath the mucous membrane of the trachea, often produced by disease

Tracheoesophageal: Pertaining to the trachea and esophagus

Tracheomalacia: Softening of the trachea and/or larynx

Tracheostomy: An artificial opening in the trachea that facilitates the passage of air or removal of secretions

Tracheotomy: The surgical operation of cutting an opening in the trachea at the level of the third and fourth tracheal rings

Tract: A path; an area of greater length than width; for example, the respiratory and digestive tracts

Transient tachypnea: Respiration rate that decreases usually three days or more after birth. Usually occurs in cesarean sections. It is caused by fluid remaining in the lungs

Transposition of great vessels: A fetal deformity of the heart in which the aorta arises from the right ventricle and the pulmonary artery arises from the left ventricle

Trauma: A wound or injury; physical damage produced by external force

Treacher Collins syndrome: Named for Edward Treacher Collins, British ophthalmologist. Mandibulofacial dysostosis characterized by hypoplasia of the facial bones; downward sloping of the palpebral tissues; defects of the ear and macrostomia. It occurs in two forms that are thought to be autosomal dominants

Tubercle bacillus: A bacterium that causes cavitation in the lungs

Tuberculosis: Infectious disease caused by the tubercle bacillus

Turbulent: Rolling, not smooth or laminar; usually describes flow of air or liquids

Turbulent flow: Non-straight line flow resulting in eddy formations. Turbulent flow results in a decreased volume of gas moved per unit of time per pressure gradient

Ultrasound: A noninvasive, safely repeatable technique that allows visualization of soft tissue and muscles; it does not penetrate bone. Stages of the oral-preparatory phase, oral phase, and tongue initiation movement for the swallow reflex can be clearly seen. Does not provide a clear picture of the bolus clearing the airway

Upper respiratory infection (URI): Any infection that involves primarily the larynx, trachea, and bronchi of the upper respiratory tract, such as the common cold, pharyngitis, laryngitis, bronchitis

Vacuum: A space from which most of the air or gas has been taken, creating a negative pressure

Vagus nerve: The tenth cranial nerve; aids in the control of respiration, most specifically the diaphragm

Vallecullar space: Space in upper part of the pharynx formed by the base of the tongue and the epiglottis. Site where food can collect when swallowing function is impaired

Vapor: Gaseous state of any substance

Vaporizer: Device for converting liquid into a vapor

Vascular: Pertaining to or composed of blood vessels

Vein: A vessel through which blood passes from various parts of the body collecting CO_2 (carbon dioxide) for removal through the lungs

Ventilation: The act of inhaling and exhaling; the movement of gas into and out of the lungs

Ventilator dependent: Requiring assistance from a mechanical device (ventilator) to breathe

Ventricular septal defect: Defect in the septum between the left and right ventricles of the heart that permits blood to be shunted between the ventricles

Videofluoroscopic swallowing evaluation (modified barium swallow): Radiologic examination that is performed using fluoroscopic equipment and recorded on videotape. This technique can be used to assess the phases of swallowing

Visceral pleura: The membranous sac that covers the lungs

Vital capacity, forced (FVC): The amount of air in a forced maximum inspiration and a forced maximum expiration; does not include residual volume; normally 4800 ml in the adult

Volume: Measurement of pulmonary capacity

Volumetric: Pertaining to the measure of volume

Web: A tissue or membrane extending across a space

Wet lung: Pathogenic condition in which the lungs have rales and other wet bubbling sounds

APPENDIX I

PULMONARY ABBREVIATIONS AND SYMBOLS*

*Adapted from American College of Chest Physicians. American Thoracic Society pulmonary terms and symbols. *Chest*, 67(5):583593, 1975.

General

↓	decrease
↑	increase
<	less than
>	greater than
Δ	change
$\dot{X}$	a dot above any symbol indicates a time derivative, (e.g., per minute)
$\bar{X}$	a dash above any symbol indicates a mean value
%X	percent sign preceding a symbol indicates percentage of the predicted normal value
X/Y%	a percent sign after a symbol indicates a ratio function with the ratio expressed as a percentage, (e.g., FEV_1/FVC% = 100 x FEV_1/FVC)

Large Capital Letters

C	concentration in blood phase; also a general symbol for compliance
F	fractional concentration of a gas
P	partial pressure or tension
Q	volume of blood
S	percent saturation in blood phase
V	gas volume, also a general term for ventilation

Small Capital Letters

A	alveolar
ALV	alveolar
ANAT	anatomic
B	barometric
D	dead space
E	expired
ET	end tidal
I	inspired
L	lung

T tidal

STPD standard temperature and pressure, dry; temperature of 0° C; pressure of 760 mm Hg, and no water vapor

BTPS body condition as follows: body temperature (37°C), ambient pressure (760 mm Hg at sea level), and saturated with water vapor

ATPD ambient temperature and pressure, dry

ATPS ambient temperature and pressure, saturated with water vapor

Lower Case Letters

a arterial blood

c capillary blood

c' pulmonary end-capillary blood

v venous blood

$\bar{v}$ mixed venous blood

an anatomic

anat anatomic

f frequency of respirations per minute

max maximum

t time

Others

ABG arterial blood gas

AIDS acquired immune deficiency syndrome

AP anteroposterior

ARC AIDS-related complex

ARDS adult respiratory distress syndrome

$AaDO_2$ alveolar-arterial oxygen pressure difference; same as $P(A\text{-}a)O_2$

a/A arterial/alveolar ratio

BPD bronchopulmonary dysplasia

$C(a\text{-}v)O_2$—arteriovenous oxygen content difference; same as Ca_{O2}— Cv_{O2}

CI cardiac index

Cdyn dynamic compliance
C_L lung compliance
Cst static compliance
COPD chronic obstructive pulmonary disease
CPAP continuous positive airway pressure
DL_{CO} diffusion capacity of the lung (measured with carbon monoxide)
DL/V_A diffusion per unit of alveolar volume
ERV expiratory reserve volume
$FEF_{25-75\%}$ forced expiratory flow over the middle half of the forced vital capacity
FEV_t forced expiratory volume, timed; (e.g., air exhaled at 1, 2, 3 seconds)
FIO_2 fractional inspired oxygen concentration
FRC functional residual capacity
FVC forced vital capacity
GPB glossopharyngeal breathing
HFV high frequency ventilation
IC inspiratory capacity
IMV intermittent mandatory ventilation
IRV inspiratory reserve volume
I:E inspiratory:expiratory ratio
IPPB intermittent positive pressure breathing
LLL left lower lobe of the lung
LUL left upper lobe of the lung
MBC maximum breathing capacity; same as MVV
MIFR maximum inspiratory flow rate
MMFR maximum mid expiratory flow rate; old term for $FEF_{25-75\%}$
MVV maximum voluntary ventilation; same as MBC
P_{aw} pressure in the airway, level to be specified
PA pulmonary artery or posteroanterior
P(A-a)o2 alveolar-arterial oxygen pressure difference; previously referred to as $A\text{-}aDO_2$
PCWP pulmonary capillary wedge pressure
PEEP positive end-expiratory pressure
PEF peak expiratory flow
PFT pulmonary function test

PIF	peak inspiratory flow
P_{pl}	pleural pressure
PSV	pressure support ventilation
P_{tc}	transcutaneous partial pressure
P_{tm}	transmural pressure of an airway or blood vessel
P_{tp}	transpulmonary pressure
P_{L}	transpulmonary pressure
PT	physical therapy
PVR	pulmonary vascular resistance
$\dot{Q}$	cardiac output per minute
$\dot{Q}_s/\dot{Q}_t$	percent intrapulmonary shunt
R	respiratory exchange ratio; also a general symbol for resistance
RLL	right lower lobe of the lung
RML	right middle lobe of the lung
RUL	right upper lobe of the lung
RQ	respiratory quotient
RV	residual volume
SIMV	synchronized intermittent mandatory ventilation
SVC	slow vital capacity
SVR	systemic vascular resistance
TB	tuberculosis
TLC	total lung capacity
$\dot{V}_{maxXX\%}$	maximum expiratory flow (i.e., instantaneous) measured at a specified volume; e.g., $V_{max75\%}$ is the maximum expiratory flow after 75% of FVC has been exhaled
$\dot{V}$	minute ventilation
V_E	minute ventilation
VC	vital capacity
V_D	dead space ventilation
V_D/V_T	dead space to tidal volume ratio
V/Q	ventilation/perfusion ratio
V_T	tidal volume
TV	tidal volume
$\dot{V}CO_2$	carbon dioxide production per minute (STPD)
$\dot{V}O_2$	oxygen consumption per minute (STPD)
$\dot{V}co/\dot{V}o_2$	respiratory exchange ratio

W general term for mechanical work of breathing
WOB general term for mechanical work of breathing
Z airway generation, e.g., Z=l (trachea) to Z=23 (alveolar sacs)

APPENDIX II

RESOURCES

AIDS

National Association of People with AIDS
P.O. Box 34056
Washington, DC 20043
(202) 898-0414

National AIDS Clearinghouse
P.O. Box 6003
Rockville, MD 20849-6003
(301) 217-0023
(800) 458-5231
(800) 243-7012 (TDD/ITY)

ALLERGY

Asthma and Allergy Foundation of America
1125 15th St. NW, Ste. 502
Washington, DC 20005
(202) 466-7643
(800)7-ASTHMA (727-8462)
(Patient Info Line)

AMYOTROPHIC LATERAL SCLEROSIS

Amyotrophic Lateral Sclerosis Association
21021 Ventura Blvd., Ste. 321
Woodland Hills, CA 91364
(818) 340-7500

APHASIA

National Aphasia Association Young People's Network
P.O. Box 1887
Murray Hill Station
New York, NY 10156-0611
(800) 922-4622

ARNOLD-CHIARI SYNDROME

Arnold-Chiari Family Network
c/o Kevin & Maureen Walsh
67 Spring Street
Weymouth, MA 02188
(617) 337-2368

ARTHRITIS

American Juvenile Arthritis Organization
1314 Spring St. NW
Atlanta, GA 30309
(404) 872-7100,
(404) 872-0457 (FAX)

Arthritis Foundation
1314 Spring St. NW
Atlanta, GA 30309
(404) 872-7100
(800) 283-7800 (Information Line)

National Arthritis & Musculoskeletal Skin Disease Information Clearinghouse
9000 Rockville Pike
Box AMS
Bethesda, MD 20892
(301) 495-4484

ARTHROGRYPOSIS

Avenues, National Support Group for Arthrogryposis Multiplex Congenita
P.O. Box 5192
Sonora, CA 95370
(209) 928-3688

BIRTH DEFECTS

Association of Birth Defect Children
Orlando Executive Park
5400 Diplomat Circle
Suite 270
Orlando, FL 32810
(407) 629-1466

March of Dimes Birth Defects Foundation
1275 Mamaroneck Ave.
White Plains, NY 10605
(914) 428-7100

National Birth Defects Center
Franciscan Children's Hospital
30 Warren St.
Boston, MA 02135
(617) 787-5958

BRAIN

American Brain Tumor Association
720 River Rd., Suite 146
Des Plaines, IL 60018
(708) 827-9910
(800) 886-2282 (patient line)
(708) 827-9918 (FAX)

Association for Brain Tumor Research
3725 N. Talman Ave.
Chicago, IL 60618
(312) 286-5571

Association of Neurometabolic Disorders
5223 Brookfield Lane
Sylvania, OH 43560-1809
(419) 885-1497

Children's Brain Diseases Foundation
350 Parnassus Ave., Suite 900
San Francisco, CA 94117
(415) 565-6259
(415) 863-3452 (FAX)

National Head Injury Foundation (NHIF)
1776 Massachusetts Ave. NW
Washington, DC 20036
(202) 296-NHIF (6443)
(800) 444-NHIF (6443)
(Family Help Line)

National Institute of Neurological Disorders and Stroke
9000 Rockville Pike, Bldg. 31
Rm. 8A-16
Bethesda, MD 20892
(301) 496-5751
(301) 402-2186 (FAX)

National Stroke Association
300 E. Hampden Ave., Ste. 240
Englewood, CO 80110-2622
(303) 762-9922

Parkinson's Disease Foundation
650 W. 168th St.
New York, NY 10032-9982
(212) 923-4700
(800) 457-6676

THRESHOLD—Intractable Seizure Disorder Support Group
26 Stavola Road
Middletown, NJ 07748-3728
(908) 957-0714

CANCER

AMC Cancer Information Center
1600 Pierce St.
Lakewood, CO 80214
(800) 525-3777

American Cancer Society
1599 Clifton Rd. NE
Atlanta, GA 30329
(404) 320-3333
(800) 227-2345

Candlelighters Childhood Cancer Foundation
7910 Woodmont Ave., Suite 460
Bethesda, MD 20814
(800) 366-2223
(301) 718-2686 (FAX)

Corporate Angel Network (CAN)
Westchester County Airport
Building 1
White Plains, NY 10604
(914) 328-1313
(914) 328-3938 (FAX)

National Cancer Institute
Cancer Information Service
Boy Scout Bldg., Rm. 340
9000 Rockville Pike
Bethesda, MD 20892
(301) 496-8664
(800)4-CANCER (422-6237)

Vital Options
Support for Young Adults with Cancer
4419 Coldwater Canyon Ave.,
Stes. A-C
Studio City, CA 91604
(818) 508-5657

CEREBRAL PALSY

United Cerebral Palsy
Washington, DC 20005
(202) 628-3630

United Cerebral Palsy Association
1522 K Street NW, #1112
Washington, D.C. 20005
(800) 872-5827
(202) 842-1266
(202) 842-3519 (FAX)

United States Cerebral Palsy Athletic Association
34518 Warren Rd., Ste. 264
Westland, MI 48185
(313) 425-8961

CHARCOT-MARIE-TOOTH DISEASE

CMT International
1 Springbank Dr.
St. Catherines, ON
Canada L2S 2K1
(416) 687-3620

CHARGE SYNDROME

CHARGE Syndrome Foundation, Inc.
Coloboma of the eye,
Heart malformations,
Atresia of the Choanae (nasal),
Retardation of growth and/or development,
Genital Hypoplasia, Ear anomalies
2004 Parkade Blvd.
Columbia, MO 65202
(314) 442-7604

CLEFT PALATE

Cleft Palate Foundation
1218 Grandview Ave
Pittsburgh, PA 15211
(800) 24-CLEFT
(412) 481-1376
(412) 481-0847 (FAX)

Prescription Parents, Inc.
P.O. Box 161
W. Roxbury, MA 02132
(617) 527-0878

CRANIOFACIAL DISORDERS

AboutFace U.S.A.
1002 Liberty Ln.
Warrington, PA 18976
(800) 225-FACE
(215) 491 -0603 (FAX)

Children's Craniofacial Association
10210 N. Central Expy./LB 37
Dallas, TX 75231
(214) 368-3590
(800) 535-3643

Hemifacial Microsomia/Goldenhar Syndrome
Family Support Network
84 Gleniffer Hill Rd.
Richboro, PA 18954
(215) 364-3199

Treacher Collins Foundation
P.O. Box 683
Norwich, VT 05055
(802) 649-3020

CYCLIC VOMITING SYNDROME

Cyclic Vomiting Syndrome
Association
13180 Caroline Court
Elm Grove, WI 53122
(414) 784-6842
(414) 821-5494 (FAX)

CYSTIC FIBROSIS

Cystic Fibrosis Foundation
6931 Arlington Rd.
Bethesda, MD 20814
(301) 951-4422
(800) 344-4823

DIABETES

American Diabetes Association
2 Reservoir Circle, #203
Baltimore, MD 21208-1309
(301) 486-5515
(800) ADA-DISC (232-3472)

Juvenile Diabetes Foundation International
432 Park Ave. South
New York, NY 10016
(212) 889-7575
(800) 223-113

DOWN'S SYNDROME

Association for Children with Down Syndrome
2616 Martin Ave.
Bellmore NY 11710
(516) 221-4700
(516) 221 -4311 (FAX)

Caring Inc.
P.O. Box 400
Milton, WA 98354
(206) 922-8607

National Down Syndrome Congress
1605 Chantilly Drive, Suite 250
Atlanta, GA 30324
(800) 232-6372, (404) 633-1555
(404) 633-2817 (FAX)

National Down's Syndrome Society
666 Broadway
New York, NY 10012
(212) 460-9330
(800) 221-4602 (24-Hour)

EXTRACORPOREAL MEMBRANE OXYGENATION

ECMO Moms and Dads International
Parent Support
P.O. Box 53848
Lubbock, TX 79453
(806) 889-3877
(806) 745-8130

GENETIC CONDITIONS

Alliance of Genetic Support Groups
35 Wisconsin Cr. #440
Chevy Chase, MD 20815-7015
(800) 336-GENE
(301) 652-5553
(301) 654-0171 (FAX)

Hereditary Disease Foundation
1427 7th Street, Suite 2
Santa Monica, CA 90401
(310) 458-4183
(310) 458-3937 (FAX)

GERIATRICS

American Association of Homes for the Aging
901 E St. NW, Ste. 500
Washington, DC 20004-2837
(202) 783-2242

American Geriatrics Society, Inc.
770 Lexington Ave., Ste. 300
New York, NY 10021
(212) 308-1414

American Society on Aging
833 Market St., Ste. 512
San Francisco, CA 94103
(415) 882-2910
(800) 537-9728

National Association of Area Agencies on Aging (NAAAA)
1112 16th St. NW, Ste. 100
Washington, DC 20036
(202) 296-8130

National Council on the Aging
409 Third St. SW
Washington, DC 20024
(202) 479-1200
(800) 424-9046

GROWTH DISORDERS

Human Growth Foundation
7777 Leesburg Pike
Falls Church, VA 22043
(800) 451-6434
(703) 883-1773
(703) 883-1776 (FAX)

GUILLAIN-BARRE SYNDROME

Guillain-Barre Syndrome
Foundation International
P.O. Box 262
Wynnewood, PA 19096
(215) 667-0131
(215) 667-7036 (FAX)

HEALTH CARE

American Association for Continuity of Care
1730 N. Lynn St., Ste. 502
Arlington, VA 22209
(703) 525-1191

American Federation of Home Health Agencies
1320 Fenwick Ln., Rrn. 100
Silver Spring, MD 20910
(301) 588-1454

American Health Care Association
1201 L St. NW
Washington, DC 20005
(202) 842-4444

Center for Consumer Healthcare Information
4000 Birch St., #112
Newport Beach, CA 92660
(714) 752-2335
(800) 627-2244

National Association for Home Care
519 C St. NE
Washington, DC 20002-5809
(202) 547-7424

National Health Information Center
P.O. Box 1133
Washington, DC 20013-1133
(301) 565-4167
(800) 336-4797

HEART, LUNG AND BLOOD DISORDERS

American Heart Association
7272 Greenville Ave.
Dallas, TX 75231 -4596
(214) 373-6300
(214) 706-1341 (FAX)

National Heart, Lung and Blood Institute
P.O. Box 30105
Bethesda, MD 20824-0105
(301) 251-1222

HYDROCEPHALUS

Hydrocephalus Association
870 Market Street, Suite 955
San Francisco, CA 94102
(415) 776-4713

National Hydrocephalus Foundation
400 N. Michigan Ave., Suite 1102
Chicago, IL 60611-4102
(815) 467-6548

IMMUNE DEFICIENCY

Immune Deficiency Foundation (IDF)
P.O. Box 586
Columbia, MD 21045
(301) 730-8837
(301) 461-3127

INTRAVENTRICULAR HEMORRHAGE

I.V.H. Parents
P.O. Box 56-1111
Miami, FL 33256 1111
(305) 232-0381
(305) 232-9890 (FAX)

LEUKEMIA

Leukemia Society of America
600 Third Ave.,4th Floor
New York, NY 10016
(212) 573-8484
(212) 856-9686 (FAX)

LUNG DISEASES

American Association for Respiratory Care
11030 Ables Ln.
Dallas, TX 75229
(214) 243-2272

American Lung Association
1740 Broadway
New York, NY 10019
(212) 315-8700
(212) 265-5642 (FAX)

NEUROFIBRAMATOSIS

National Neurofibromatosis Foundation
141 Fifth Avenue, Suite 7-S
New York, NY 10010-7105
(800) 323-7938
(212) 460-8980
(212) 529-6094 (FAX)

NEUROLOGICAL AND NEUROMUSCULAR DISORDERS

Dystonia Medical Research Foundation
One East Wacker Drive, Suite 2900
Chicago, IL 60601-2001
(312) 755-0198
(312) 321-5710 (FAX)

Huntington's Disease Society of America
140 W. 22nd Street 6th Fl.
New York, NY 10011-2420
(212) 242-1968
(212) 243-2443 (FAX)

Muscular Dystrophy Association
3300 E. Sunrise Drive
Tucson, AZ 85718-3208
(602) 529-2000
(602) 529-5300 (FAX)

Myasthenia Gravis Foundation (MGF)
53 W. Jackson Blvd., Suite 660
Chicago, IL 60604
(800) 541-5454
(312) 427-6252
(312) 427-8437 (FAX)

National Ataxia Foundation
15500 Wayzata Blvd.
Ste. 750
Wayzata, MN 55391
(612) 473-7666

National Multiple Sclerosis Society
733 Third Ave., 6th Fl.
New York, NY 10017-5706
(212) 986-3240
(800) 624-8236 (24-Hour Info Resource Center)
(212) 986-7981 (FAX)

ORTHOPEDIC AND BURN PROBLEMS

International Shriners Headquarters
2900 Rocky point Drive
Tampa, FL 33607
(800) 282-9161 (in FL)
(800) 237-5055 (US)
(800) 361-7256 (CAN)
(813) 281-0300
(813) 287-8214 (FAX)

REHABILITATION

National Rehabilitation Association
1910 Association Dr., #205
Reston, VA 22091
(703) 715-9090 (Voice)
(703) 715-9209 (TDD)

National Rehabilitation Information Center
8455 Colesville Road, Ste. 935
Silver Spring, MD 20910
(301) 588-9284
(800) 227-0216 (Voice/TDD)
(800) 368-3513

Project Magic
Kansas Rehabilitation Hospital
1504 SW 8th St.
Topeka, KS 66606
(913) 232-8515

Rehabilitation International (RI)
25 E. 21st St.
New York, NY 10010
(212) 420-1500

Research and Training Center on Independent Living
4089 Dole Bldg.
University of Kansas
Lawrence, KS 66045
(913) 864-4095 (Voice/TDD)

SHORT STATURE

Little People of America, Inc.
P.O. Box 9897
Washington, DC 20016
(800) 24D-WARF

SPINAL CORD DISORDERS

American Paralysis Association
500 Morris Avenue
Springfield, NJ 07081
(800) 225-0292
(201) 379-2690 (in NJ)
(201) 912-9433 (FAX)7465
(800) 886-1762
(708) 432-5551 (phone/FAX)

American Paraplegia Society
75-20 Astoria Blvd.
Jackson Heights, NY 11370-1178
(718) 803-3782

American Spinal Injury Association
2020 Peachtree Rd. NW
Atlanta, GA 30309
(404) 355-9772

Families of S.M.A. (Spinal Muscular Distrophy)
P.O. Box 1465
Highland Park, IL 60035-7465
(800) 886-1762
(708) 432-5551 (phone/FAX)

Foundation For Spinal Cord Injury Prevention
1546 Penobscot Bldg.
Detroit, Ml 48226
(313) 963-1600

National Paraplegia Foundation
3400 Hulen
Ft. Worth, TX 76107
(817) 737-6661

National Scoliosis Foundation
72 Mount Auburn St.
Watertown, MA 02172
(617) 926-0397
(617) 926-0398 (FAX)

National Spinal Cord Injury Association
600 W. Cummings Park, Ste. 2000
Woburn, MA 01801
(617) 935-2722
(800) 962-9629 (Hot Line only)
(800) 342-0330
(617) 932-8369 (FAX)

Paralyzed Veterans of America (PVA)
801 18th St. NW
Washington, DC 20006
(202) 872-1300
(800) 424-8200

Spina Bifida Association of America
4590 MacArthur Blvd. NW #250
Washington, DC 20007-4226
(800) 621-3141
(202) 944-3285
(202) 944-3295 (FAX)

Spina Bifida Association of Canada
220-388 Donald Street
Winnipeg, MB Canada R3B 2J4
(204) 957-1794

Spinal Cord Society
Rte. 5 Box 22A
Fergus Falls, MN 56537
(218) 739-5252

SUPPORT GROUPS

A.M.E.N.D. (Aiding Mothers & Fathers Experiencing Neonatal Death)
4324 Berrywick Terrace
St. Louis, MO 63128
(314) 487-7582

Children's Hospice International
901 N. Washington Street, Suite 700
Alexandria, VA 22314
(800) 242-4453
(703) 684-0330

Christian Council on Persons with Disabilities
1324 Yosemite Blvd.
Modesto, CA 95354
(209) 524-7993

Compassionate Friends
P.O. Box 3696
Oak Brook, IL 60522-3696
(708) 990-0010
(708) 990-0246 (FAX)

Council on Family Health
225 Park Avenue S
17th Floor
New York, NY 10003
(212) 598-3617

Families of Children Under Stress (FOCUS)
P.O. Box 1058
Conyers, GA 30207
(404) 483-9845

MUMS (Mothers United for Moral Support, Inc.)
c/o Julie Gordon
150 Cluster Street
Green Bay, WI 54301
(414) 336-5333

Parent Care, Inc.
9041 Colgate St.
Indianapolis, IN 46268-1210
(317) 872-9913

Parents of Chronically Ill Children
1527 Maryland St.
Springfield, IL 62702
(217) 522-6810

Sick Kids Need Involved People (SKIP)
216 Newport Drive
Severna Park, MD 21146
(410) 379-0999

GENERAL

ACCESS: The Foundation for Accessibility by the Disabled
P.O. Box 356
Malverne, NY 11564-0356
(516) 887-5798

American Occupational Therapy Association
1383 Piccard Dr.
P.O. Box 1725
Rockville, MD 20849-1725
(301) 948-9626

American Orthotic & Prosthetic Association
1650 King St., Ste. 500
Alexandria, VA 22314
(703) 836-7116

American Physical Therapy Association
1111 N. Fairfax St.
Alexandria, VA 22314
(703) 684-APTA (2782)

American Red Cross
431 18th St. NW
Washington, DC 20006
(202) 737-8300

American Speech-Language-Hearing Association
10801 Rockville Pike
Rockville, MD 20852
(301) 897-5700 (Voice/TDD)
(800) 638-6868 (Consumer Action Line)

Americans with Disabilities Act
For information related to the Americans with Disabilities Act.
(800) USA-ABLE

Association for Retarded Citizens (ARC)
P.O. Box 300649
Arlington, TX 76010
(817) 261-6003
(800) 433-5255

Association on Higher Education and Disability (AHEAD)
P.O. Box 21192
Columbus, OH 43221
(614) 488-4972 (Voice/TDD)

Canadian Rehabilitation Council for the Disabled
45 Sheppard Ave. East, Ste. 801
Toronto M2N 5W9
CANADA
(416) 250-7490

Council for Learning Disabilities (CLD)
P.O. Box 40303
Overland Park, KS 66204
(913) 492-8755

DIRECT LINK for the disABLED, Inc.
P.O. Box 1036
Solvang, CA 93464
(805) 688-1603 (Voice/TT)

Disabled American Veterans
P.O. Box 14301
Cincinnati, OH 45250
(606) 441-7300

Family Survival Project
425 Bush St., Ste. 500
San Francisco, CA 94108
(415) 434-3388

Fifty-Two Association for the Handicapped
350 Fifth Ave., Ste. 1829
New York, NY 10118
(212) 563-9797

Gazette International Networking Institute (GINI)
5100 Oakland Ave., #206
St. Louis, MO 63110
(314) 534-0475

IBM National Support Center for Persons with Disabilities
P.O. Box 2150
Atlanta, GA 30301-2150
(800) 426-2133 (Voice)
(800) 284-9482 (TDD)

Independent Living Research Utilization (ILRU)
2323 S. Shepherd, Ste. 1000
Houston, TX 77019
(713) 520-0232 (Voice)
(713) 520-5136 (TDD)

Information Center for Individuals with Disabilities
Fort point Place
27-43 Wormwood St.
Boston, MA 02210-1606
(617) 727-5540
(800) 462-5015 (in MA only)

Institute for the Advancement of Prosthetics (IAP)
4424 S. Pennsylvania Ave.
Lansing, MI 48910-5695
(517) 394-5850

International Center for the Disabled
340 E. 24th St.
New York, NY 10010
(212) 679-0100

International Foundation for the Handicapped
P.O. Box 409
Solvang, CA 93463
(805) 686-4287
(800) 444-3339

Job Accommodation Network (JAN)
West Virginia University
P.O. Box 6123
809 Allen Hall
Morgantown, WV 26506
(800) 526-7234 (USA) (Voice/TDD)
(800) 526-4698 (W.V.) (Voice/TDD)
(800) 526-2262 (Canada) (Voice/TDD)
(800) DIAL-JAN (Bulletin Bd)
(800) ADA-WORK (Questions on Law)

Joni & Friends (Networking Resource)
P.O. Box 3333
Agoura Hills, CA 91301
(818) 707-5664

Learning Disabilities of America
4156 Library Rd.
Pittsburgh, PA 15234
(412) 341-1515

Living Bank
P.O. Box 6725
Houston, TX 77265
(713) 528-2971
(800) 528-2971

Mainstream
3 Bethesda Metro Center, Ste. 830
Bethesda, MD 20814
(301) 654-2400 (Voice/TDD)

March of Dimes Birth Defects Foundation
1275 Mamaroneck Ave.
White Plains, NY 10605
(914) 428-7100

Medical Frontiers
750 Park Ave.
New York, NY 10021
(212) 744-6370

Medical Information Service
Palo Alto Medical Foundation
400 Channing Ave.
Palo Alto, CA 94301
(415) 853-6000
(800) 999-1999

Mobility International U.S.A. (MIUSA)
P.O. Box 3551
Eugene, OR 97403
(503) 343-1284 (Voice/TDD)

NICHCY
(National Information Center for Children and Youth with Disabilities)
P.O. Box 1492
Washington, DC 20013
(703) 893-6061
(800) 999-5599
(703) 893-8614 (TDD)
(703) 893-1741 (FAX)

NISH (Creating Employment Opportunities For People With Severe Disabilities)
2235 Cedar Ln.
Vienna, VA 22182-5200
(703) 560-6800 (Voice)

NPND (National Parent Network on Disabilities)
1600 Prince Street,
Suite 115
Alexandria,VA 22314
(703) 684-NPND
(703) 684-6763 (Voice/TDD)

National Association for the Physically Handicapped (NAPH)
440 Lafayette Ave., #117
Cincinnati, OH 45220-1000
(513) 961-8040

National Association of Driving for the Disabled (NADD)
87 Main St.
Fort Plain, NY 13339
(518) 993-4092

National Association of Medical Equipment Suppliers (NAMES)
625 Slaters Ln., Ste. 200
Alexandria, VA 22314-1171
(703) 836-6263

National Association of Protection and Advocacy Systems
900 Second Street NE, Suite 221
Washington, DC 20002
(202) 408-9514
(202) 408-9520 (FAX)

National Catholic Office for Persons with Disabilities
P.O. Box 29113
Washington, DC 20017
(202) 529-2933 (Voice/TDD)
(202) 529-4678

National Center for Youth with Disabilities
University of Minnesota
420 Delaware Street SE
Box 721
Minneapolis, MN 55455-0392
(612) 626-2825
(800) 333-6293
(612) 626-2134 (FAX)

National Council of Guilds for Infant Survival
P.O. Box 3586
Davenport, IA 52808
Mailing address only.

National Council on Communicative Disorders
10801 Rockville Pike
Rockville, MD 20852
(301) 493-4914
(800) 638-8255

National Council on Disability
800 Independence Ave. SW, Ste. 814
Washington, DC 20591
(202) 267-3846 (Voice)
(202) 267-3232 (TDD)

National Council on Independent Living (NCIL)
c/o Troy Resource Center for Independent Living
Troy Atrium
Broadway & 4th St.
Troy, NY 12180
(518) 274-0701

National Easter Seals Society
70 East Lake Street
Chicago, IL 60601
(312) 726-6200
(312) 726-4258 (TDD)
(800) 221-6827

National Handicapped Sports
451 Hungerford Dr., # 100
Rockville, MD 20850
(800) 966-966-4647

National Information Center for Children and Youth with Disabilities
P.O. Box 1492
Washington, DC 20013
(703) 893-6061
(800) 999-5599

National Information System and Clearinghouse Center for Developmental Disabilities
University of South Carolina
Benson Building
Columbia, SC 29208
(800) 922-9234 Ext. 201
(800) 922-1107 (in SC)
(803) 777-6058 (FAX)

National Information System for Vietnam Veterans and their Children
University of South Carolina Center for Developmental Disabilities
Benson Bldg.
Columbia, SC 29208
(800) 922-9234 Ext. 401
(800) 922-1107 Ext. 401 (in SC)

National Mobility Equipment Dealers Association
909 E. Skagway Ave.
Tampa, FL 33637
(813) 932-8566
(800) 833-0427

National Organization for Rare Disorders (NORD)
P.O. Box 8923
New Fairfield, CT 06812
(203) 746-6518
(800) 999-NORD (6673)

National Organization on Disability (NOD)
910 16th Street NW, Suite 600
Washington, DC 20006
(202) 293-5960 (Voice)
(202) 229-1187 (in MD)
(202) 293-5968 (TDD)
(800) 248-ABLE (2253)

National Parent Network on Disabilities
1600 Prince St., Ste. 115
Alexandria, VA 22314
(703) 684-6763

Osteogenesis Imperfecta Foundation
P.O. Box 24776
5005 W. Laurel St., Ste. 210
Tampa, FL 33607
(813) 282-1161

PRIDE Foundation
(Promote Real Independence for the Disabled & Elderly)
391 Long Hill Rd.
Groton, CT 06340
(203) 445-1448

Polio Survivors Association
12720 La Reina Ave.
Downey, CA 90242
(213) 862-4508

President's Committee on Employment of People With Disabilities
1331 F St. NW
Washington, DC 20004-1107
(202) 376-6200 (Voice)
(202) 376-6205 (TDD) (703) 560-6512 (TDD)

Sensory Access Foundation
385 Sherman Ave., Ste. 2
Palo Alto, CA 94306
(415) 329-0430

Special Olympics International
1350 New York Ave. NW, Ste. 500
P.O. Box 11749
Memphis, TN 38111-0749
(901) 452-7343
(800) 992-9392

Special Recreation
362 Koser Ave.
Iowa City, IA 52246-3038
(319) 337-7578

TASH: The Association for Persons with Severe Handicaps
11201 Greenwood Ave. N.
Seattle, WA 98133
(206) 361-8870
(206) 361-0113 (TTY)

Technical Aids & Assistance (TAAD)
1950 W. Roosevelt Rd.
Chicago, IL 60608
(312) 421-3373
(800) 346-2939 (in IL only)

Travel Companion Exchange
Box 833
Amityville, NY 11701
(516) 454-0880

United Way of America
701 N. Fairfax St.
Alexandria, VA 22314
(703) 836-7100

Well Spouse Foundation
P.O. Box 28876
San Diego, CA 92198
(619) 673-9043

Wilderness Inquiry
1313 Fifth St. SE/P.O. Box 84
Minneapolis, MN 55414
(612) 379-3858 (Voice/TTY)
(800) 728-0719

World Institute on Disability
510 16th St., Ste. 100
Oakland, CA 94612
(510) 763-4100 (Voice/TDD)

HOTLINES

AIDS 24-Hour Hotline:
(800) 342-AIDS; (800) 344-SIDA (in Spanish); (800) AIDS-TTY (for the hearing impaired)

American Paralysis Spinal Cord Hotline:
2201 Argonne Drive
Baltimore, MD 21218
(800) 526-3456

Lung Line Information Service:
(800) 222-LUNG

Medicare Information:
(800) 462-9306

INDEX

NOTE: Page numbers followed by *f* contain figures. Page numbers followed by *t* contain tables.

D

END INDEX